MALARIA AND BABESIOSIS

W0016681

NEW PERSPECTIVES IN CLINICAL MICROBIOLOGY

Brumfitt W, ed Hamilton-Miller JMT, assist. ed: New perspectives in clinical microbiology. 1978. ISBN 90-247-2074-5

Tyrrell DAJ, ed: Aspects of slow and persistent virus infections. 1979.
ISBN 90-247-2281-0

Brumfitt W, Curcio L, Silvestri L, eds: Combined antimicrobial therapy. 1979.
ISBN 90-247-2280-2

van Furth R, ed: Developments in antibiotic treatment of respiratory infections. 1981.
ISBN 90-247-2493-7

van Furth R, ed: Evaluation and management of hospital infections. 1982.
ISBN 90-247-2754-5

Kuwahara S, Pierce NF, eds: Advances in research on cholera and related diarrheas 1.
1983. ISBN 089838-592-X

Ristic M, Ambroise-Thomas P, Kreier J, eds: Malaria and babesiosis: Research findings
and control measures. 1984. ISBN 0-89838-675-6

Kuwahara S, Pierce NF, eds: Advances in research on cholera and related diarrheas 2.
1984. ISBN 089838-680-2

Takeda Y: Bacterial diarrheal diseases. 1984. ISBN 089838-681-0

MALARIA AND BABESIOSIS

Research findings and control measures

edited by

MIODRAG RISTIC, DVM, PhD
Department of Pathobiology, College of Veterinary Medicine
University of Illinois
Urbana ILL 61801, USA

PIERRE AMBROISE-THOMAS, MD, DSc
Department of Parasitology, School of Medicine
University of Grenoble
38700 La Tronche, France

JULIUS KREIER, DVM, PhD
Department of Microbiology, College of Biological Sciences
Ohio State University
Columbia OH 43210, USA

1984 **MARTINUS NIJHOFF PUBLISHERS**
a member of the KLUWER ACADEMIC PUBLISHERS GROUP
DORDRECHT / BOSTON / LANCASTER

Distributors

for the United States and Canada: Kluwer Academic Publishers, 190 Old Derby Street, Hingham, MA 02043, USA
for the UK and Ireland: Kluwer Academic Publishers, MTP Press Limited, Falcon House, Queen Square, Lancaster LA1 1RN, England
for all other countries: Kluwer Academic Publishers Group, Distribution Center, P.O. Box 322, 3300 AH Dordrecht, The Netherlands

Library of Congress Cataloging in Publication Data

Main entry under title:

Malaria and babesiosis.

　　(New perspectives in clinical microbiology)
　　Papers from the Second International Conference on
Malaria and Babesiosis held in Annecy, France, Sept.
1983.
　　Includes bibliographical references and index.
　　1. Malaria--Congresses.　2. Babesiosis--Congresses.
3. Domestic animals--Parasites--Congresses.　I. Ristic,
Miodrag, 1918-　　.　II. Ambroise-Thomas, Pierre.
III. Kreier, Julius P.　IV. International Conference on
Malaria and Babesiosis (2nd : 1983 : Annecy, France)
V. Series.
　RC156.M38　1984　　　616.9'362　　　　84-1207
　ISBN-13:978-94-009-6044-2　　　e-ISBN-13:978-94-009-6042-8
　DOI: 10.1007/978-94-009-6042-8

ISBN-13:978-94-009-6044-2 (this volume)

Copyright

© 1984 by Martinus Nijhoff Publishers, Dordrecht.
Softcover reprint of the hardcover 1st edition 1984

All rights reserved. No part of this publication may be reproduced, stored in a retrieval system, or transmitted in any form or by any means, mechanical, photocopying, recording, or otherwise, without the prior written permission of the publishers,
Martinus Nijhoff Publishers, P.O. Box 163, 3300 AD Dordrecht,
The Netherlands.

Annecy: Charles Mérieux's dedication to Miodrag Ristic

En hommage au professeur Ristic
après l'inoubliable congrès d'Annecy

28. 4. 84

Table of contents

Preface

Annecy in September 1983 to provide an organization to assist in the achievement of this objective.

The conference also presented a meritorious award to Dr. James M. Erickson in recognition of his outstanding contribution of behalf of USAID toward the organization, development and implementation of research programs in malaria.

Each major division of the scientific program of the Annecy meeting was preceeded by a keynote presentation. These presentations outlined the major research developments in the study area covered in the division. The present volume contains papers developed by the keynote speakers from their presentations, the papers given at the meeting and relevant information drawn from the scientific literature.

It is the hope of the editors of this book that the scientific community and public in general will gain from reading it, as we gained from its preparation.

Miodrag Ristic D.V.M. Ph.D.
Pierre Ambroise-Thomas M.D. DSc
Julius P. Kreier V.M.D. Ph.D.

1. Malaria and babesiosis: similarities and differences

MIODRAG RISTIC AND J.P. KREIER

Department of Pathobiology, College of Veterinary Medicine, University of Illinois, Urbana, Illinois 61801, and the Department of Microbiology, The Ohio State University, Columbus, Ohio 43210.

1. Introduction

This inaugural paper presented by the senior author at the Second International Conference on Malaria and Babesiosis was chosen by the organizers of the conference to consider common features of the two diseases and their causative agents and thereby suggest the advantage of a comparative research approach. Our awareness of the similarities between the two diseases prompted us to plan the first conference in Mexico City in May of 1979. The proposal for this first conference arose during a review of babesiosis vaccine trials in Mexico among Drs. J.P. Kreier, Professor and malariologist of The Ohio State University; J.A. Pino, Director of the Agricultural Sciences of the Rockefeller Foundation and the senior author. At this meeting we concluded that findings from babesiosis research should be of interest to malariologists and that comparative analysis of many other aspects of the two diseases would be advantageous to each research group.

Aside from their biologic resemblance, malaria and babesiosis are of equal importance to human health and to the agricultural economy, respectively. Mortality and morbidity reports indicate that malaria remains one of the most important and inadequately controlled infectious disease of man [1, 2]. The distribution of babesiosis depends on the distribution of its arthropod vector, the tick, and *Babesia* species cause disease in various domestic animals with bovine babesiosis being economically the most important. Only a few places in the world are free of ticks. Consequently, babesiosis is also widely distributed and is an infectious disease of global importance [3].

The traditional concept that there is almost absolute specificity of individual *Babesia* species for their respective hosts is no longer valid. Beginning in 1957, many human cases of clinical and subclinical babesiosis have been reported with bovine, equine, and rodent species of *Babesia* as etiologic agents [4]. While not all the factors which govern human susceptibility to babesiosis are known at this time, splenectomy or other factors causing immunological deficiency appears to

Ristic, M. et al. (eds.) *Malaria and babesiosis.*
© 1984, Martinus Nijhoff Publishers, Dordrecht/Boston/Lancaster.

be important. The occurrence of babesiosis in man adds another link between the two diseases.

The principal objective of these malaria and babesiosis conferences is to review recently acquired knowledge about the two diseases so that information gained by each group of researchers will be shared. The subsequent papers in this volume consider, in great detail, the most recent findings relevant to the control of these diseases. This first paper is limited to the evaluation of various features common to the two diseases in an effort to emphasize the advantages of comparative studies which may benefit both research groups. The common and unique characteristics of each disease and their respective etiologic agents will become evident in the course of this discussion.

2. History

The history of malaria starts earlier and is, by far, better documented than that of babesiosis. The existance of malaria in prehistoric man many centuries B.C. has been suggested. Hippocrates, in the fifth century B.C., is considered to be the first physician to describe the clinical features of malaria and relate its occurrence to the seasons of the year [5]. Malaria is also unique among infectious diseases in that the cure was recognized many years before the etiologic agent and the mode of its transmission were fully understood. The most important historic events which contribute to our knowledge of malaria and babesiosis occurred during the last 20 years of the 19th century. It is during this period that the etiologic agents of both diseases were first recognized and the mode of their transmission by an arthropod vector was described. It was Alphonso Laveran, a French Army surgeon in Algeria, who in 1880 was the first to describe malaria parasites in the red blood cells of man. A few years before the end of the 19th century, the mosquito was recognized as the vector of malaria by Ronald Ross working in India and Amico Bignami and his coworkers in Italy [6].

The classic work of Smith and Kilbourne, which was underway in the United States at approximately the same time, signified the beginning of the scientific history of babesiosis. It is through their work that the tick was recognized for the first time to be the vector of babesiosis and subsequently to be the biologic vector of a protozoan agent, *Babesia bigemina* [7]. For several decades thereafter, the disease known as Texas cattle tick fever caused serious losses among the US cattle population. While the disease was gradually eliminated from the US by eradication of the tick vector, *Boophilus annulatus*, it remained one of the most important infectious diseases of cattle in all tropical and semitropical regions of the world. It is estimated today that one-half billion cattle throughout the world may be endangered by the disease caused by one or more babesias.

In 1957, the World Health Organization initiated a global campaign against malaria. This effort and earlier national efforts resulted in eradication of malaria from the United States, much of Europe and the Middle East and many areas in Central and South America. In general, the campaign produced reduction of malaria incidence in many other areas of the world. But today, a tragic resurgence of malaria is taking place, particularly in Asia and in certain Central and South American regions. It is estimated that the current incidence of malaria in the world is as high today as it was half a century ago [6].

Problems associated with the control of malaria are numerous. Poorly organized public health programs and the lack of trained personnel are primary difficulties for implementing malaria control in certain countries. These difficulties are augmented by resistance of plasmodia or anophelines in localized areas to chemical compounds. There is a widespread appearance of strains of *Plasmodium falciparum* that are resistant to the 4-amino quinoline drugs, including chloroquine (see chapter 10).

While drug resistance to *Babesia* app. does not seem to be a problem, implementation of chemotherapy under field conditions is nevertheless difficult and often impractical. The more serious problem with the control of babesiosis is the complicated nature of the life cycle of the organism. Transovarial transmission of Babesia (Fig. 1) and the wide range of hosts for many species of ticks provide practically indefinite survival of the organism away from its natural host.

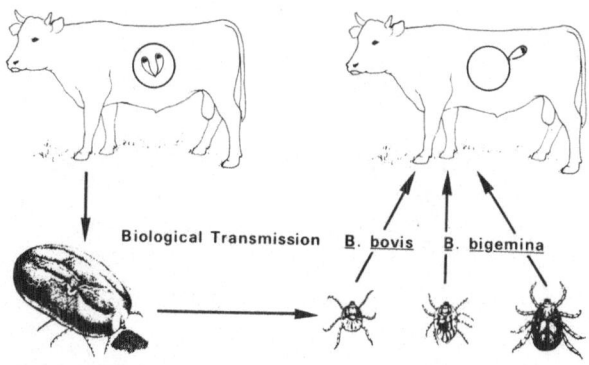

Figure 1. Biological transmission of *Babesia bovis* and *Babesia bigemina* by *Boophilus microplus*. The infection is acquired during engorgement of the adult tick. *Babesia bovis* is transmitted by larvae while *B. bigemina* is transmitted by nymphs and adults.

3. Cycle of development

Two major distinguishing features in the cycle of development of *Plasmodium* and *Babesia* are the lack of a mammalian tissue phase in the latter organism and the mode of growth and development of this organism in the host erythrocyte. A

6

simplified life cycle of *Babesia* with some possible homologies to *Plasmodium* is outlined in Figure 2. There are certain morphologic resemblances between plasmodial sporozoites and babesial vermicules. It is possible that the pre-erythrocytic phase in *Babesia* which takes place in the tick vector in the form of a continuous reproduction of vermicules may be analogous to the mammalian liver phase of *Plasmodium*. Vaccination with babesial vermicules as with malaria sporozoites, does not induce immunity to the blood phase although there may be some antigenic sharing between vermicules and erythrocytic forms.

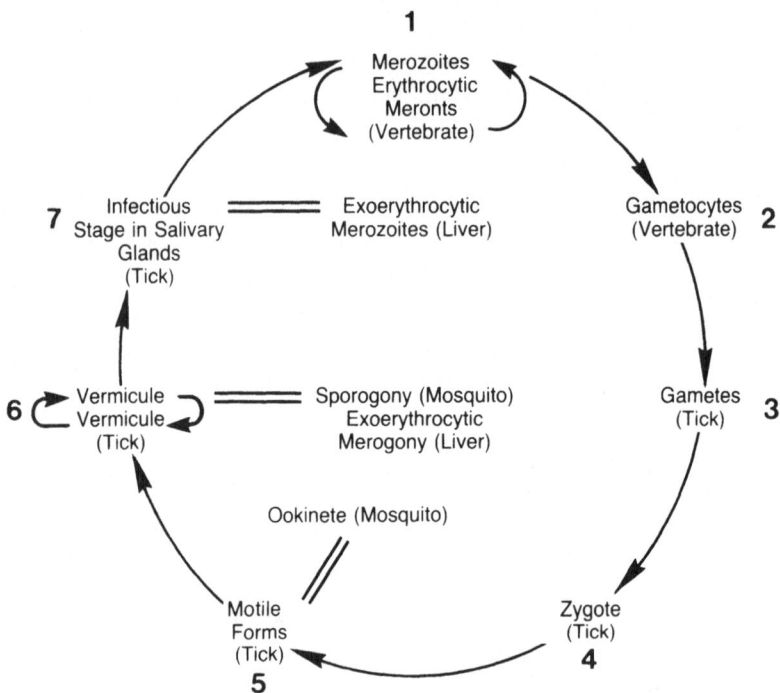

Figure 2. Simplified life cycle of *Babesia* with some possible homologies to *Plasmodium*.

In the erythrocytes, babesias form merozoites by a process of 'budding'. The process is not synchronous, there being mainly two with a maximum of four offspring produced at one time (Figs. 3a and b). At the time of their development in the erythrocyte, merozoites of malaria and babesia synthesize a surface coat antigen that seems to be essential for attachment to and subsequent entry into erythrocytes. The exit of babesial merozoites is random as opposed to plasmodium in which there is characteristic periodicity of erythrocytic schizont rupture resulting in a synchronous release of merozoites [8].

The feeding mechanisms of babesia and plasmodia during the erythrocytic growth phase are similar, although apparently not identical. The parasite engulfs large droplets of erythrocytic cytoplasm by phagotrophy, leading to the formation of food vacuoles. With babesia, unlike plasmodium, there is no residual pigment

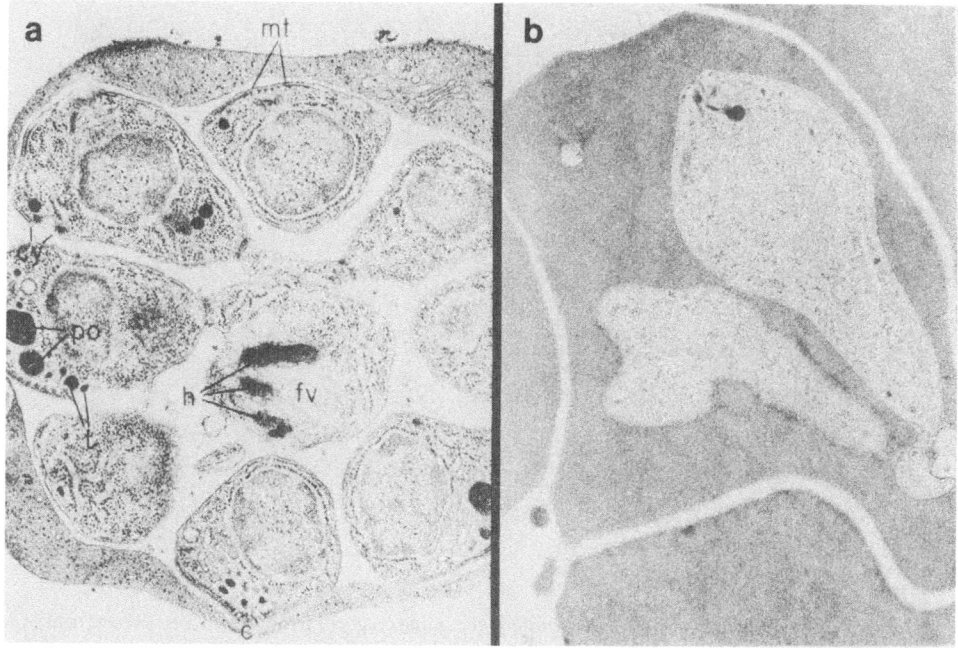

Figure 3. Mode of multiplication of *Plasmodium cathemerium* (a) and *Babesia canis* (b) in their respective host erythrocytes. Unlike the *Plasmodium* parasite which undergoes the process of merogony and a multiple release of merozoites, *Babesia* multiplies by binary fission or a process of 'budding' with a maximum of four progenies. (a – from M.A. Rudziska and K. Vickerman, *Inf. Blood Dis. of Man and Animals,* Vol. 1, D. Weinman and M. Ristic eds. 1968. p. 265).

(hemozoin) detectable in the cytoplasm following digestion of the contents of food vacuole.

4. Kinetics of merozoites

After contact has been established between the erythrocyte membrane and the anterior end of the merozoite, the next step, invagination of the host cell membrane, is effected. Attachment following contact is mediated through recognition by the merozoite surface coat of receptors on the erythrocyte membrane (Fig. 4). Removal of the merozoite surface coat from the babesia by extraction in cold saline eliminates the ability of the organism to attach to the erythrocyte and function in the Merozoite Serum Neutralization (MSN) test. With some variations among plasmodia, removal of erythrocyte receptors by various enzymes greatly reduces or eliminates infection [9]. The need for a specific erythrocyte receptor for the infection to take place is best illustrated by the dependence of *P. vivax* on recognition of Duffy blood group factors as the receptor for the merozoite [10, 11].

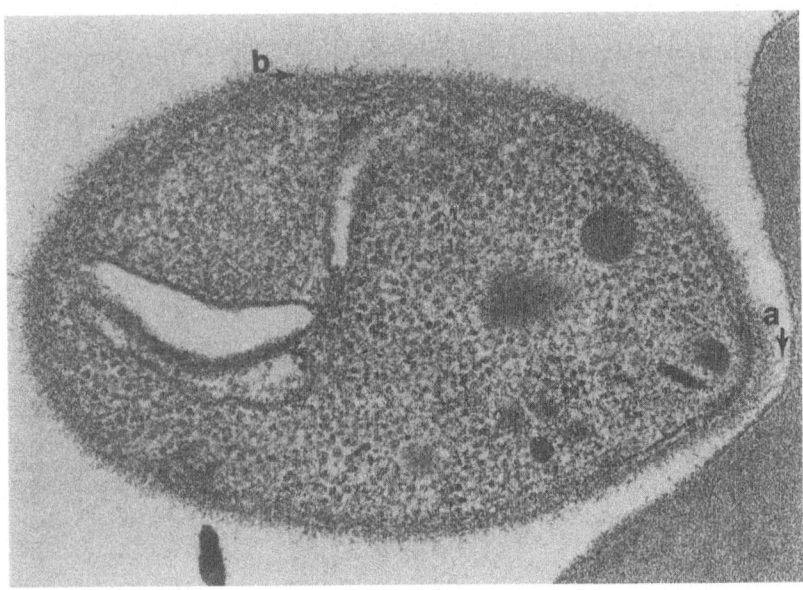

Figure 4. Plasmodium falciparum merozoite at the initial contact (arrow a) between the merozoites apical end and erythrocyte. The contact is preceeded through recognition by the merozoite surface coat (electron light layer surrounding the outer merozoite membrane – arrow b) of specific receptors on the erythrocytic membrane. (From Dr. Masamichi Aikawa, Institute of Pathology, Case Western Reserve University, Cleveland, Ohio).

There is evidence that the invagination of the host membrane by invading merozoites is assisted by lytic enzymes associated with rhoptries and micronemes. In babesia, unlike plasmodia, the parasitophorous vacuole only surrounds the parasite for a brief period after penetration and then gradually disappears by fusing with the plasma membrane of the parasite (Figs. 5a and b). After fusion the babesial merozoite can leave the host cell and re-enter other erythrocytes. Babesia retain their viability for up to 16 hours outside the erythrocytes and, may penetrate several erythrocytes before finally settling in one for growth and development. In plasmodium, on the other hand, all the merozoites from one meront are kept together by the parasitophorous membrane which is not incorporated into the forming merozoites. This parasitophorous bag keeps the new merozoites together until they leave the host cell which takes place when the cell is destroyed. This property in plasmodium may be responsible for the occurrence of synchrony of exit in malaria and the lack of such a phenomenon in babesias. The survival of the plasmodial merozoite in the extracellular environment seems to be of very short duration (Table 1).

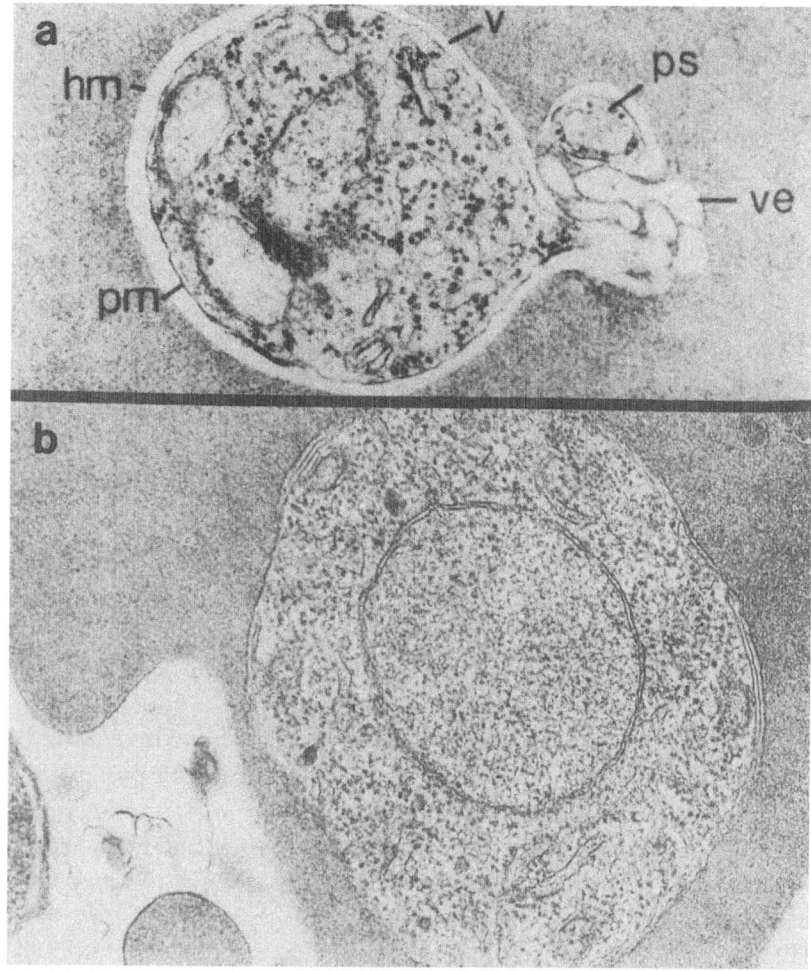

Figure 5. An early (a) and a more advanced stage of development (b) of a *Babesia* parasite. During the initial stage the organism is clearly separated from the erythrocyte by a parasitophorous vacuole. In the more advanced stage of development the membrane of the parasitophorous vacuole becomes closely apposed to the parasite and eventually disintegrates. (a – from M.A. Rudzinska, *Babesiosis,* M. Ristic and J.P. Kreier, eds. 1981:97.

Table 1. Comparative kinetics of babesial and plasmodial merozoites

Parameter	Babesia	Plasmodium
Development	Asynchronous budding 1–4	Synchronous budding 10–25
Viability	Multiple penetration survival up to 16 h	Single penetration survival 10–15 min; max 1 hr
Parasitophorous vacuole	Lost during development	Retained

5. *In vitro* cultures

The development of methods for continuous *in vitro* propagation of *P. falciparum* and *B. bovis* was a major achievement in the century long research efforts on malaria and babesiosis. These accomplishments initiated a new era in the study of the two diseases and have opened a vast horizon of possibilities for easier and more accurate studies of the properties of the organisms, their antigens, and, consequently, for the development of effective immunoprophylactic and sero-diagnostic methods for the control of these diseases.

It was the pioneering work of Trager in 1943 who, using short-term cultures of *P. lophurae* and *P. knowlesi*, started defining the specific nutritional require-ments of plasmodia [12]. Most striking was the discovery that these organisms require p-aminobenzoic acid (PABA). Studies which followed led to the develop-ment of the first continuous *in vitro* culture of *P. falciparum* by Trager and Jensen in 1976 [13]. The prototype culture method was called the petri dish candle jar system. A 50% cell suspension consisting of infected and uninfected human erythrocytes was diluted to an 8% cell suspension with RPMI medium containing 10% normal human serum and placed in petri dishes. Once a day, or more often if needed, the cultures were provided with fresh medium. Using this method, the 0.1% parasitemia in the cultures at the start increased to 2–5% after 96 hours of incubation.

This development prompted further investigations on improvements of the above cultivation method which would provide for a larger-scale production of *P. falciparum* [14]. These new procedures include: flask cultures, continuousflow methods, 'tipping vessel' or automated medium changer, and more recently, a semi-automated and computer controlled unit designed for the production of large quantities of *P. falciparum* material [15, 16]. In general, the culture substrate used in most of these procedures was RPMI medium supplemented with 10–15% human serum in the presence of low O_2 tension, usually 2–6%. Gentamicin was found useful as an antibacterial agent.

The development of methods for *in vivo* propagation of *P. falciparum* provided an opportunity for various studies of the organism and its properties which were not possible or were difficult with the organisms derived from infected animals. These new studies and accomplishments include, among others: detailed obser-vations on the morphology and kinetics of the organism, evaluation of efficacy of various chemotherapeutic agents, and the development of an inhibition assay for examining the effect of anti-*P. falciparum* antibodies on the invasion of host erythrocytes by this organism.

The successful *in vitro* cultivation of *P. falciparum* encouraged our group to engage in a long-term study of techniques for cultivation of babesia. However, attempts to adapt the method for cultivation of *P. falciparum* to the cultivation of *B. bovis* were unsuccessful. The first *in vitro* method for short-term cultivation of *B. bovis*, called the spinner flask method, was developed by Erp et al. in 1978 [17].

Subsequently, the technique was modified and adapted into a continuous culture system for *B. bovis* [18]. Levy and Ristic radically modified the spinner flask method into a microaerophilous stationary phase (MASP) culture system [19]. The latter method fulfilled the requirements of *B. bovis* for low oxygen tension. The method provided for a continuous generation of massive quantities of merozoites and soluble antigens for use as immunogens and serodiagnostic reagents. In addition, the method was found useful for the evaluation of anti-babesial drugs and for determination of the role of blood factors in resistance to *B. bovis* [20]. The principal requirements for the propagation of *B. bovis* in the MASP culture system are: medium 199, depth of medium 0.6 cm, 5% CO_2 in air and 40% bovine serum. A streptomycin – penicillin combination may be used to control bacterial contamination.

Deprivation of CO_2 in the MASP cultures causes the merozoites to exit erythrocytes and accumulate in the medium rather than invade new erythrocytes. This indicates that this gas is essential for invasion and growth of the organism in the erythrocytes. Exploitation of this phenomenon provided a method for collection of cell-free merozoites and for study of host cell-parasite interaction. Finally, the finding led to the development of the first *in vitro* merozoite neutralization (MN) test for a hemotropic parasite [21]. In the MN test, measured quantities of immune babesia serum are used to inhibit invasion of erythrocytes by the extracellular merozoites. Consequently, the MN test provided a means for quantitation of protective antibodies in babesiosis. Soluble antigens presumably originating from the surface of merozoites were shown to interact with specific antibodies and prevent the inhibition of merozoites by antibody. The latter test is known as the merozoite neutralization inhibition (MNI) test.

6. Pathobiology

A common feature of malaria and babesiosis and, for that matter, all other hemotropic diseases, is the continuous presence of the causative agent in the blood. While anemia is a characteristic feature of the two diseases, the mechanism of induction of anemia and its intensity in the course of the disease may depend on the nature of the causative agent. Using certain pathohematologic and clinical parameters as criteria, one may distinguish a disease syndrome caused by *P. falciparum* and *B. bovis* from that caused by *P. vivax* and *B. bigemina* (Table 2). In the disease caused by the latter two agents, the appearance of a moderate parasitemia and anemia usually coincides with the onset of the first clinical signs of the disease. The disease caused by *P. falciparum* and *B. bovis* on the other hand, may commence in the absence of appreciable parasitemia and anemia.

We should first discuss the pathogenesis of anemia along with other pathologic manifestations typical of the disease syndrome caused by *P. vivax* and *B. bigemina*. From a strictly mechanical point of view, the anemia caused by these agents

Table 2. Malaria and babesiosis: two similar disease syndromes

Parameter	P. falciparum	B. bovis	P. vivax	B. bigemina
Adhesion to endothelial cells	Yes	Yes	No	No
Pathogenicity	High	High	Moderate	Moderate to high
Signs of toxicity	Yes	Yes	No	No
Parasitemia at first clinical eigns	Low	Low	High	High
Anemia at first clinical sings	Slight	Slight	Moderate to high	Moderate to high

is due to intravascular hemolysis which results in a profound anemic anoxia that may cause death of the host. Immunologic factors, however, can also contribute to the anemia. Prominent among these factors are: opsonins or auto-antibody-like globulins to erythrocyte antigens; antibodies to soluble antigens on the surface of infected and normal erythrocytes; binding of immune complexes to normal erythrocytes: and erythrophagocytosis by activated macrophages [1, 22, 23].

Utilizing an *in vitro* system consisting of rat erythrocytes, mouse peritoneal exudate cells, and serum from normal and infected animals, it was demonstrated that opsonins occur in the serum of *B. rodhaini* and *P. berghei*-infected rats [23, 24]. The opsonins were heat stable and sensitized normal uninfected autologous and homologous erythrocytes to phagocytosis by macrophages of the RES [24, 25]. The appearance and titers of the opsonins were related to the onset, degree, and duration of anemia in infected animals [23]. This finding is in accord with the observation that the sera of patients with acute malaria agglutinate papain-treated erythrocytes [26]. However, eluates from Coombs-positive erythrocytes did not appear to react with normal erythrocytes, thus giving no support for an autoimmune haemolytic component in the malaria.

Studies utilizing soluble plasma antigens obtained during the acute phases of babesial or plasmodial infections have shown that these may be nonspecifically adsorbed to the surfaces of normal erythrocytes. This process brings about the secondary binding of antibodies to the antigens and triggers complement or cell-dependent effector mechanisms resulting in removal of the erythrocytes. This observation was further substantiated by the finding that inoculation of soluble plasma antigens into normal uninfected animals induces anemia and a degree of protection against subsequent challenge of these animals. These and other findings prompted us to suggest the protective role of soluble plasma antigens in infections caused by *Plasmodium* and *Babesia* spp. [27, 28, 29, 30, 31, 32, 33, 34]. Utilizing this principal, latex particles coated with avian, rodent, simian, and human serum antigens were used to detect antibodies against the human plasmodia [35].

Immune complex glomerulonephritis has been demonstrated in rats infected with *B. rodhani* [36]. The extent of immunopathology with renal complications in domestic animals is not clearly understood. However, hemoglobinemia of cattle affected by *B. bigemina* is frequently followed by hemoglobinuria suggesting an impaired renal function. In human and rodent malaria, circulating immune complexes have been detected by the Clq assay [37, 38, 39]. These immune complexes are apparently instrumental in the development of anemia and glomerulonephritis characteristic of malaria.

Finally, nonspecifically activated cells of the reticuloendothelial system and immunologically activated macrophages play an equally important role in the development of pathologic manifestations and protection in malaria and babesiosis. The histiocytes lining the sinuses of the spleen, lymph nodes, and the liver undergo remarkable hyperplastic and hypertrophic changes during babesiosis and malaria. This cellular response in the spleen is a major factor in the splenomegaly syndrome of the two diseases [40]. A massive and persistent splenomegaly known as Tropical Splenomegaly Syndrome is a characteristic pathologic feature in certain malaria-endemic areas [41]. In rodent malaria, spleen macrophages of infected animals were found more efficient in the ingestion of parasitized reticulocytes than those of normal animals, indicating immunologic activation. There is an indication that an interaction between T-lymphocytes and macrophages is involved in the activation of the latter cells and the ensuing erythrophagocytosis [42].

Characteristic features of the disease caused by *P. falciparum* and *B. bovis* are relatively low levels of parasitemia and anemia at the onset of clinical signs (Table 2). It is known that these organisms are able to avoid destruction by the splenic filter by sequestration of infected erythrocytes in the small capillaries of the brain and other organs. The mechanism by which sequestration occurs and which frequently leads to the development of thrombic anoxia was not clearly understood until recently. It was through electron microscopy study that electron dense cone-shaped protrusions described as knobs were recognized in the membrane of erythrocytes infected with *P. falciparum* [43]. It was then shown that these knobs contain at least one malaria antigen and that they mediate binding to receptors on the surface of endothelial cells lining certain blood capillaries [44]. An examination in similar fashion of sequestered bovine erythrocytes infected with *B. bovis* showed that these cells have stellate projections on their surfaces. These projections mediate attachment to the endothelial cells in a manner similar to that by which the knobs of the *P. falciparum* infected erythrocytes mediate attachment [44]. Recent studies described the elliptical protrusions on the membranes of *B. bovis* infected erythrocytes in greater detail. These protrusions measured about 320 nm in the long axis and about 160 nm in the short axis with erythrocyte cytoplasm beneath the protrusions appearing slightly more electron dense than the remainder of the erythrocyte cytoplasm [45]. Very recently, sections of cerebral blood vessels from a calf infected with *B. bovis* were examined by electron microscopy. There was clear evidence of spike-like projections on the surface of infected erythrocytes. These projections extended between erythrocytes and from erythrocytes to endothelial cell membranes [46] (Fig. 6).

In vitro studies revealed that the virulent form of *B. bovis* has more protrusions on the erythrocyte membrane than the avirulent form produced by frequent passage in splenectomized calves [45]. This suggests that the number of protrusions which appear on the membrane of infected erythrocytes may have a direct relationship to the virulence of the parasites. Similar studies on *P. falciparum* revealed that the knobless clone of the organism was less virulent than the knobbed counterpart [47]. In both malaria and babesiosis, the knobless parasite populations were shown to be capable of inducing immunity against the knobbed-virulent type [48] (see chapter 7).

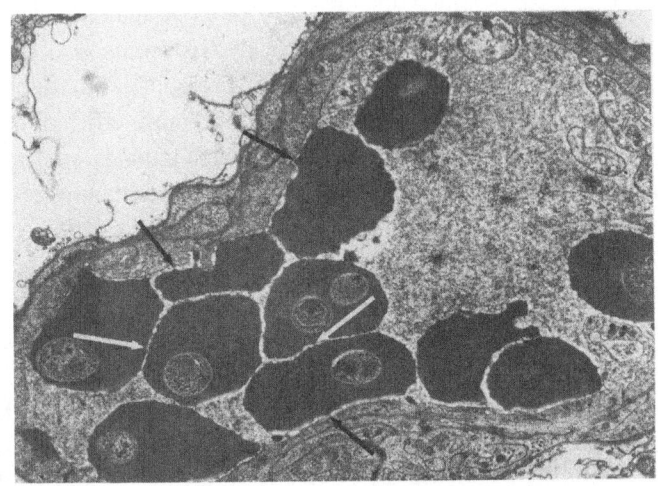

Figure 6. Cerebral blood vessel from calf infected with *Babesia bovis*. Erythrocytes are irregularly shaped and have numerous 'spikes' that extend between erythrocytes (white arrow) or from erythrocytes to endothelial cell membranes (black arrows). From Shadduck *et al.*, Ref. No. 46.

7. Immune responses and antigens

Immune responses to *Babesia*, particularly those responsible for protection, appear to be limited to the erythrocytic phase of development. On the other hand, host-parasite interactions in malaria must be considered separately for each of the three developmental phases of the organism.

7.1. *Sporozoite Immunity*

Sporozoite-induced immunity in malaria is strictly stage specific. Both humoral and cell-mediated (CMI) immune response play a role in sporozoite-induced immunity [42]. Major progress in the study of humoral immune responses to plasmodial sporozoites started with the development of a monoclonal antibody against *P. berghei* sporozoites which produced circumsporozoite precipitates and reacted specifically with the surface antigen Pb44 [49]. The protective role of this antibody is evident by its ability to prevent the attachment and penetration of *P. berghei* sporozoites into target cells *in vitro*. Preincubation of sporozoites with the antibody to the surface antigen results in a reduction and/or neutralization of sporozoite infectivity. Subsequent studies have demonstrated the applicability of these early findings to other malaria parasites including *P. knowlesi*, *P. falciparum* and *p. vivax* [50]. Most recently, the cloning and expression in *E. coli* of a gene coding for *P. knowlesi* sporozoite surface antigen has been achieved [51].

Acquired resistance to sporozoite infection is thymus dependent. There is an indication that CMI effector mechanisms may act against sporozoites in the absence of antibody]48].

Unlike malaria, in babesiosis the pre-erythrocytic form of parasite development takes place in the tick vector rather than in the mammalian host [52]. This form of babesia is termed the vermicule and bears a significant morphologic resemblance to plasmodial sporozoites (Fig. 7a and b). There is no demonstrable immunity to challenge with erythrocytic babesis following immunization with vermicules [3].

7.2. *Merozoite immunity*

The major thrust of the humoral immune response in both malaria and babesiosis is directed against blood phase antigens, particularly against those of the merozoite. Numerous antigens, some of which may be involved in the induction of immunity, have been variously identified as being associated with the organism, the host cell membrane, or free in the blood plasma or supernatant culture medium. In view of the magnitude of literature on immune responses to blood phase antigens, this discussion will be limited to a comparative analysis of immune responses to major protective antigens of *P. falciparum* and *B. bovis*. The three antigens apparently intimately associated with the induction of protective immunity against these agents are: merozoite surface coat, knobs in the membrane of infected erythrocytes and soluble proteinaceous moieties (exoantigens) naturally liberated in culture supernatant medium. Exoantigens should be distinguished from solubilized antigens which may be obtained by physical and/or biochemical degradation of the organism and infected erythrocytes. Exoantigens of *P. falciparum* and *B. bovis* and their role in induction of protective immunity will be reviewed in the next section.

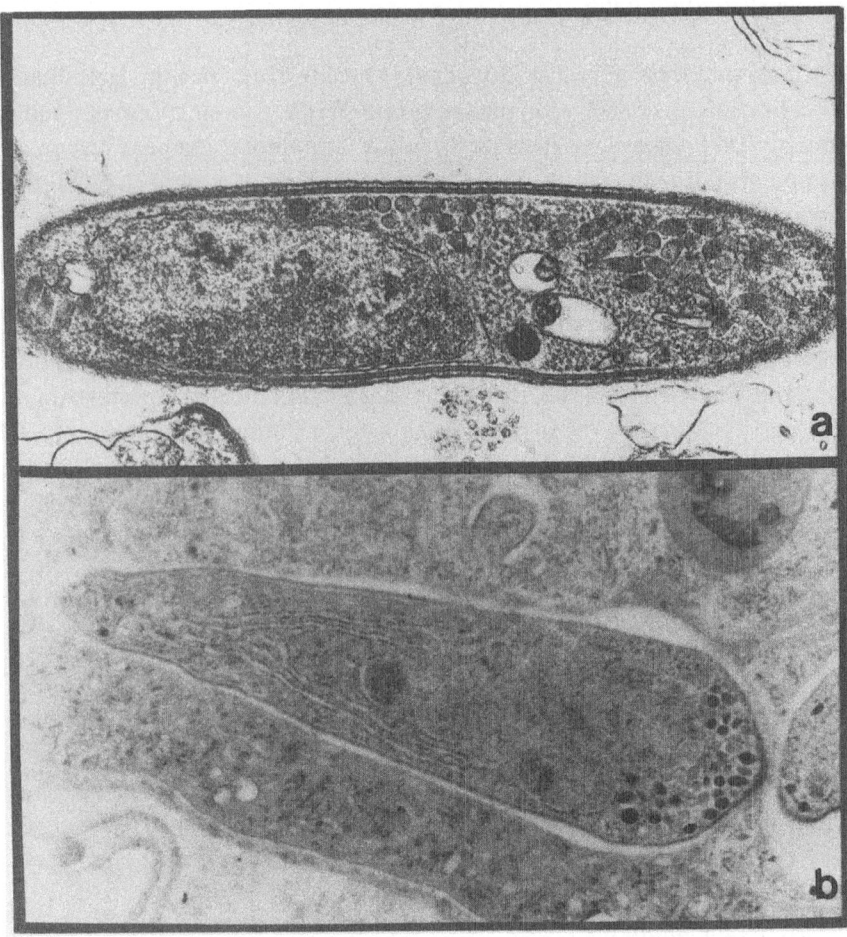

Figure 7. The appearance of malarial sporozoite (a) and babesial vermicule (b). The latter organism shares many morphologic features with the infective malaria sporozoite, however, it is non-infective for the mammalian host.

Merozoite surface coat antigen appears to be intimately associated with the recognition of and attachment to specific erythrocyte receptors, thus contributing to the process of parasite entry into the host cell [9, 10]. In anology with surface components of other microbes, the surface coat serves to protect the merozoite against constitutive (normal) immune mechanisms. Being poorly immunogenic, surface coat antigen promotes slow induction of specific immune responses in an infected and usually immunosuppressed host. However, in an immunologically competent susceptible host, inoculation of surface coat antigens in combination with appropriate adjuvants shortens the time required for the development of a specific immune response. In this way, all immunized animals can overcome the parasite's defense mechanisms more rapidly [21]. The knobs in the membranes of erythrocytes harboring *P. falciparum* and *B. bovis* also aid these parasites in protecting themselves against splenic filtration. This is a mechanical form of protection. Plasma antigens, on the other hand, complex with anti-parasite-antibodies and in this fashion shield the merozoite during invasion of erythrocytes. Jointly, surface coat, knobs, and exoantigens are not there to put the parasite at risk, rather their role is to frustrate the hosts' defense mechanisms and promote survival of the parasite.

The immune mechanisms by which the host controls the development of asexual blood stages of the two organisms include those directed against; (a) merozoites during the passage from one erythrocyte to another, (b) antigens of infected erythrocytes, i.e., knobs and other antigens intimately associated with the host cell membrane, and (c) organisms inside the erythrocytes.

Antibodies to merozoites include those directed against the surface coat which, by interacting with this antigen, may prevent the merozoite's attachment to and penetration of erythrocytes [21, 52, 53, 54, 55]. Similarly, cytophilic and opsonizing antibodies may invite phagocytosis as an efficient anti-parasitic mechanism [56, also see chapter 7]. Antibodies to infected erythrocytes include those directed against antigens on or in the erythrocytic membrane and those against altered erythrocytic surface (auto-antibodies and normal serum opsonins) [23, 57]. Deposit of plasma exoantigens on the surface of both infected and noninfected erythrocytes may also instigate an anti-erythrocyte antibody effect.

Immune mechanisms directed against the intraerythrocytic parasite may involve CMI forces, including lymphokines and monokines. The role of T cells in protective immunity to malaria and babesiosis includes cooperation in antibody synthesis by B cells and production of mediators that recruit and activate the monocyte-macrophage system. Another indicator of the CMI response is delayed cutaneous hypersensitivity which has been reported in both malaria and babesiosis [58, 59].

7.3. *Gamete immunity*

For babesia, the word gamete must still be used with reservation. While forms typical of gametes have been described by several investigators and occasionally a close connection between cytoplasms of two gametes was found, suggesting fusion, thus far there have been no reports attesting the actual fertilization of gametes [8].

In malaria, rapid and considerable advances have been made toward the recognition and understanding of immunity against gametes. Earlier studies on the definition of protective gamete-specific antigens in *P. galinaceum* and *P. knowlesi* have now been expanded to include *P. falciparum*. By use of monoclonal antibodies, at least three proteins have been identified in *P. falciparum* gametes. Monoclonal antibodies to these antigens seem to block the infectivity of gametes for the mosquito [60].

8. Vaccines

The idea of using vaccines as a means of prevention and control of malaria and babesiosis has evolved as a logical sequence after realization that chemotherapy and vector control are not sufficiently effective and the results frequently unpredictable. The development of systems for continuous *in vitro* propagation of *P. falciparum* and *B. bovis* and the availability of hybridoma and genetic engineering technologies, all realized during the last decade, are the most significant elements which triggered scientifically sound efforts on vaccine research in malaria and babesiosis.

Research on malaria vaccines is divided according to the growth stage of the organism. Extracellular stages of the parasite, i.e., sporozoites, erythrocytic merozoites and microgametes have been the principal targets of vaccine research.

In babesiosis, the focus of the research has been on live or inactivated organisms, or their components, derived from the blood of an infected animal or *in vitro* cultures. A most recent and thus far most promising approach to vaccination against babesiosis is the use of cell culture-derived soluble 'exoantigens' as immunogens in combination with appropriate adjuvants. This immunogen appears safe, effective, and practical to produce and dispense. It is because of these and other qualities that it is being used for commercial production of the first protozoan vaccine, namely that against *Babesia canis* (see chapter 9).

The literature on vaccines for malaria and babesiosis is very voluminous. There are some recent excellent reviews on the subject which include those in this book [1, 3, 48, 61]. Consequently, only a comparative overview of essential findings will be covered in this communication. In view of the fact, however, that the soluble exoantigen vaccination approach, originally developed for *B. bovis*, has also been found applicable to *P. falciparum*, a synopsis of findings with the two agents and their interpretation will be covered in this section.

8.1. *Sporozoite vaccines*

Research on a sporozoite vaccine has involved the use of whole live or irradiated sporozoites and specific surface antigen (circumsporozoite antigens) as potential immunogens. To be immunogenic, sporozoites must be obtained at a specific stage of their development in the vector's salivary gland, and must be administered intravenously. Challenge studies indicated that protective immunity lasted three to six months and was species specific [48]. In another study, no immunity was demonstrated against a natural exposure [62].

The use of hybridoma technology has led to the identification of a family of circumsporozoite antigens serving as candidate vaccines against infection caused by sporozoites. In most instances, the role of the isolated antigens in immunity has been ascertained by *in vitro* neutralization and *in vivo* growth inhibition tests using monoclonal antibodies and isolated sporozoites. The recent cloning and expression in *E. coli* of a gene coding for *P. knowlesi* sporozoite surface antigen may lead to the production of an antigen useful for active immunization studies (see chapter 6).

8.2. Merozoite vaccines

Immunization studies in malaria using various preparations of cell free merozoites have generally produced good results indicating that protection against this blood stage is possible. Various adjuvants including Freund's complete adjuvant (FCA), saponin, Muramyl dipeptide derivatives, and liposomes were found effective [48]. In one study using *P. knowlesi* merozoites in FCA, over 90% of vaccinated rhesus monkeys were protected against a lethal homologous challenge or challenge with a heterologous variant [63]. On challenge, vaccinated animals developed a low grade parasitemia of short duration. Subinoculation of blood from vaccinated animals after the end of parasitemia revealed that the vaccination method induced sterile immunity. These encouraging results, however, are complicated by the technical difficulties of a large scale production of *P. falciparum* merozoites by means of culture techniques. Other equally difficult problems include the availability of methods for collection of merozoites and assuring their freedom from contaminating erythrocytic blood group antigens. To circumvent these difficulties, current efforts are being directed toward isolation of specific protective blood stage antigens as potential vaccine candidates [53, 54, 55].

Over the years, many live and inactivated vaccines have been used to control bovine babesiosis under laboratory and field conditions. Among the live vaccines, best results have been obtained with an 'avirulent' *B. bovis* vaccine [64]. This vaccine strain, produced by rapid passage of the organism through splenectomized calves, has been used to control bovine babesiosis in Australia since 1965. Recent studies on the mechanism of attenuation of *B. bovis* showed that the rapid passage through splenectomized calves results in the selection of a parasite population which lacks the ability to become sequestered in blood capillaries, thereby being susceptible to splenic filtration. This phenomenon seems to be associated with a lack of knob markers on erythrocytes harboring high calf passage parasites (see chapter 7).

Aside from the practical difficulty of dispensing the live vaccine, such a vaccine establishes and maintains bovine reservoirs of infection and occasionally may bring about adverse reactions in vaccinated animals. These and other difficulties prompted researchers to investigate the usefulness of inactivated vaccines which induce sterile immunity.

All early inactivated vaccines used corpuscular babesia immunoges derived from erythrocytes of infected animals at the peak of parasitemia. The immunogens were partially purified, lyophilized or used fresh, and inoculated emulsified in an adjuvant. While partial protection was evident in vaccinated cattle, the development of antibodies to blood group antigens following immunization constituted one of several serious obstacles to use of these preparations. Following a similar course to that followed by those working on malaria, the researchers studying babesiosis then focused on isolation of purified soluble *B. bovis* antigens as immunogens. Monoclonal antibodies were used to identify and isolate protective antigens [65, 66].

The most recent method for immunization against *B. bovis* and *B. canis* was made possible by availability of *in vitro* cultures for these organisms. Soluble exoantigens present in supernatant culture medium are being used in combination with a new saponin adjuvant (Quil-A) for immunization of cattle and dogs against infections with *B. bovis* and *B. canis*, respectively [21, 67]. The vaccine against the latter agent is expected to be available through commercial sources [68] in the very near future (see chapter 9).

8.3. *Gamete vaccines*

Injection of gametes of plasmodia uncontaminated with blood forms of the parasites induce the immunocompetent host to produce stage specific antibodies. These antibodies have no effect upon the asexual forms present in the vertebrate host but inhibit gametes of rodent, avian, and simian malaria parasites after their release from erythrocytes in the mosquito gut [48]. The actual protective mechanism involves agglutination of emerging microgametes which inhibits fertilization [69]. Future successes in research on gamete vaccines will require the development of methods for efficient production of essential gamete antigens. Hybridoma and recombinant DNA technologies seem to be the most appropriate for this purpose.

8.4. *Soluble exoantigen vaccines*

Exoantigens are soluble proteinaceous moieties naturally released in the blood plasma of animals infected with plasmodia and babesia or in the supernatant medium of *in vitro* cultures of these organisms. Plasmodial antigens from human plasma have been grouped and characterized according to their heat stability, molecular weight, enzyme sensitivity, and antigenicity [70]. Exoantigens derived from the plasma of animals acutely infected with various plasmodial and babesial species have been used for the induction of protective immunity in their respective natural hosts [21, 27, 32, 70, 71]. While the protective potential of exoantigens was clearly recognized in the course of the above studies, it was also recognized that the immunogenicity of these antigens was not great possibly due to immune complex formation and enzymatic degradation [21].

8.4.1. *Research in babesiosis*

The development of methods for continuous *in vitro* propagation of *B. bovis* renewed our interest in soluble exoantigens as potential antigens for immunization against bovine babesiosis [19]. In most vaccination experiments, culture-derived exoantigens were used as lyophilized preparations which were emulsified with saponin adjuvant shortly before administration. Two doses of vaccine spaced at 21-day intervals and administered subcutaneously were used in all studies [21].

Well controlled vaccination experiments against bovine babesiosis caused by *B. bovis* were conducted in the United States, Mexico, Venezuela, and Australia. Evidence of protection was demonstrated against virulent homologous and heterologous *B. bovis* using infected ticks or infected blood as the source of challenge material. The challenge periods after vaccination varied from three weeks to six months. Humoral immune responses to vaccination and challenge were measured by the IFA, CF, and ELISA systems. In one instance, the lymphocyte transformation (LT) test was used to measure CMI responses in vaccinated animals (see chapter 7).

The principle of vaccination with exoantigen was successfully adapted for formulation of an immunogen against *B. canis*. Large scale field trials recently completed with this vaccine yielded most satisfactory results (see chapter 9).

Based upon results of various immunochemical studies, it is evident that many of the exoantigens originate from the merozoite surface coat [21, 52, 72]. Most of this antigen is shed in the culture medium at the time of parasite entry into the host erythrocytes, although a portion of the antigen mass may be liberated at the time of merozoite exit from these cells. Appreciable quantities of exoantigens are found adsorbed onto the surfaces of cultured erythrocytes (Fig. 8). Exoantigens have been isolated and generally characterized as being proteinaceous moieties, 30–40,000 molecular weight, which are degraded by papain and trypsin, are stable at 60° C for 30 minutes, have fast electrophoretic mobility and an isoelectric point at pH 5.0–5.5 [72]. Location of these antigens with reference to the host erythrocyte was determined [73].

The use of the *in vitro* babesia merozoite serum neutralization (SN) test has contributed greatly toward the understanding of the mechanism of protection induced by anti-exoantigen antibodies [21]. Aside from preventing or retarding penetration of erythrocytes by the organism, the opsonizing effect of these antibodies and the ensuing phagocytosis present a powerful anti-parasite effect. The production of cytophilic antibodies by immunization with exoantigens, which are capable of binding cell-free babesia onto the surfaces of activated marcophages presents an additional protective element. More recently, it was found that bovine macrophages, sensitized *in vitro* with exoantigens, produce a

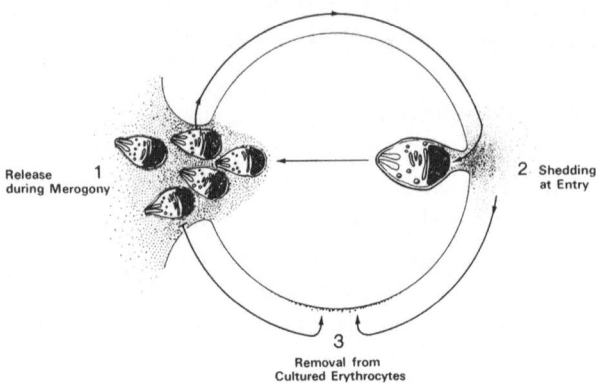

Figure 8. Hypothetical consideration of the origin of culture-derived plasmodial and babesial exoantigens. It is proposed that most of these antigens are liberated in the culture supernatant medium at the time the organisms enter and exit host erythrocytes. A portion of these antigens may be found adsorbed on the surface of both infected and non-infected erythrocytes.

soluble factor capable of inhibiting the growth of babesia in cell cultures and causing development of 'crisis' parasite forms. (see chapter 7).

8.4.2. *Research in malaria*

Successful use of culture-derived soluble babesia exoantigens as immunogens under laboratory and field conditions and the close resemblance between *B. bovis* and *P. falciparum* and the diseases they cause stimulated us to explore vaccination with plasmodial exoantigens. For this purpose, we selected *P. falciparum* Indochina I strain and the squirrel monkey for which this strain is highly pathogenic. A total of 32 Bolivian squirrel monkeys divided in several smaller groups were used to examine the immunogenicity of culture-derived soluble *P. falciparum* exoantigens. All experiments included susceptible negative and known positive (carrier) controls. Challenge doses consisting of 1×10^6 to 2.0×10^7 *P. falciparum* parasitized erythrocytes contained in the whole blood of acutely infected monkeys were administered intravenously at two to nine months after the first vaccine dose.

In order to avoid contaminating antigenic material of human origin, an early trial utilized exoantigens derived from *P. falciparum* culture in squirrel monkey erythrocytes and serum. Prior to injection, saponin (Quil-A) adjuvant was added to the exoantigen preparations. Subsequent studies utilized exoantigens derived from standard human cultures with aluminum hydroxide incorporated as the adjuvant [74, 75]. Crude or partially purified exoantigens concentrated 10-fold by ultrafiltration were administered subcutaneously, in two doses on days 1 and 21. Partially purified exoantigens from cultures of Indochina I and African *P. falciparum* strains were obtained using ion exchange chromatography [76, 77]. The presence of *P. falciparum* antigens in the fractions was determined by means of the ELISA technique using monoclonal antibodies or specific IgG fractions derived from human placentas. An analysis of these fractions by SDS-PAGE and Western Blot techniques revealed the presence of *P. falciparum* moieties of approximately 43 and 95.000 M.W. [78].

All vaccinated animals showed evidence of a specific immune response by the IFA and ELISA tests. These responses commenced approximately two weeks after the first dose of vaccine and were considerably augmented following the second dose. On challenge, typical anamnestic humoral responses were noted in all vaccinated animals. These responses were particularly evident in animals challenged at four or more months after the second dose of vaccine [79].

The negative control monkeys were the only ones to develop signs of *P. falciparum* malaria and die following challenge. These signs were most pronounced approximately one week prior to death and included elevated temperatures, low hematocrit levels and high parasitemia. Pathologic examination of the animals revealed abnormalities typical of *P. falciparum* malaria including clogging of brain capillaries and a hyperplastic spleen. None of the vaccinated and positive control carrier monkeys showed clinical signs of the disease following challenge. Moreover, their eating habits and general behavior remained normal following challenge. All vaccinated animals, however, contracted the infection as they developed a low level and relatively transitory peripheral blood parasitemia. Their hematocrit levels remained stable and their humoral immune responses were much greater than those of the controls. Following challenge, many of the parasites in the vaccinated animals were deformed. These deformed parasites occurred intra- and extraerythrocytically and appear similar to 'crisis' forms seen in immune humans.

Further corroborative evidence of the efficacy of the vaccine was the protective capacity of sera collected from the vaccinated animals prior to challenge. This was established by *in vitro* growth inhibition studies. Of special interest in these studies was the evidence of growth inhibition by serum between Indochina I and African *P. falciparum* strains [80, 81]. Recent findings by Jepsen render strong support to these preliminary findings [80]. In a search for candidate molecules for a malaria vaccine, he demonstrated that affinity-purified human IgG antibodies to soluble exoantigens inhibited the growth *in vitro* of both homologous and heterologous *P. falciparum* antigens. These and other findings by Jepsen indicate that acquired immunity in man to *P. falciparum* is associated with anti-exoantigen IgG and that these antigens may play an important role in the induction of protective immunity. The author concluded that exoantigens are potential candidate molecules for malaria vaccine and suggested that 'since soluble antigens are easily obtainable from *in vitro* cultures, these results open new possibilities for the development of a malaria vaccine'. [82].

The patterns of protection induced in squirrel monkeys by injection of exoantigens appear similar to those previously shown to develop following use of whole merozoites as immunogens [1, 48, 63]. In considering that the major protective antigens of the malaria merozoite are associated with its surface coat and that a good portion of these antigens are liberated in the supernatant medium during merozoite entry into erythrocytes, one may conclude that similar plasmodial immunogens were instrumental in the induction of protective immunity in vaccination experiments using whole merozoites and exoantigens [63]. The use of exoantigens as a malaria vaccine introduces a refinement over that obtained with the whole merozoite immunogen, which is suitable for wider application not only in primates but also in man. The only impurity in culture-derived exoantigen preparation is human serum. Various effective techniques are now available for isolation and purification of malaria associated antigens from the culture supernatants. Moreover, new well-defined synthetic growth supplements that may be useful as a serum substitute are now becoming available. Finally, identification, isolation, and characterization of these molecules may produce information needed for generating these antigens by methods other than from cultures.

With very few exceptions, most of the previous malaria vaccine experiments have used adjuvants which are either not suitable or not acceptable for use in man. The majority of the animals in our study were vaccinated with exoantigens fortified by aluminum hydroxide which is the only adjuvant permitted for human use. None of the animals inoculated with the exoantigens in aluminum hyroxide developed clinical side effects or local tissue damage. Yet, on challenge, nine months after vaccination, a strong immune response and protection was noted in vaccinated animals. These results suggest that exoantigens in aluminum hydroxide induce an immune response that can be recalled rapidly by challenge enabling the animal to efficiently cope with the subsequent infection.

Various observations on the protective mechanisms in babesiosis and now in malaria induced by injection of exoantigens suggest that specific antibodies generated in response to these antigens are the principal effectors [10, 52, 83]. It is apparent that in a nonimmune animal an excess of plasma exoantigens in relationship to antibodies during the patent phase of the disease results in the removal of available antibodies by complex formation, thereby degrading any protective immune responses of the host by allowing undisturbed merozoite cell to cell passage. In contrast, in an immunized animal, the excess of antibodies to soluble exoantigens enables the animal to reduce and gradually overcome various detrimental effects during the critical phase of the disease and allows for recovery without evidence of gross clinical manifestations (Fig. 9).

Assuming that the pattern of response to exoantigens demonstrated in this study by use of primates is that which will occur in man, one may anticipate that a vaccine prepared from exoantigens should prevent severe disease and mortality in the recipients. The results at present observed with this type of the vaccine appear to be in general agreement with the realistic view of what a human malaria vaccine will be. Having a full understanding of the intricate host-parasite-vector relation in malaria, and being a proponant of a vaccine against that disease, but

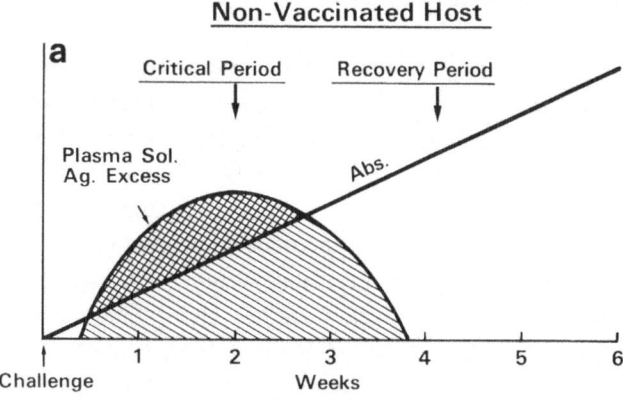

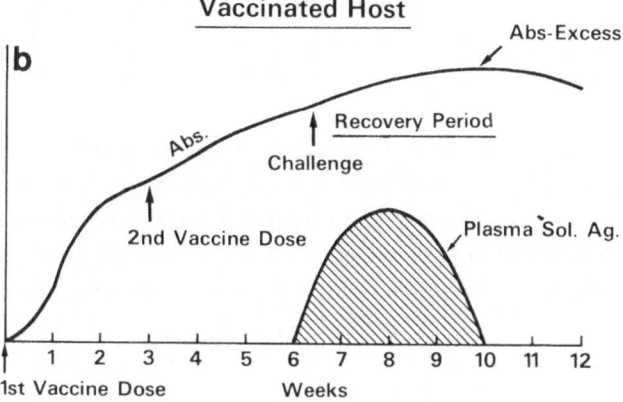

Figure 9. Proposed mechanism of protection induced by immunization with culture-derived soluble plasmodial and babesial exoantigens. In a susceptible animal an excess of plasma exoantigens in relationship to specific antibodies during the patent phase of the disease results in the removal of available antibodies by complex formation, thus degrading protective immune competence of an infected host (a). In contrast, in an immunized animal the excess of anti-exoantigens antibodies in relationship to the plasma exoantigens enables the host to overcome various pathohematological effects of the critical phase of the disease and allows its gradual recovery without the evidence of gross clinical manifestations (b).

recognizing certain limitations of such an immunogen, the late Professor Zuckerman wrote . . . 'This procedure might permit the vaccinated patient in an endemic area to survive the most dangerous period of the disease, primary infection, while establishing acquired immunity associated with progressively increasing resistance to superinfection with the local strains of plasmodia to which he is constantly being exposed' [84].

9. Detection of antibodies and antigens

Microscopic detection of the parasites in stained blood films remains the method of choice for the diagnosis of malaria and babesiosis during the acute phase. In a suspected case of human babesiosis, lack of the pigment in the intraerythrocytic protozoan is a helpful means of differentiation from malaria. In the absence of microscopically visible parasites, the detection of circulating soluble antigens and/or antigen-antibody complexes in the plasma of patients would be a useful means for diagnosis of a current infection. While such antigens have been demonstrated in both diseases, further studies and refinements of detection techniques of these antigens are necessary before such methods can be used routinely for diagnosis of malaria and babesiosis [52, 70]. Continuous efforts for isolation and characterization of serum antigens occurring in individuals with malaria and babesiosis and production of monospecific and monoclonal antibodies to these antigens may soon bring about the development of satisfactory procedures based on antigen detection for the diagnosis of plasmodial and babesial infections.

Soluble and corpuscular antigens from the blood of infected hosts, and from continuous cultures have been used in various serologic tests for diagnosis of malaria and babesiosis. The tests most frequently used for epidemiologic studies and as indicators of the disease in a population are: indirect fluorescent antibody (IFA), indirect hemagglutination (IH), and enzyme-linked immunosorbent assay (ELISA) tests. For the diagnosis of malaria, anti-immunoglobulin conjugates are available from the WHO and these can be used to standardize IFA tests for this disease.

Since parasitemia and disease may appear before antibodies are detectable, a negative test may not mean that the subject is free of infection. Also, the tests will not revert immediately to a negative status after an infection has terminted spontaneously or by chemotherapy. These and other limitations of serologic procedure for the two diseases must be taken into consideration in the analysis of disease data.

The commercial availability of fluorescein-labelled antiglobulin and the fact that IFA tests for babesiosis can utilize eluate from blood samples dried on filter paper as a source of antibody make the collection and transport of serum samples feasible under tropical field conditions. Although considerable efforts have been made to purify *Babesia* antigens, some serologic cross-reaction has been observed among the various *Babesia* and *Plasmodium* species.

Reviews by Sulzer and Wilson [85] and by Cohen and Lambert [1] provide information regarding the advantages and limitations of various serodiagnostic procedures for malaria. Similarly, a comprehensive review by Todorovic and Carson [86] provides information on the subject of babesiosis.

The two test procedures useful for analysis of the immune responses to malaria and babesiosis are the *in vitro* growth inhibition and merozoite neutralization tests, respectively. These tests are recognized as the only available laboratory procedures for detection and measurement of protective antibodies directed aganist erythrocytic forms of *P. falciparum* [1, 87] and *B. bovis* [21, 88].

10. Chemotherapy

It is evident that different sets of compounds are effective against the two agents. The matter is best reflected by the fact that quinine sulfate and chloroquine, the two traditional anti-malaria compounds, are generally ineffective in the treatment of human babesiosis. Chemotherapy of babesiosis in animals, however, is not a simple matter as there is no compound available that is effective against all species of babesia. The chemotherapeutic agents most commonly used for treatment of babesiosis are the diamidine, quinoline, and acridine derivatives. The efficacy of a given drug is determined by the *Babesia* species involved and the tolerance to the drug of the animal being treated.

Experimental induction of drug resistance against various *Babesia* has been documented, however, drug resistance has not yet evolved into an important constraint under field conditions. On the contrary, the phenomenon of drug resistance in malaria is reaching alarming proportions and poses serious problems for the future of chemotherapeutic control of this disease. The most important problem is resistance of *P. falaciparum* to chloroquine which may be associated with resistance to compounds such as pyrimethamine, pyrimethamine-sulphonamide combinations, and quinine also.

Research on the mechanisms of resistance of *Plasmodium* to chemical compounds and the formulation of therapies based on drug combinations, which may inhibit or retard induction of drug resistance, are urgently needed (see chapter 10 and 11).

11. Summary and conclusions

The history of human malaria and bovine babesiosis documents the pioneering discovery of the transmission of protozoan pathogens by the arthropod vectors respectively mosquitos and ticks. In these vectors, *Plasmodium* and *Babesia* undergo a sexual phase of development. In their vertebrate hosts they cause similar clinicopathologic abnormalities, with the resemblances being particularly pronounced in the two groups of diseases caused respectively by *P. vivax-B. bigemina*, and *P. falciparum-B. bovis*.

There is no tissue phase of development in babesia in its vertebrate host, however, a strong morphologic resemblance exists between plasmodial sporozoites and babesial vermicules. It is therefore possible that in babesia the phase equivalent to the plasmodial pre-erythrocytic phase takes place in the tick in the form of a continuous reproduction of vermicules which eventually give rise to forms directly invading the erythrocytes. Blood phase merozoites of plasmodia and babesia appear structurally similar and both invade erythrocytes in a like manner characterized by specific recognition between merozoite and host cell receptors. In babesia, unlike in malaria, the parasitophorous vacuole only temporarily surrounds the babesia in the erythrocyte and then gradually disappears by fusion with the plasma membrane leaving this organism free in the erythrocyte cytoplasm. The babesial merozoite unlike the plasmodial merozoite is free to leave the host cell. On the other hand, the persistence of a parasitophorous vacuole in malaria may keep the merozoites together and contribute to the occurence of synchrony in development.

Diagnostic methods for both diseases are similar and a common pathologic manifestation of the two diseases is anemia. One of the unique pathologic effects of infections with *P. falciparum* and *B. bovis* is sequestration of infected erythrocytes in blood capillaries of the brain and other tissues. Recent studies revealed the presence of knob-like structures in the membranes of human and bovine erythrocytes infected with these agents. These knobs which apparently constitute virulence markers appear to be antigenetically specific and interact with receptors on endothelial cells of the blood vessels.

Acquired immunity in malaria is stage and species specific and is based upon antibodies which block attachment of sporozoites to hepatocytes or inhibit entry of merozoites into erythrocytes. In both malaria and babesiosis, cytophilic and opsonizing antibodies may facilitate phagocytosis as an anti-parasite mechanism. Antibody action against gametes in the vectors probably does not occur normally in nature. The roles of cell-mediated immunity and nonspecific immunity including autoimmune mechanisms in the pathogenesis of these diseases are not clearly defined.

The development of methods for continuous *in vitro* propagation of *P. falciparum* and *B. bovis* has opened a vast horizon of opportunities for more definitive characterization of the two agents. Culture has made immunochemical studies of their antigens and eventual selection of candidate vaccine molecules possible. The three antigens apparently intimately associated with the induction of immunity to the blood phase of these agents are: merozoite surface coat, erythrocytic knobs and plasma exoantigens. Some of the latter antigens originate from the surfaces of merozoites while others are found loosely associated with the organisms in the host erythrocyte. Consequently, these antigens are liberated in the blood plasma and culture medium at the time of merozoite entry into and exit from host cells.

In an actual infection, the abundance of undesirable antigens and tissue products exert an excessive demand (immunosuppression) on the host's reticuloendothelial system and so may interfere with prompt recognition of protective antigens and antiparasite activity. Hence, the induction of natural protective immunity is slow and generally requires repeated infections. The induction of sterile immunity with the appropriate antigens fortified with suitable adjuvants in a susceptible, immunologically competent host, results in the host's generating a maximum specific immune effector response and enables the host to survive the most dangerous period of the disease, the primary infection.

The availability of *in vitro* cultures for plasmodium allows the identification of protective blood phase antigens and evaluation of their immunogenic properties in appropriate primate species. Unfortunately, those engaged in the development of malaria sporozoite and gamete vaccines do not have culture technique available to them. Nevertheless, by the use of hybridoma technology and monoclonal antibodies, those workers have been able to develop and isolate what appear to be stage specific antigens. These antigens, however, must first be demonstrated to induce protective immunity in a primate model before it will be possible to proceed further with their use as vaccine candidates.

This comparative overview of malaria and babesiosis indicates many common features of the two diseases and their causative agents and suggests the advantage of an interdisciplinary research approach. By virtue of its enormous importance to human health, the research in malaria has been better funded and thus more prolific and more profound than that in babesiosis. The availability of the natural host, however, for study of the various infectious and immunologic parameters in babesiosis should be of interest to malariologists and serve as a basis for comparative evaluation of essential findings.

Some of the studies described in this communication have been made possible by senior author's research contracts from the United States Agency for International Development, Washington, DC; and the Institute Mérieux of Lyon, France.

12. References

1. Cohen S and Lambert PH: Malaria. In: Immunology of Parasitic Infections. KS Warren (ed). Blackwell Scientific Publ., 2nd Edition, Oxford. 1982, p. 422–474.
2. Wernsdorfer WH: The importance of malaria in the world. In: Malaria. JP Kreier (ed). Academic Press, New York, NY. 1980, p. 1–79.
3. Ristic Miodrag and Kreier JP: Babesiosis. Academic Press Publishers, New York, NY, 1981.
4. Ristic Miodrag and Healy GR: Babesiosis. In: Parasitic Zoonoses. L. Jacobs, P. Arambulo (eds.). CRC Press, Inc., Boca Raton, FL. 1982, p. 151–165.
5. Jones WHS: Malaria and Greek History. Manchester University Press, Manchester. 1909.
6. Bruce-Chwatt LJ: Essential Malariology. William Heineman Med Books, Ltd., London. 1980.
7. Smith T and Kilbourne FL: Investigation into the Nature, Causation, and Prevention of Texas or Southern Cattle Fever. US Department Agri Bur Anim Ind Bull 1:1–301, 1893.
8. Rudzinskia MA: Morphologic Aspects of Host-Cell-Parasite Relationships in Babesiosis. In:

Babesiosis. M Ristic and JP Kreier (eds.). Academic Press, Publ., New York, NY. 1981, p. 87–141.

9. Miller LH: Hypothesis on the mechanism of erythrocyte invasion by malaria merozoites. Bull WHO 55:157–162, 1977.

10. Miller LH , Aikawa M and Dvorak JA: Malaria (*Plasmodium knowlesi*) merozoites: immunity and the surface coat. J Immunol 114:1237–1242, 1975.

11. Miller LH, McAuliffe FM and Mason SJ: Erythrocyte receptors for malaria merozoites. Am J Trop Med Hyg Supp 26:204–208, 1977.

12. Trager W: Further studies on the survival and development *in vitro* of malaria parasite. J Expt Med pp. 411–420, 1943.

13. Trager W and Jensen JB: Human malaria parasites in continuous culture. Science 193:673–675, 1976.

14. Trager W and Jensen JB: Cultivation of erythrocytic and exoerythrocytic stages of plasmodium. In: Malaria Vol. 3. JP Kreier (ed.). Academic Press, Inc., New York, NY 1980, p. 271–319.

15. Palmer K, Hui GSN, Siddiqui WA and Palmer EL: A large-scale *in vitro* production system for *Plasmodium falciparum*. J Parasit 68:1180–1183, 1982.

16. Palmer K, Hui GSN, Siddiqui WA and Palmer EL: A large scale semi-autometed cellular system for production of *Plasmodium falciparum* antigen (Abstract). Proc 2nd Int Conf Malaria and Babesiosis, Sept. 18–22, 1983. Annecy, France. p. 19.

17. Erp EE, Gravely SM, Smith RD, Ristic M, Osorno BM and Carson CA: Growth of *Babesia bovis* in Bovine Erythrocyte Cultures. Am J Trop Med Hyg 27:1061–1064, 1978.

18. Erp EE, Smith RD, Ristic M, Osorno BM: Continuous *in vitro* cultivation of *Babesia bovis*. Am J Vet Res 41:1141–1142, 1980.

19. Levy MG and Ristic M: *Babesia bovis*: Continuous cultivation in microaerophilous stationary phase culture. Science (207) (No. 4426):1218–1220, 1980.

20. Levy MG, Erp E and Ristic M: Cultivation of babesia. In: *Babesiosis*. M Ristic and JP Kreier (eds.) Academic Press, Inc., New York, NY.1981, p. 207–223.

21. Ristic M and Levy MG: A new era of research toward solution of bovine babesiosis. In: Babesiosis. M Ristic and JP Kreier (eds.). Academic Press, Inc., New York, NY. 1981, p. 509–544.

22. Seed TM and Kreier JP: Erythrocyte destruction mechanisms in malaria. In: Malaria, Vol. 2. JP Kreier (ed.). Academic Press, Inc., New York, NY. 1980, p. 1–46.

23. Schroeder WF and Ristic M: Autoimmune response and pathogenesis of blood parasite disease. In: Infectious Blood Disease of Man and Animals. D Weinman and M Ristic (eds.). Academic Press, Inc., New York, NY. 1968, p. 63–77.

24. Zuckerman A: A review: current status of the immunology of blood and tissue protozoan. II. Plasmodium. Expt Parasit 42:374–446, 1977.

25. Zuckerman A and Ristic M: Blood parasite antigens and antibodies. In: Infectious Blood Diseases of Man and Animals. D Weinman and M Ristic (eds.). Academic Press, Inc., New York, NY. 1968, p. 79–122.

26. Facer CA, Bray RS and Brown J: Direct Coombs antiglobulin reaction in Gambian children with *Plasmodium falciparum* malaria. I. Incidence and class specificity. Clin Exp Immunol 35:119–127, 1979.

27. Sibinovic KH: Immunogenic properties of purified antigens isolated from the serum of horses, dogs, and rats with acute babesiosis. PhD Thesis, University of Illinois, Urbana, IL. 61801, 1966.

28. Sibinovic KH, Sibinovic S, Ristic M and Cox HW: Immunogenic properties of babesial serum antigens. J Parasitol 53:1121–1129, 1967.

29. Sibinovic KH, Milar R, Ristic M and Cox HW: *In vivo* and *in vitro* effects of serum antigens of babesial infection and their antibodies on parasitized and normal erythrocytes. Ann Trop Med Parasitol 63:327–336, 1969.

30. Smith AR, Karr LJ, Lykins JD and Ristic M: Serum soluble antigens of malaria: a review. Exp Parasit 31:120–125, 1972.

31. Smith AR, Lykins JD, Voss EW and Ristic M: Identification of an antigen and specific antibody in the sera of chickens infected with *Plasmodium gallinaceum*. J Immunol 103:6–14, 1969.

32. Todorovic R, Ferris D and Ristic M: Immunogenic properties of serum antigens from chicken infected with *Plasmodium gallinaceum*. Ann Trop Med Parasit 61:117–124, 1967.

33. Todorovic R, Ferris D and Ristic M: Antigens of *Plasmodium gallinaceum*. I. Biophysical and biochemical characterization of explasmodial antigen. Am J Trop Med Hyg 17:685–694, 1968.

34. Todorovic R, Ferris D and Ristic M: Antigens of *Plasmodium gallinaceum*. II. Immunoserological characterization of explasmodial antigens and their antibodies. Am J Trop Med Hyg 17:695–701, 1968.

35. Todorovic R, Ristic M and Ferris D: A tube latex agglutination test for the diagnosis of malaria. Trans R Soc Trop Med Hyg 62:51–57, 1968.

36. Annable CR and Ward RA: Immunopathology of the renal complications of babesiosis. J Immunol 112:1–8, 1974.

37. Perrin LH, Mackey L, Aguado T, Lambert PH and Mieschber PA: Demonstration d'antigens parasitaires solubles d'anticorps correspondant et de complexes immuns lois du traitement de la malaria. Schweizerische med Wochenschr 109:1832–1834, 1979.

38. Willson RJM, McGregor IA and Williams K: Occurrence of S-antigens in serum in *Plasmodium falciparum* infections in man. Trans R Soc Trop Med Hyg 69:453–459, 1975.

39. June CH, Contreres E, Perrin LH, Lambert PH and Miescher PA: Circulating and tissue bound immune complex formation in murine malaria. J Immunology 122:2154–2161, 1979.

40. Hildebrandt PK: Organ and vascular pathology of babesiosis. In: Babesiosis. M Ristic and JP Kreier (eds.). Academic Press, Inc., New York, NY. 1981, p. 459–473.

41. Lowenthal MW, Hutt MSR, Jones IG, Mohelski K, and Riordan EC: Massive splenomegaly in northern Zambia. I. Analysis of 344 cases. Trans R Soc Trop Med Hyg 74:91–98, 1980.

42. Roberts DW and Neidanz WP: Splenomegaly, enhanced phagocytosis and anemia are thymus-dependent response to malaria. Infec Immunity 20:728–731, 1978.

43. Aikawa M, Rabbege J, Udeinya I and Miller LH: Electron microscopy of knobs in *P. falciparum*-infected erythrocytes. J Parasitology 62:435–437, 1983.

44. Aikawa M, Miller LH and Ristic M: Morphologic modification of erythrocyte membrane associated with malaria and babesia infection. (Abstract) Proc 2nd Int Conf Malaria and Babesiosis. Sept. 18–22, 1983. Annecy, France. p. 28.

45. Aikawa M, Rabbege J, Ristic M and Miller LH: Structural alterations of the membrane of erythcoytes infected with *Babesia bovis*. In Press. Am J Trop Med and Hyg, 1984.

46. Shadduck JA, Everitt J, Ristic M and Miller LH: Pathology of bovine babesiosis. (Abstract) Proc 2nd Int Conf Malaria and Babesiosis. Sept. 18–22, 1983. Annecy, France. p. 18.

47. Langreth SG and Peterson E: Pathogenicity of knobless clone of *Plasmodium falciparum* in Aotus monkeys. (Abstract) Proc 2nd Int Conf Malaria and Babesiosis, Sept. 18–22, 1983. Annecy, France. p. 117.

48. Deans JA and Cohen S: Immunology of malaria. Ann Rev Microbiol 37:25–49, 1983.

49. Yoshida N, Potonanjak P, Nussenzweig V, Nussenzweig RS: Biosynthesis of Pb44, the protective antigen of sporozoites of *Plasmodium berghei*. J Exp Med 154:1225–1236, 1981.

50. Santoro F, Cochrane AH, Nussenzweig V, Nardin E, Nussenzweig RS, Gwadz RW and Ferreirz A: Structural similarities among the protective antigens of sporozoites from different species of malaria parasites. J Biol Chem (258):3341–3345, 1983.

51. Ellis J, Ozzki LS, Gwadz RW, Cochrane AH, Nussenzweig V, Nussenzweig RS, Godson GW: Cloning and expression in *E. coli* of the malaria sporozoite surface antigen gene from *Plasmodium knowlesi*. Nature 302:536–538, 1983.

52. Ristic M, Smith RD, Kakoma I: Characterization of babesia antigens derived from cell culture and ticks. In: Babesiosis. M Ristic and JP Kreier (eds.). Academic Press, Inc., New York, NY. 1981, p. 337–380.

53. Hudson DE, Miller LH, Richard RL, David PH, Alving CR and Gitler C: The malaria merozoite

surface: a 140,000 M.W. protein antigentically unrelated to other surface components in *Plasmodium knowlesi*. J Immunol 130:2886–2890, 1983.

54. Deans JA, Thomas AW, Alderson T and Cohen S: Biosynthesis of a putative protective *Plasmodium knowlesi* merozoite antigen (Abstract). Proc 2nd Int Conf Malaria and Babesiosis, Sept. 18–22, 1983. Annecy, France. p. 101.

55. Miller LH, David PH and Hadley TJ: The surface membranes of *Plasmodium*: events leading to invasive merozoites (Abstract). Proc 2nd Int Conf Malaria and Babesiosis, Sept. 18–22, 1983. Annecy, France. p. 29.

56. Khusmith S, Druilhe P: Specific arming of monocytes by cytophilic IgG promotes *Plasmodium falciparum* merozoite ingestion. Roy Soc Trop Med Hyg 76:423–424, 1982.

57. Kreier JP, Shapiro H, Dilly D, Szilvessy IP, Ristic M: Autoimmune reactions in rats with *Plasmodium berghei* infection. Exp Parasit 19:155–162, 1966.

58. Finerty JF, Krehl EP: Cyclophosphamide pretreatment and protection against malaria. Inf and Immun 14:1103–1105, 1976.

59. Banerjee DP, Sing B, Gaulam OP and Sarup S: Cell-mediated immune response in equine babesiosis. Trop Anim Health Prod 9:153–158, 1977.

60. Rener J, Graves PM, Carter R, Williams JL, Burkot TR: Identification of target antigens of malaria transmission blocking monoclonal antibodies on gametes of *Plasmodium falciparum*. J Exp Med. In Press. 1983.

61. Kreier JP: Malaria. Vols. 1, 2, 3. Academic Press, Inc., New York, NY. 1980.

62. Bray RS: Vaccination against *Plasmodium falciparum* a negative result. Trans R Soc Trop Med Hyg 70:250, 1976.

63. Richards WHG, Michell GH, Butcher GA and Cohen S: Merozoite vaccination of rhesus monkeys against *Plasmodium knowlesi* malaria immunity to sporozoite (mosquito transmitted) challenge. Parasitology 74:191–198, 1977.

64. Callow LT: Vaccination against bovine babesiosis. Adv Exp Med Biol 93:121–149, 1977.

65. Mahoney DF, Wright IG and Goodget BV: Bovine babesiosis: the immunization of cattle with fractions of erythrocytes infected with *Babesia bovis* (syn. *B. argentina*). Vet Immun and Immunopath 2:145–156, 1981.

66. Wright IG, White M, Tracey-Patte PD, Donaldson RA, Goodger BV, Waltisbuhl DJ and Mahoney DF: *Babesia bovis*: isolation of a protective antigen by using monoclonal antibodies. Inf and Immun 41:244–250, 1983.

67. Molinar E, James MA, Kakoma I, Holland C, Ristic M: Antigenic and immunogenic studies on cell culture-derived *Babesia canis*. Vet Parasit 10:29–40, 1982.

68. Laurent N, Moreau V, Levy MG, Ristic M: A vaccine against canine babesiosis using a soluble antigen derived from cell culture of *Babesia canis*. (Abstract). Proc 2nd Int Conf Malaria and Babesiosis, Sept. 18–22, 1983. Annecy, France. p. 106.

69. Mendis KN and Targett GAT: Immunization to produce a transmission blocking immunity in *Plasmodium yoelii* malaria infections. Trans R Soc Trop Med Hyg 75:158–159, 1981.

70. Hamburger J and Kreier JP: The isolation of malaria parasites and their constituents. In: Malaria Vol. 1. JP Kreier (ed.). Academic Press, Inc., New York, NY. 1980. p. 1–65.

71. Collins WE, Cantacos PL, Harrison AJ, Staufill PS, Skinner JC: Attempts to immunize monkeys against *Plasmodium knowlesi* by using heat stable serum soluble antigens. Am J Trop Med and Hyg 26:373–376, 1976.

72. James MA, Levy MG and Ristic M: Isolation and partial characterization of culture-derived soluble *Babesia bovis* antigens. Infec and Immun 31:358–361, 1981.

73. Montenegro-James S, James MA and Ristic M: Localization of culture-derived soluble *Babesia bovis* antigens in the infected erythrocyte. Vet Parasit 13:311–316, 1983.

74. Chilbert ML, Ristic M, Ambroise-Thomas P: Development of *Plasmodium falciparum* vaccine: use of culture-derived soluble antigens in squirrel monkey system (Abstract) Proc 2nd Int Conf Malaria and Babesiosis, Sept. 18–22, 1983. Annecy, France. p. 126.

75. Chilbert ML, Ristic M and Ambroise-Thomas P: Malaria vaccination using soluble *Plasmodium falciparum* exoantigens I: clinical and immunologic findings. Manuscript in Preparation, 1984.

76. Thelu J, Ambroise-Thomas P, Contat M, Kupka P: Antigenes excretès-sécrétés par *Plasmodium falciparum* en cultures *in vitro*. Etude Comparée avec les antigènes Somatiques et les antigènes figurés. WHO Bulletin 60 (No. 5):761–766, 1982.

77. Thelu J, Ambroise-Thomas P, Contat M, Kupka P and Dodadille A: Purification and immunochemical study of *Plasmodium falciparum* exoantigens produced by *in vitro* culture (Abstract). Proc 2nd Int Conf Malaria and Babesiosis, Sept. 18–22, 1983. Annecy, France. p. 107.

78. Shamansky L, James M, Hager L and Ristic M: Purification and characterization of culture-derived *Plasmodium falciparum* exoantigens. Manuscript in Preparation, 1984.

79. James M, Kakoma I, Ristic M and Cagnard MY: Induction of Protective immunity to *Plasmodium falciparum* in squirrel monkeys using partially purified exoantigens. Manuscript in Preparation, 1984.

80. Chilbert ML, Ristic M, Ambroise-Thomas P and Cagnard MY: Development of *Plasmodium falciparum* vaccine: immunobiologic properties of soluble antigen-antibody systems. (Abstract). Proc 2nd Int Conf Malaria and Babesiosis, Sept. 18–22, 1983. Annecy, France. p. 127.

81. Chilbert ML and Ristic M: Malaria vaccination using soluble *Plasmodium falciparum* exoantigens II: serum antiparasite effect *in vitro*. Manuscript in Preparation, 1984.

82. Jepsen S: Inhibition of *in vitro* growth of *Plasmodium falciparum* by purified antimalarial human IgG antibodies. Scand J Immunology (Supplement) 18:863-1 to 863-5, 1983.

83. Smith RD, James MA, Ristic M, Aikawa M, Vega CA: Bovine babesiosis: protection of cattle with culturederived soluble *Babesia bovis* antigen. Science 212:335–338, 1981.

84. Zuckerman A: Vaccination against *Plasmodia*. Isr J Med Sci 5:429–434, 1969.

85. Sulzer AJ and Wilson M: Fluorescent antibody test for malaria. CRC – critical reviews in laboratory services 2:601–619, 1971.

86. Todorivic RA, Carson CA: Methods for measuring the immunological response to *Babesia*. In: Babesiosis. Academic Press, Inc., New York, NY. 1981, p. 381–410.

87. Green TJ, Morhardt M, Brackett RG, Richard L: Serum inhibition of merozoite dispersal from *Plasmodium falciparum* schizonts: indicator of immune status. Inf and Immun 31:1203–1208, 1981.

88. Levy MG and Ristic M: Cultivation and *in vitro* studies of *Babesia*. In: *In vitro* Cultivation of Protozoan Parasites. JB Jensen (ed.). CRC Press, Inc., Boca Raton, FL. 1983, p. 221–241.

2. Immunology of malaria

JULIUS P. KREIER AND MIODRAG RISTIC

Department of Microbiology, The Ohio State University, Columbus, Ohio 43210.
College of Veterinary Medicine, University of Illinois, Urbana, Illinois 61801.

1. Introduction

Plasmodium species which cause malaria have a complex life cycle part of which is spent in the invertebrate host and part in the vertebrate. The invertebrate host has a constitutive defense against infection which includes physical and biochemical barriers, phagocytic and humoral deterring elements but appears to lack an inducible system comparable to that present in higher vertebrates. In general, mosquitoes of various strains are either susceptible or resistent to infection with a given plasmodium but unfortunately infection of mosquitoes does not result in disease and death of the vector. The infection of the invertebrate by the plasmodium is not generally considered to invoke an immunological response and will thus not be considered further in this assay.

Plasmodial infection in the vertebrate involves several distinct stages. Accordingly, for the sake of convenience and because of the unique features of the host-parasite interaction at each stage of development, the analyses of these processes will be made by stage [1]. The sequence of presentation will be host reaction to: (1) sporozoites, (2) exoerythrocytic meronts (schizonts) and exoerythrocytic merozoites, (3) asexual erythrocytic plasmodia, which will be discussed from the standpoint of, (a) the erythrocyte plasmodium complex, (b) the plasmodium in the erythrocyte, and (c) blood stage merozoites, and (4) sexual stages.

Features common to all plasmodial-host interactions will be stressed and unique features of particular plasmodial-host pairs will be considered. The data discussed will be primarily drawn from the presentations and abstracts of the 2nd International Conference on Malaria and Babesiosis held in Annecy, France 18–22, September 1983. Other literature will be cited where needed to aid in understanding of the subject being discussed. No attempt will be made to cite all sources or indicate precedence in publication. The interested reader should consult the publications in a set of three volumes entitled 'Malaria' published following the 1st International Conference on Malaria and Babesiosis, held in Mexico City in 1979 for a complete review of the literature then extant [2].

Ristic, M. et al. (eds.) *Malaria and babesiosis.*
© 1984, Martinus Nijhoff Publishers, Dordrecht/Boston/Lancaster.

The host-parasite interaction is best understood if considered both from the plasmodium's and the host's points of view. The parasite posesses its own defenses necessary for evading and neutralizing the host's constitutive defense systems. The difference between a parasite and a harmless saprophyte resides precisely in the ability of the parasite to enter and grow in the nonimmune host by circumventing the constitutive defenses which rapidly destroy saprophytes when they enter the body.

An immune animal treats a parasite as a nonimmune animal treats a saprophyte. Thus one may consider that the induced immune response specifically overcomes the parasites defences against the hosts constitutive immune system. Because this is so the structures on the parasite which protect it from the host's constitutive defenses must be the structures to which the induced response is directed, and one may consider the induced response a system for enhancing the constitutive defenses.

Glycocalyxes, slime layers, capsules, and surface coats of various compositions are common defenses of microorganisms against deleterious environmental influences [3]. Immunological control of an organism, like other chemically mediated control systems requires contact between the effector molecules and the target. In general it is true that while the parasite is alive and intact the host can act only against it's external portions [4]. This is probably because effector molecules such as antibodies cannot penetrate intact plasmalemmas nor penetrate freely through capsules. The cellular elements of the host defense also exert their detrimental effects by direct contact although some may act in part through relatively small molecular weight soluble substances which they secrete.

In the remaining part of this assay on host-parasite interaction an attempt will be made to summarize the date on the hosts mechanisms for overcoming the plasmodia's defenses. In interpreting this assay it is crucial to remember that the structures on the parasite against which the immune responses are directed are there to protect the parasite and not to aid the host in limiting the parasites growth. Because this is so we should not be surprised if what we carelessly refer to as 'protective antigens' are often poorly immunogenic.

2. Plasmodium-host interaction

2.1. *Sporozoites*

The portion of the plasmodial life cycle in the vertebrate is initiated when the mosquito injects sporozoites into a host blood capillary at the time of feeding. Within an hour or less the sporozoites leave the blood and enter their target cells, hepatocytes in mammalian malaria and vascular endothelium in bird malaria. Sporozoites of plasmodia of mammals appear to reach hepatocytes through

Kupffer cells [5, 6, 7], although *in vitro* direct invasion of cultered host cells, i.e., human embyonic lung (w138) fibrobasts and human hepatoma (Hep G2-A16) cells may occur [8].

Entry into and passage through Kupffer cells requires an intact surface coat and homologous plasma proteins [5, 6, 7]. Entry into Kupffer cells does not require phagocytosis, but rather an active penetration by sporozoites [5, 6, 7]. Antibody from animals immune to sporozoite infection binds to the parasite surface coat; and antibody treated sporozoites are taken up by Kupffer cells, but instead of passing through the phagocyte on their way to hepatocytes, antibody coated sporozoites are destroyed in the phagocytes [5]. Specific antisporozoite antibodies also block entry into cultered cells [9]. Monoclonal antibodies against sporozoites have been raised [10]. Monoclonal antibodies against the circumsporozoite proteins block entry into host cells [9]. These antibodies bind to a 42000 mw protein on the surface of the sporozoite [11]. Studies with panels of monoclonal antibodies to circumsporozoite (cs) proteins indicate that the cs proteins contain a single immunodominant region with two or more identical epitopes and that this region is highly antigenic [13].

A synthetic peptide of cs protein induces production of antibodies that bind to sporozoites [13] but it is not yet clear whether these antibodies will protect from infection. There is antigenic diversity among cs proteins of *Plasmodium cynomolgi*; whether this is the case with other cs proteins is not at present known [14]. Antisporozoite antibodies occur in individuals living in malarious areas [15, 16], but their importance in antimalarial immunity is not properly understood.

In summary the data available suggests that the surface coat of the sporozoite plays a role in recognition of the host cell. Antibody to surface coat antigen interferes with its function, although to what degree this occurs in nature is unclear. Antibody coated sporozoites enter phagocytes, possibly by mechanisms different from those by which unopsonized sporozoites enter phagocytes, where they are destroyed and thus prevented from reaching hepatocytes. These results indicate that the surface coat of the sporozoite is both a parasite defense against destruction by phagocytes and an aid to the parasite in host cell recognition. The surface coat thus makes constitutive clearance mechanisms ineffective. The antibody component of the induced response apparently helps the host to block the parasite defense and recognition mechanisms. There is no information on the role of macrophage activation in host defense against sporozoites.

It is surprising that the sporozoite surface coat is highly antigenic. Possibly the highly specific uptake of sporozoites by the liver phagocytes, which appear to degrade antigenic materials rather than use them to initiate an immune response has made selection for poor immunogenicity irrelevant. A study regarding the identity of phagocytes, splenic or hepatic, which process sporozoite vaccines would possibly help us understand the role of the surface coat antigen in protection against the sporozoite.

2.2. *Exoerythrocytic meronts (schizonts) and merozoites*

Little or no pathology and no clinical signs are associated with infection by the exoerythrocytic stages of mammalian plasmodia. The site of the exoerythrocytic meront in the liver tissues shows little reaction until after the meront releases its crop of merozoites at which time there is infiltration by phagocytic cells which remove debris. On the other hand there may be considerable disturbance caused by the exoerythrocytic forms of avian plasmodia which reproduce extensively in the vascular endothelial cells and may cause blockage, for instance, of brain capillaries and severe clinical disease.

Immunity to exoerythrocytic avian malaria does develop and is probably directed against stage specific components of merozoites in mature meronts [reviewed by Seed and Manwell (17); Kreier and Green (18)].

Fluorescent antibody studies show that at low dilutions antibodies in polyclonal sera from individuals with natural *P. falciparum* infection bind diffusely to exoerythrocytic *P. falciparum* meronts in liver sections and interact only with peripheraly situated meront antigens at higher dilution. Polyclonal sera from individuals infected with *P. falciparum* by blood transfusion and sera from people with heterologous plasmodial infections only give the diffuse pattern of binding at low dilutions. None of 26 monoclonal antibodies specific for blood stages reacted with exoerythrocytic forms [19].

These results suggest that there are common somatic antigens between blood and exoerythrocytic stages of plasmodium and that some of these may be shared with many members of the genus. The stage specific antigens on the other hand appear to be limited to the periphery of the organism and are species specific [19].

Immunity to infection can be generated in mice by treatment of sporozoite infected mice with difluoromethylornithine, a drug which inhibits exoerythrocytic merogony. The mice are not immune to blood stage challange, accordingly, the immunity is stage specific [20]. These results and those of Druilhe et al. [199] suggest that the induced immune response is directed to stage specific components of the exoerythrocytic plasmodia which are located in the outer membranes of the meront. If antibody based immunity is directed against the outer layers of the more mature exoerythrocytic meronts then the mechanism of protection is probably due to the interference with functions of the surface coat of the exoerythrocytic merozoites.

2.3. *Asexual erythrocytic stages of plasmodia*

2.3.1. *The erythrocyte-plasmodium complex*
It is probable that plasmodia inside erythrocytes are sheltered against some of the effector mechanisms of the immune system since neither antibodies nor phagocytes readily pass the intact erythrocyte plasmalemma. The intracellular plas-

modium is, however, at risk of destruction if its host cell is destroyed.

Elimination of parasites by destruction of host erythrocytes requires that there be some modification of the host cell detectable by the host defense systems. In malaria these modifications could include reduced flexability of the erythrocyte and changes in the erythrocyte membrane.

Schmidt-Ullrich et al. [21] described a 74KD Glycoprotein of plasmodial origin in the membranes of *P. knowlesi* infected erythrocytes. This glycoprotein appears to be produced by cleavage of larger molecules of up to 230KD. Immunization with the 74KD molecule induced immunity. The parasite origin proteins in the membranes of asexual stages of *P. knowlesi* [22] and *P. falciparum* [23] are variant antigens. One group of these parasite origin proteins are components of electron-dense structures called 'knobs' found in the erythrocyte membranes of *P. falciparum* infected erythrocytes [24, 25]. The 'knobs' serve to bind the erythrocytes containing maturing asexual *P. falciparum* to the vascular endothelium. Knobless clones of *P. falciparum* are not pathogenic in spleen intact monkeys but produce virulent infection in splenectomized monkeys [26].

These results suggest that the function of the 'knob' proteins is to protect the developing asexual plasmodium by keeping it from passage through the splenic filter. Induced antibodies to the 'knob' proteins could block binding to the vascular endothelium and put the parasite at risk of destruction in the spleen.

In view of the fact that a knobless clone of *P. falciparum* induces immunity to knobbed clones [27], it would appear that immunity due to blockage of adhesion to the vascular endothelium is not the sole mechanism of protective immunity to malaria.

That autoantibodies specific for erythrocyte membrane components are present during malaria has been known for many years [28, 29, 30]. Cold type anti-I autoantibodies occur frequently in people with malaria [31]. Tolerance to self may be broken by insertion of parasite derived components into the erythrocyte membrane. In mice this may result in enhancement of parasitemia [32].

In support of a role for autoantibody mediated clearance of infected erythrocytes is the observation that mice genetically lacking the ability to produce autoantibodies to enzyme modified erythrocytes develop more severe infections than normal mice; both normal and defective mice ultimately control their infections, however when they develop antibody specific to the plasmodia [33].

Complement is consumed during malaria; some may be bound on antibody coated erythrocytes [34]. Bound complement does not appear to regularly cause erythrocyte lysis but may enhance opsonization [35]. Opsonic activity of ascitic fluids from *P. falciparum* infected *Saimiri* monkeys correlates with protection induced in passive transfer studies [36]. Soluble immune complexes block phagocytosis of erythrocytes derived from malarious subjects [37]. These results indicate a role for antibody mediated phagocytosis in removal from the blood of infected erythrocytes and suggest that soluble immune complexes may protect the plasmodia from destruction by phagocytic mechanisms. Nonantibody mediated mechanisms may also shorten the erythrocyte life span during malaria. Lipid metabolism is abnormal and erythrocyte morphology is grossly distorted during periods of high parasitemia [38].

The relative degree of benefit to the host or parasite of the much accelerated erythrocyte destruction which occurs in malaria is an unanswered question. It is an appealing hypothesis that the host benefits itself by destroying parasites when it destroys host cells. Most of us would like to believe that the process of natural selection would eliminate all pointless or even mutually destructive aspects of the host-parasite relationship. There is some evidence in favor of this belief. The protection afforded to asexual stages of *P. falciparum* by adhesion to the vascular endothelin [27], for example, indicates that the splenic filter can destroy infected host cells in a sufficiently selective way to benefit the host. Jayawardena's [33] observation that ability to produce autoantibodies to modified erythrocytes helps mice to control acute malaria also indicates benefit to the host from selective erythrocyte destruction.

2.3.2. *The plasmodium in the erythrocyte*
At the end of the period of rapid increase in parasitemia the condition known as the crisis may occur. During crisis there is a rapid fall in packed erythrocyte volume, a rapid fall in parasitemia and pycnotic and degenerating parasites appear in erythrocytes [39, 40, 41, 42].

Products released by mononuclear cells can destroy plasmodia inside erythrocytes. Mononuclear cells release these substances when stimulated by antigen, probably complexed with antibody [43] and when stimulated with various substances having mitogenic potential [44, 45]. A variety of products are released by the activated mononuclear cells including interleukin 2, tumor necrosis factor and various reactive oxygen compounds. The reactive oxygen compounds (including H_2O_2) are known to be able to enter erythrocytes and kill plasmodia [46, 47]. Nonantibody mediated mechanisms for killing intracellular plasmodia are present in sera of Sudenese immune to malaria at levels capable of preventing plasmodial growth in cultures but appear to be absent from the sera of immune Indonesians [48].

Membranes of erythrocytes containing *P. falciparum* develop pores; presence of these pores is necessary for plasmodial growth [49]. If coating of erythrocytes by antibodies results in blockage of nutrient transport, this could be another means of action against the intraerythrocytic stages of plasmodia.

2.3.3. *Blood stage merozoites*
The blood stage merozoite is perhaps the stage most vulnerable to immunological control of any of the erythrocytic stages of plasmodia. It is the only erythrocytic stage in which extracellular merozoites come in direct contact with the humoral and cellular defense elements of the host. The merozoites' sole function is to carry the plasmodial genome from one host cell into another. There are a variety of

points at which the immune system may interfere with this merozoite function. (1) Antibody may clump the merozoites at exit by crosslinking the capsular material while the merozoites are still in the parasitophorous vacuole or possibly just at the point of release [50, 51], (2) Antibody may interfere with the initial adherance of the merozoite to the erythrocyte membrane. In support of this possibility is the observation that monoclonal antibodies which bind diffusely to the merozoite surface block invasion [52]. In addition, the observation that the initial recognition contact of the erythrocytes and ensuing distortion of the erythrocyte membrane preceedes apical attachment indicates that this initial merozoite-erythrocyte interaction is a general surface phenomenon [53, 3] Antibody could interfere with apical complex function. In support of this mechanism is the observation that a monoclonal antibody which protects mice from *P. yoelii* infections combines exclusively with the rhopteries of *P. yoelii* merozoites [54, 4] Complement activated by the classical pathway could cause lysis of merozoites. Evidence presently available does not support this mechanisms [reviewed by Kreier and Green (18), and (5)]. Immune phagocytosis could eliminate merozoites. The encapsulated merozoite is not bound nor engulfed by phagocytes unless it is opsonized by specific antibody to the capsular material [55, 56, 57], and thus the merozoite is effectively shielded by its capsule from the constitutive host defenses. This observation should not be taken to indicate that antibody mediated phagocytosis of merozoites is necessarily the means of control of blood stage plasmodia. The other antibody mediated mechanisms such as inhibition of dispersion of merozoites from the meront by cross linking of capsular material by antibody [50, 51] or antibody mediated modification of the merozoite capsule so as to interfere with merozoite attachment to the red cells [53] or interference by antibody with rhoptry function [54] may neutralize the merozoite. If these humoral defense mechanisms are truly operational, then the act of phagocytosis would be a scavenging function.

Many studies on the mechanisms by which the host controls plasmodia are conducted on intact (spleen *in situ*) animals or in complex *in vitro* systems. In such studies it is often difficult to determine which stage of the parasite is being inhibited and what mechanisms are operating; control may in fact be by a variety of means acting together or alone.

There are many observations that indicate the importance of antibody in control of plasmodia. For example, certain genetic lines of poor antibody responder mice do not control *P. berghei* as well as do otherwise congeneric lines that are good responders [58]. Moreover, the mechanism of antibody action may be more complex than simple neutralization. Correlation between the results of passive protection studies against *P. falciparum* in *Saimiri* monkeys and *P. falciparum* growth inhibition in culture is poor. Some sera are both protective and inhibitory, some only one or the other [59].

In *in vitro* growth inhibition studies antibody to *P. falciparum* is more effective in association with monocytes than alone [60]. Opsonization of merozoites is required for phagocytosis [55], but phagocytosis as noted earlier may not be an important antibody mediated effector mechanisms in malaria [61].

Ingestion of immune complexes is known to activate monocytes [62]. Hence, it is posssible that the greater inhibition of growth in cultures containing antibodies and monocytes than in cultures containing antibody alone may be due to macrophage activation by immune complex ingestion with release of monokines [44, 45, 46, 60] which kill the intracellular plasmodia rather than by enhanced antibody mediated phagocytosis of merozoites.

Soluble antigens and immune complexes inhibit phagocytosis of opsonized merozoites [56]. *In vivo* such soluble complexes can inhibit protection by antibody [63]. This can be demonstrated by passive protection tests in mice (Fig. 1). Mice given acute phase serum (Fig. 1APS) had higher parasitemias eight days after challenge than did mice given normal rat serum (Fig. 1-c). After fractionation, the antibody fraction (Fig. 1-Ab) of the acute phase serum protected the

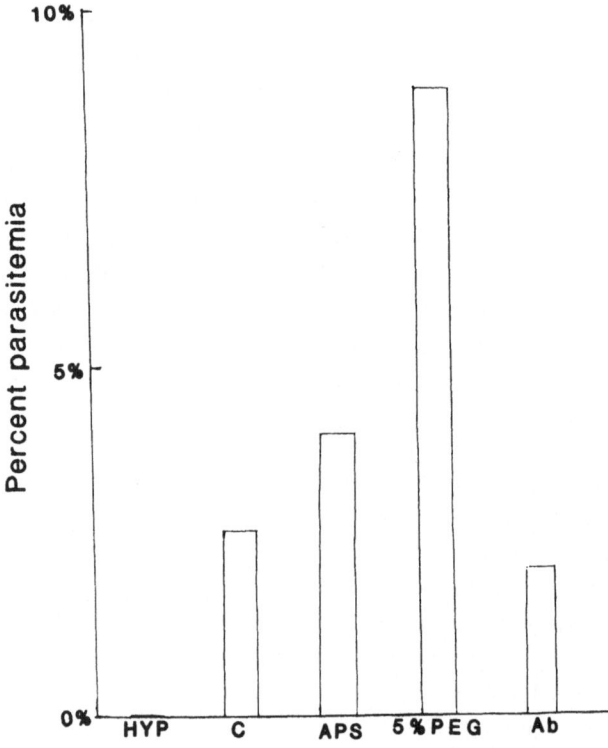

Figure 1. Plasmodium berghei parasitemias 8 days following infection in mice given serum and various fractions of serum collected 26 days after challenge from nonvaccinated rats. In this test the mice given acute phase serum (APS) developed higher parasitemias at 8 days than did the control (C) mice given normal serum. The mice given the complex containing fraction (5% PEG) of the serum developed very high parasitemias while the mice given the antibody fraction of the serum (Ab) developed parasitemias lower than did the mice given the negative control (C) serum but higher than did the mice given the positive (HYP) control. i.e., hyperimmune serum.

mice while the complex contaminating fraction separated from the antibody by 5% polyethylene glycol precipitation (Fig. 1–5% PEG) aggravated the infections. Since soluble immune complexes block phagocytosis of opsonized merozoites *in vitro* [57], it is possible that they may function similarly *in vivo*. As noted earlier, however, not everyone believes phagocytosis of opsonized merozoites contributes to control of plasmodia [61].

Acute phase serum and hyperimmune serum injections also effect the course of parasitemias in rats (Fig. 2). Three injections of 1/2 ml of acute phase serum, administered one day before, on the day, and one day after infection, respectively, enhanced parasitemia and delayed recovery. Hyperimmune serum injection initially protected the rats, then enhanced parasitemias and delayed recovery.

It is probable that the immune complexes in the acute phase serum inhibited the induction of the immune response and thus delayed the development of immunity. The antibodies in the immune serum could have directly delayed

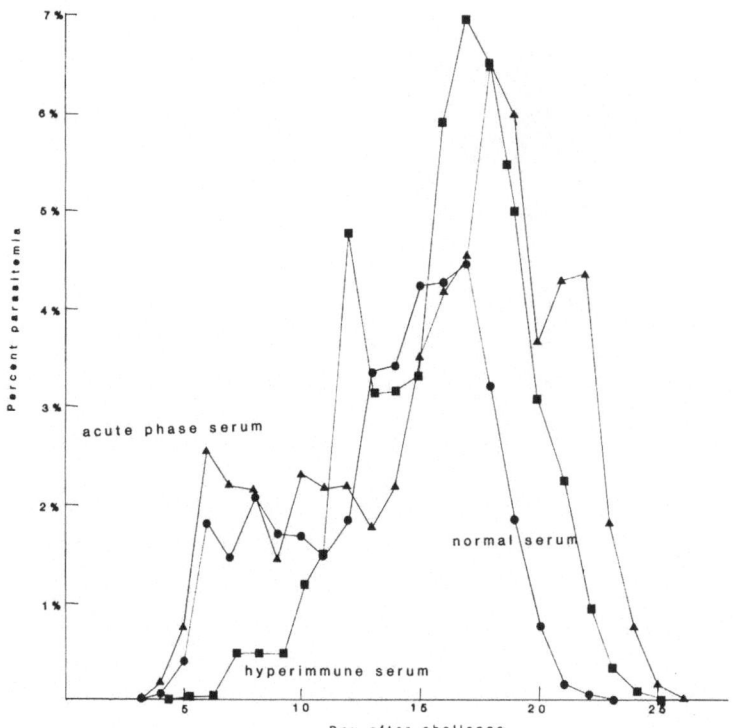

Figure 2. Course of parasitemia in rats given three IP injections of 0.5 ml of acute phase serum, normal serum, or hyperimmune serum the day before, the day of, and the day after infection by intravenous injection of 1×10^3 *P. berghei* infected erythrocytes. Hyperimmune serum initially inhibited the development of the parasitemia but then delayed recovery. Acute phase serum aggravated the development of parasitemia and also delayed recovery.

44

development of immunity by a feedback system or could have complexed with plasmodial antigens and affected induction of immunity as complexes. Low density lypoproteins in acute phase serum inhibit induction of immunity to malaria [64] and could have contributed to the effects observed.

Macrophages meeting plasmodial antigens in the presence of specific antibody degrade it more rapidly than do macrophages which encounter antigens in the presence of normal serum (Fig. 3).

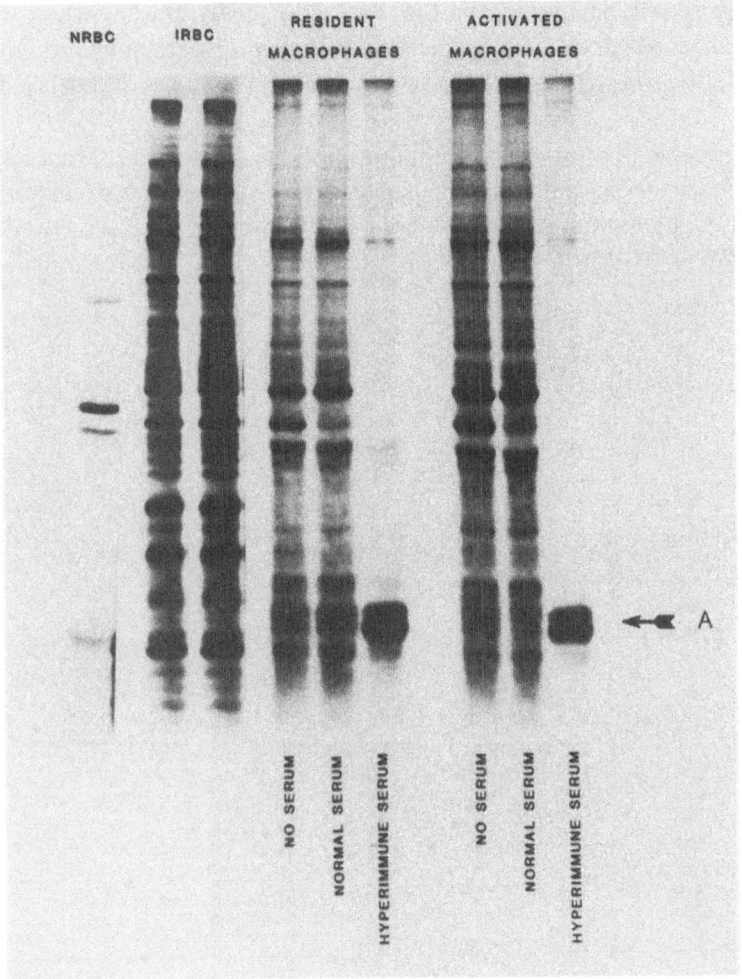

Figure 3. Autoradiograph of a polyacrylamide gel showing degradation by macrophages of the proteins of *P. berghei*. The array of *P. bergei* antigens retained by macrophages in the presence of normal serum or in the absence of serum is not identical to the array in the antigen preparation but the differences are small in comparison to those which occur if the macrophages encounter the antigen in the presence of hyperimmune serum. In this latter situation most of the macrophage associated antigen is degraded to relatively small (i.e., 24–25 KO) molecular weight components (arrow A).

Rapid antigen degradation could adversely affect antigen presentation and thus induction of immunity.

These few observations on the effects of antibody and immune complexes on immune effector mechanisms and induction of immunity clearly show how difficult it is to analyze the complex sequence of events involved in immunological control of plasmodia. How antibody operates in control of plasmodial merozoites is unclear. We know that the macrophage is a part of the effector phase of control, but little is known regarding the relative importance of monokines and phagocytosis in control. The targets of antibody are surely both surface coat and rhoptory contents and may also be some other portions of the merozoite. It is probable that antibodies of a variety of specificities all contribute to control but whether control can be obtained by antibodies of only a few specificities is still unclear. There is at present active debate about the relative degree of importance of control mechanisms directed against the merozoite as opposed to mechanisms active against other asexual stages. It is most likely that a variety of mechanisms operate to control plasmodia. The present evidence certainly supports this conclusion.

2.4. *Sexual stages*

Immune mechanisms directed against sexual stages can be considered in two parts; (1) Mechanisms directed against gametocytes in the vertebrate blood and, (2) Mechanisms directed against the gametes in the mosquitoes gut. It is possible that some of the mechanisms active against intracellular asexual stages of plasmodia are also active in destruction of the sexual stages. We know that gametocytes remain in the blood for some days and then are removed; little more is known [65].

Anti-gamete effects exerted in the mosquito gut are probably experimental artifacts. Under normal conditions the vertebrate host never encounters gamete specific antigens and thus never produces antibodies capable of blocking fertilization in the blood meal in the mosquitoes gut. To induce this type of immune response gamete preparations must be made and injected into the vertebrate [66, 67, 68, 69, 70, 71]. Consequently, this type of research is more a part of the studies on immunization than immunity. The observation, however, that it is surface components of gametes [67, 69], which are acted against in this system as in systems for control of sporozoites [72] and possibly merozoites [55, 73, 74] does support the assertion that immune control of parasites operates on physically accessible portions of the parasite.

3. Summary and conclusions

When one looks at the literature on the relationships between plasmodia and their vertebrate hosts which has just been reviewed, one sees complexity. Each stage of the parasite invades different host cells. In the nonimmune mammal the sporozoites may enter liver phagocytes but are not trapped there and destroyed, rather they pass on to liver parenchyma cells where they are able to complete their development. The exoerythrocytic merozoites produced by the exoerythrocytic meront enter erythrocytes where they continue asexual reproduction. Some of the merozoites from this asexual cycle may initiate the sexual phase. These develop into gametocytes capable of initiating infection in the mosquito but quite incapable of continuing infection in the vertebrate. The uninhibited development in the nonimmune host of these various stages of the plasmodium indicates that they are well equipped to evade the hosts constitutive defenses.

In the susceptible nonimmune vertebrate asexual erythrocytic infection proceeds with little restraint until the induced immune response develops. There is little pathology and no disease associated with the exoerythrocytic development in the mammal, not because the host restrains the parasite, but because the cycle of development of the organism of this stage is self-limited.

In avian malaria, on the other hand, where exoerythrocytic forms reproduce without self-imposed limits, disease may occur at this stage of the infection. The absence of disease following infection in the mosquito may also be related to the self-limiting nature of reproduction of the stages in the mosquito.

The sporozoite appears to be well shielded from the constitutive defenses of the host. Sporozoites actually need normal serum proteins for efficient entry into liver phagocytes. It is only following immune opsonization that phagocytes destroy sporozoites. The merozoite also is well shielded from the constitutive defenses of the host. However, immune opsonization is required for their entry into phagocytes. It may be that the surface coats of merozoites and sporozoites actually have dual roles, one being recognition of host cells and the other inhibition of constitutive defenses. In the former role, recognition of host cells, the merozoite surface coat assists the organisms in recognition of, and binding to, the erythrocyte before entry and the sporozoite surface coat modulates initial aspects of sporozoite entry into the Kuppfer cells. The latter role, inhibition of constitutive defenses, becomes apparent when it is overriden by the induced response. The opsonized merozoite is readily phagocytized and the antibody coated sporozoite is destroyed in the Kuppfer cell. The dual role of the surface coat of the sporozoite is more difficult to percieve than the dual role of the surface coat of merozoites because Kuppfer cells are involved in both functions of the sporozoite surface coat. We know that the fate of the opsonized sporozoite in the phagocyte is death while that of the sporozoite in the presence of normal serum is survival. It is probable, but not demonstrated, that the mechanisms of entry differ in each case, the opsonized sporozoite being taken up by phagocytosis following fc and c' mediated binding and the entry of the sporozoite in the presence of normal serum by sporozoite determined processes. The opsonized sporozoite in any event is destroyed in a fully functional phagosome while the unopsonized sporozoite passes into its definitive host cell, the liver parenchyma cell.

Antibody probably acts in several ways against asexual stages of plasmodia in addition to facilitation of phagocyte function. Inhibition of dispersion of merozoites, and inhibition of host cell recognition by merozoites and sporozoites being probably the most important. In addition, antibody reaction with plasmodial components on the erythrocyte surface may facilitate host cell and parasite destruction either by erythrocyte lysis or phagocytosis. With *P. falciparum* malaria the action of antibody with plasmodial components in the erythrocyte membrane may also be indirect, by blocking 'knob' mediated adhesion to the vascular endothelium and thus subjecting the parasitized erythrocyte to the action of the splenic filter.

Non-antibody mediated means of destruction of plasmodia have been given a physical basis with the identification of oxygen mediated killing mechanisms and with the demonstration that sera of many immune Africans is capable of inhibiting intracellular development of plasmodia by means other than antibody. It is probable that under normal conditions plasmodia are controlled by both antibody mediated and nonantibody mediated means and that both systems operate in a variety of ways. The relative importance of one or the other of the systems may differ in different host-plasmodial pairs and at different times in the same pair. This should not, however, confuse us nor involve us in nonproductive arguments regarding the true nature of the mechanisms used by the host to control plasmodia; rather we should continue to strive for a complete understanding of the complex of systems involved in antimalarial immunity and particularly those which are invoked by immunization.

An acknowledgement is due to Jeffrey Alder for the data presented in figures 1 and 2, and Kathryn Brown for the data presented in figure 3.

4. References

1. Kreier JP: A review of immune responses and regulation in malaria. (Abstract). Proc 2nd Int Conf Malaria and Babesiosis, September 18–22, 1983. Annecy, France. p 4.
2. Kreier JP: Malaria. Academic Press, New York, N.Y. Vol. 1: 416 pages; Vol. 2: 328 pages; Vol. 3: 346 pages, 1980.
3. Costerton JW, Irvin RT and Cheng K-J: The bacterial glycocalyx in nature and disease. Annual Review of Microbiology 35:299–324, 1981.

48

4. Mims CA: The pathogenesis of infectious disease. 2nd *ed*. Academic Press, London. 297 pages, 1982.
5. Danforth HD, Aikawa M, Cochrane AH and Nussenzweig RS: Sporozoites of mammalian malaria: Attachment to, interiorization and fate within macrophages. The Journal of Protozoology 27:193–202, 1980.
6. Meis J, Verhave JP, Jap P and Meuwissen J: The role of Kuppfer cells in the trapping of malarial sporozoites in the liver and the subsequent infection of hepatocytes. In: Sinusoidal Liver Cells. D.L. Knock and E. Weisse (eds). Elsevier Biomedical Press. 1982, p 429–436.
7. Meis JFGM, Verhave JP, Meuwissen JHETh: Electron microscopic observations on the entry of sporozoites of *Plasmodium berghei* into rat kuppfer cells *in vivo*. (Abstract). Proc 2nd Int Conf Malaria and Babesiosis, September 18–22, 1983, Annecy, France. p 64.
8. Hollingdale MR: *In vitro* invasion of cultured cells by sporozoites of primate and human species. (Abstract). Proc 2nd Inter Conf Malaria and Babesiosis, September 18–22, 1983. Annecy, France. p 74.
9. Hollingdale MR, Zavala F, Nussenzweig RS and Nussenzweig V: Antibodies to the protective antigen of *Plasmodium berghei* sporozoites prevent entry into cultured cells. The Journal of Immunology 128:1929–1930, 1982.
10. Cochrane AH, Santoro F, Collins WE, Gwadz RW, and Nussenzweig RS: Monoclonal antibodies against sporozoites of *Plasmodium malariae*. (Abstract) Proc 2nd Inter Conf Malaria and Babesiosis, September 18–22, 1983. Annecy, France. p 135.
11. Fine E, Aikawa M, Cochrane A and Nussenzweig R: Ultrastructural localization of the protective antigens of *Plasmodium knowlesi* sporozoites. (Abstract). Proc 2nd Inter Conf Malaria and Babesiosis, September 18–22, 1983. Annecy, France. p 134.
12. Zavala F, Cochrane AH, Nardin EH, Nussenzweig RS and Nussenzweig V: Circumsporozoite proteins of malaria parasites contain a single immunodominant region with two or more identical epitopes. (Abstract). Proc 2nd Inter Conf Malaria and Babesiosis, September 18–22, 1983. Annecy, France. p 112.
13. Gysin J, Nussenzweig V, Schlesinger D and Nussenzweig RS: Synthetic peptide of circumsporozoite antigen induces antibodies to malaria parasites. (Abstract). Proc 2nd Inter Conf Malaria and Babesiosis, September 18–22, 1983. Annecy, France. p 122.
14. Cochrane AH, Ojo-Amaize E, Hii J, Santoro F, Ferreira A, Gwadz RW and Nussenzweig RS: Antigenic diversity among the circumsporozoite proteins of three strains of *Plasmodium cynomolgi*. (Abstract). Proc 2nd Inter Conf Malaria and Babesiosis, September 18–22, 1983. Annecy, France. p 113.
15. Nardin EH, Nussenzweig RS, McGretor IA and Bryan JH: Antibodies to sporozoites: their frequent occurrence in individuals living in an area of hyperendemic malaria. Science 206:597–599, 1979.
16. Tapchaisri P, Chomcharn Y, Poonthong C, Asavanich A, Limsuwan S, Maleevan O, Tharavanij S, Harinasuta ST: Anti-sporozoite antibodies induced by natural infection. (Abstract). Proc 2nd Inter Conf Malaria and Babesiosis, September 18–22, 1983. Annecy, France. p 208.
17. Seed TM and Manwell RD: Plasmodia of birds. In: Parasitic Protozoa Vol III. Kreier JP (ed). Academic Press, New York. 1977, p 311–357.
18. Kreier JP and Green TJ: The vertebrate hosts immune response to plasmodia. In: Malaria, Vol 3. Kreier JP (ed). Academic Press, New York. 1980, p 111–162.
19. Druilhe P, Puebla RM, Miltgen F, Perrin L and Gentilini M: Demonstration of species and stage-specific antigens in *Plasmodium falciparum* hepatic stages. (Abstract). Proc 2nd Inter Conf Malaria and Babesiosis, September 18–22, 1983. Annecy, France. p 105.
20. Bone G, Gillet J, Lowa P, Charlier J and Rona AM: Immunity against the exoerythrocytic schizogony of plasmodium induced by difluoromethylornithine in mice inocluated with *Plasmodium berghei* sporozoites. (Abstract). 2nd Inter Conf Malaria and Babesiosis, September 18–22, 1983. Annecy, France. p 42.

21. Schmidt-Ullrich R, Millni E and Monroe MTM: A protective 74 000 Mr *Plasmodium knowlesi* antigen in the membrane of schizont-infected rhesus erythrocytes. (Abstract). Proc 2nd Inter Conf Malaria and Babesiosis, September 18–22, 1983. Annecy, France. p 116.

22. Howard RJ and Barnwell JW: Antigenic variation of a malarial protein expressed on the surface of *Plasmodium knowlesi*-infected erythrocytes. (Abstract). Proc 2nd Inter Conf Malaria and Babesiosis, September 18–22, 1983. Annecy, France. p 151.

23. Hommel M: *P. falciparum*: antigenic variation and antigenic diversity of erythrocyte-associated surface antigens. (Abstract). Proc 2nd Inter Conf Malaria and Babesiosis, September 18–22, 1983. Annecy, France. p 6.

24. Aikawa M, Miller LH and Ristic M: Morphological modification of erythrocyte membrane associated with malaria and babesia infection. (Abstract). Proc 2nd Inter Conf Malaria and Babesiosis, September 18–22, 1983. Annecy, France. p 28.

25. Gorenflot A, Marchais H, Le Bras J and Savel J: *Plasmodium falciparum*: Etude en microscopie electronique a balayage de la formation *in vitro* des microprotuberances (knobs) et des modifications antigeniques, a la surface des hematies parasitees. (Abstract). Proc 2nd Inter Conf Malaria and Babesiosis, September 18–22, 1983. Annecy, France. p 62.

26. Langreth SG and Peterson E: Pathogenicity of a knobless clone of *Plasmodium falciparum* in *aotus* monkeys. (Abstract). Proc 2nd Inter Conf Malaria and Babesiosis, September 18–22, 1983, Annecy, France. p 117.

27. Peterson E and Langreth SG: The immune response of *aotus* monkeys to the D3 knobless clone of *Plasmodium falciparum*. (Abstract). Proc 2nd Inter Conf Malaria and Babesiosis, September 18–22, 1983. Annecy, France. p 118.

28. Zuckerman A: Autoimmunity in rats with *Plasmodium berghei*. Nature 185:189–190, 1960.

29. Seed TM and Kreier JP: Autoimmune reaction in chickens with *Plasmodium gallinaceum* infection: the isolation and characterization of a lipid from trypsinized erythrocytes which reacts with serum from acutely infected chickens. Military Medicine 134:1220–1227, 1969.

30. Kreier JP, Shapiro H, Dilley D, Szilvassy IP and Ristic M: Autoimmune reactions in rats with *Plasmodium berghei* infection. Experimental Parasitology 19:155–162, 1966.

31. Penalba C, Simonneau M, Autran B, Bouvet E, Vroclans M, Coulaud JP, Saimot AG and Vachon F: Autoimmunisation anti-erythrocytaire anti-i au cours du paludisme. (Abstract). Prod 2nd Inter Conf Malaria and Babesiosis, September 18–22, 1983. Annecy, France. p 54.

32. Jarra W and Brown KN: Protective immunity to rodent malaria and anti-erythrocyte autoimmunity. (Abstract). Proc 2nd Inter Conf Malaria and Babesiosis, September 18–22, 1983. Annecy, France. p 41.

33. Jayawardana AN, Janeway CA and Kemp JD: Experimental malaria in the CBA/N mouse. Journal of Immunology 123:2532–2539, 1979.

34. Omanga U: Mecanisme immunologique possible de l'anemie hemolytique de l'aces palustre. (Abstract). Prod 2nd Inter Conf Malaria and Babesiosis, September 18–22, 1983. Annecy, France. p 88.

35. Schetters ThPM, Van Lent P, Van Run JHJ, Van Breda and Eling WMC: Complement dependent defense mechanisms against intraerythrocytic *Plasmodium berghei* parasites. (Abstract). Proc 2nd Inter Conf Malaria and Babesiosis, September 18–22, 1983. Annecy, France. p 12.

36. Michel JC, Fandeur T, Neuilly G, Roussilhon C and Dedet JP: Opsonic activity of ascitic fluids from *Plasmodium falciparum* infected *saimiri* monkeys: positive correlation with protection in passive transfer assay. (Abstract). Proc 2nd Inter Conf Malaria and Babesiosis, September 18–22, 1983. Annecy, France. p 47.

37. Shear HL: Malarial immune complexes inhibit phagocytosis by normal macrophages and monocytes. (Abstract). Prod 2nd Inter Conf Malaria and Babesiosis, September 18–22, 1983. Annecy, France. p 51.

38. Maurios P, Dei Cas E, Feo C, Pessah M, Alcindor JL: Anaemia during rodent malaria: relationships with the impairment of lipoprotein matabolism. (Abstract). Prod 2nd Inter Conf Malaria and Babesiosis, September 18–22, 1983. Annecy, France. p 89.

50

39. Taliaferro WH and Taliaferro LG: The effect of immunity on the asexual reproduction of *Plasmodium brasilianum*. Journal of Infectious Diseases 75:1–32, 1944.
40. Taliaferro WH and Taliaferro LG: Asexual reproduction of *Plasmodium cynomolgi* in rhesus monkeys. Journal of Infectious Diseases 80:78–104, 1947.
41. Thompsom PE: Changes associated with acquired immunity during initial infections in simian malaria. Journal of Infectious Diseases 75:138–149, 1944.
42. Zuckerman A and Yoeli M: Age and sex as factors influencing *Plasmodium berghei* infections in intact and splenectomized rats. Journal of Infectious Diseases 94:225–236, 1954.
43. Brown J and Greenwood BM: Killing of *Plasmodium falciparum* by human mononuclear cells. (Abstract). Proc 2nd Inter Conf Malaria and Babesiosis, September 18–22, 1983. Annecy, France. p 248.
44. Lelchuk R, Rose G and Playfair JHL: Changes in interleukin production during murine malaria infection. (Abstract). Proc 2nd Inter Conf Malaria and Babesiosis, September 18–22, 1983. Annecy, France. p 49.
45. Taverne J, Depledge P, Playfair JHL, Matthews N, Wozencraft A and Targett GAT: Macrophage-derived factors cytotoxic for tumour cells and for malaria parasites. (Abstract). Proc 2nd Inter Conf Malaria and Babesiosis, September 18–22, 1983. Annecy, France. p 73.
46. Dockrell HM, Playfair JHL, Targett GAT and Wozencraft AO: Killing of malaria parasites by reactive oxygen intermediates. (Abstract). Proc 2nd Inter Conf Malaria and Babesiosis, September 18–22, 1983. Annecy, France. p 71.
47. Ockenhouse CF, Schulman S and Shear HL: Oxidative killing of *Plasmodium falciparum* by human monocytes and lymphokine-activated monocyte-derived macrophages. (Abstract). Proc 2nd Inter Conf Malaria and Babesiosis, September 18–22, 1983. Annecy, France. p 36.
48. Jensen JB and Hoffman SL: Comparison between Indonesian and Sudanese immune response to malaria. (Abstract). Proc 2nd Inter Conf Malaria and Babesiosis, September 18–22, 1983. Annecy, France. p 40.
49. Ginsburg H, Drugliak M, Kutner S and Cabantchik ZI: A new permeation pathway appearing in *Plasmodium falciparum* infected red cell membranes displays pore-like properties. (Abstract). Proc 2nd Inter Conf Malaria and Babesiosis, September 18–22, 1983. Annecy, France. p 61.
50. Green TJ, Morhandt M, Brachett RG and Jacobs RL: Serum inhibition of merozoite dispersal from *Plasmodium falciparum* schizonts: indicator of immune status. Infection and Immunity 31:203–1208, 1981.
51. Packer BJ and Green TJ: *Plasmodium falciparum* malaria: examination of *in vitro* schizont inhibition using the parasite inhibition test. (Abstract). Prod 2nd Inter Conf Malaria and Babesiosis, September 18–22, 1983. Annecy, France. p 159.
52. Miller LH, David PH and Hadley TJ: The surface membrane of plasmodium: events leading to invasive merozoites. (Abstract). Proc 2nd Inter Conf Malaria and Babesiosis, September 18–22, 1983. Annecy, France. p 29.
53. Enders B, Neunziger G and Hermentin P: Erythrocyte invasion by *Plasmodium falciparum in vitro*: video pictures obtained upon interference microscopy. Presented at the Proc 2nd Inter Conf Malaria and Babesiosis, September 18–22, 1983. Annecy, France. (no abstract).
54. Oka M, Aikawa M, Holder A and Freeman R: Ultrastructural localization of protective antigens of *Plasmodium yoelii* by the use of monoclonal antibodies and ultrathin cryomicrotomy. (Abstract). Proc 2nd Inter Conf Malaria and Babesiosis, September 18–22, 1983. Annecy, France. p 146.
55. Brooks CB and Kreier JP: Role of surface coat on *in vitro* attachment and phagocytosis of *Plasmodium berghei* by peritoneal macrophages. Infection and Immunity 20:827–835, 1978.
56. Brown K and Kreier JP: *Plasmodium berghei* malaria: Blockage by immune complexes of macrophage receptors for opsonized plasmodia. Infection and Immunity 37:1227–1233, 1982.
57. Brown KM, Kreier JP: Recognition of the erythrocytic stages *Plasmodium berghei* by *corynebacterium parvum* activated macrophages. (Abstract). Proc 2nd Inter Conf Malaria and Babesiosis, September 18–22, 1983. Annecy, France. p 48.

58. Stiffel C, Bucci A and Heumann AM: Role des anticorps et du fond genique dans la resistance postvaccinale des souris a l'infection par *Plasmodium berghei*. (Abstract). Proc 2nd Inter Conf Malaria and Babesiosis. Annecy, France. p 160.

59. Fandeur T, Dubois P, Gysin J, Dedet JP and Pereira Da Silva L: *In vitro* and *in vivo* studies on protective and inhibitory antibodies against *Plasmodium falciparum* produced in blood induced infection of the *saimiri* monkey. (Abstract). Proc 2nd Inter Conf Malaria and Babesiosis, September 18–22, 1983. Annecy, France. p 156.

60. Khusmith S and Druilhe P: Demonstration of a cooperative effect between human blood monocytes and malarial antibodies effective upon *in vitro* proliferation of *P. falciparum*. (Abstract). Proc 2nd Inter Conf Malaria and Babesiosis, September 18–22, 1983. Annecy, France. p 44.

61. Deans JA and Cohen S: Immunology of malaria. Annual Review of Microbiology 37:25–49, 1983.

62. Unanue ER: The regulatory role of macrophages in antigenic stimulation. Adv Immunology 31:1–136, 1981.

63. Alder JD and Kreier JP: Characterization of the role of immunocomplexes during the immune response of rodents to *Plasmodium berghei*. (Abstract). Proc 2nd Inter Conf Malaria and Babesiosis, September 18–22, 1983. Annecy, France. p 267.

64. Camus D, Van Dac N, Goumard P and Maurois P: Immunopathologic disorders induced by lipoproteins during malaria. 2. Immunoregulation of a pre-existing antibody response to heterologous antigens. (Abstract). Proc 2nd Inter Conf Malaria and Babesiosis, September 18–22, 1983. Annecy, France. p 53.

65. Vanderberg JP and Gwatz RW: The transmission by mosquitoes of plasmodia in the laboratory. In: *Malaria*, Vol 2. Kreier JP (ed). 1980, p 153–234.

66. Targett GAT, Rogers N and Harte PG: Mechanisms of transmission blocking immunity in mice. (Abstract). Proc 2nd Inter Conf Malaria and Babesiosis, September 18–22, 1983. Annecy, France. p 161.

67. Kumar N, Grotendorst CA, Carter R: Biosynthesis of antigens on the surface of the transforming zygote and mature ookinete of *Plasmodium gallinaceum*. (Abstract). Proc 2nd Inter Conf Malaria and Babesiosis. September 18–22, 1983. Annecy, France. p 136.

68. Verhave JP, Van Nhan V, Dung PH, Meuwissen JGET: Vaccination with micro- and macrogametes of *Plasmodium berghei*. (Abstract). Proc 2nd Inter Conf Malaria and Babesiosis, September 18–22, 1983. Annecy, France. p 131.

69. Carter R, Rener J, Kaushal DC, Graves PM, Miller LH, Grotendorst CA, Williams JL and Burkot TR: Antigenic targets of transmission blocking immunity in malaria. (Abstract). Proc 2nd Inter Conf Malaria and Babesiosis, September 18–22, 1983. Annecy, France. p 130.

70. Vermeulen AN, Ponnudurai T, Beckers PJA and Meuwissen JHETh: Antigens of macrogametes/zygotes of *Plasmodium falciparum*. (Abstract). Proc 2nd Inter Conf Malaria and Babesiosis, September 18–22, 1983. Annecy, France. p 114.

71. Ponnudurai T, Feldmann AM, Vermeulen AN, Beckers PJ and Meuwissen JHETh: The transmission of cultured *Plasmodium falciparum* to *Anopheles stephensi* and its blockade by antigamete antibodies. (Abstract) Proc 2nd Inter Conf Malaria and Babesiosis, September 18–22, 1983, Annecy, France. p 84.

72. Cochrane AH, Santoro F, Nussenzweig V, Gwadz RW and Nussenzweig RS: Monoclonal antibodies identify the protective antigens of sporozoites of *Plasmodium knowlesi*. Proc National Academy of Sciences, USA 79:5651–5655, 1982.

73. Miller LH, Aikawa M and Dvorak JA: Malaria (*Plasmodium knowlesi*) merozoites: immunity and the surface coat. Journal of Immunology 114:1237–1242, 1975.

74. Saul K and Kreier JP: *Plasmodium berghei*: immunization of rats with antigens from a population of free parasites rich in merozoites. Zeitschrift fur Tropenmedizin and Parasitologie 28:302–318, 1977.

3. Immunology of Babesia infections

MARK A. JAMES

College of Veterinary Medicine, University of Illinois, 2001 S. Lincoln Ave., Urbana, Illinois 61801.

1. Introduction

Immunity to *Babesia* infection depends on general innate characteristics of the host in addition to its responsiveness to specific babesial antigens. The specific immune response includes both humoral and cellular components. Protective antibodies related to thymus-dependent lymphocyte activity probably damage extracellular merozoites and promote phagocytosis of free parasites and parasitized erythrocytes. There is now evidence that recovery from experimental *Babesia* infections in rodents is T-lymphocyte dependent with natural killer cells also participating in protective immune responses. *Babesia bovis* antigens derived from culture supernatant fluids or from infected erythrocyte lysates have recently been characterized as to their immunologic properties. These antigens are being effectively utilized as immunogens for vaccination against bovine babesiosis and also as reagents in newly-developed immunodiagnostic techniques.

2. Innate resistance

The ability of the host to overcome a babesial infection is determined not only by immunologic mechanisms but also by certain innate characteristics of the host. In a series of publications by Jack and Ward [1, 2, 3], they reported that complement C3 and the C3b receptor may facilitate *B. rodhaini* infections in the rat. Complement apparently induces modifications in either the erythrocytes or parasites, thereby enabling subsequent penetration of erythrocytes. In addition, the ability of *B. rodhaini* to penetrate erythrocytes may depend on factors of the alternate complement pathway (properdin and factor B) as well as ionic magnesium and the fifth (C5) component of complement [4]. Mahoney et al. [5] found that hemolytic activity of serum complement in cattle during *B. bovis* infection decreases significantly after five days post-infection and is absent during the acute phase of the disease. Complement C3 and C4 levels and hemolytic activity have

Ristic, M. et al. (eds.) *Malaria and babesiosis.*
© 1984, Martinus Nijhoff Publishers, Dordrecht/Boston/Lancaster.

been shown to be suppressed in acute-phase sera from humans infected with *B. microti* [6]. It has been suggested that decreases in the first three components of complement during acute infection are due to their involvement in the intravascular sludging of infected erythrocytes within the microcirculation [7]. Actually, the principle mechanism of the hypocomplementemia may be the depletion of the classical complement components C1 to C9 by immune complexes.

It has previously been reported that nonspecific resistance to *Babesia* spp. may be conferred by killed bacterial agents [8,9]. Clark [10] has demonstrated that a commercially available extract of *Coxiella burnetii* protects mice against *B. microti* and *B. rodhaini*, possibly by activating interferon production or natural killer cells.

In vitro cultivation of *B. bovis* in erythrocyte cultures [11] showed that blood from young animals contains a factor(s) responsible for their resistance to severe babesiosis. Levy et al. [12] found this factor to be independent of antibody and dialyzable. The presence of this factor results in inhibition of parasite multiplication and the eventual death of the parasite while inside the erythrocyte.

3. Role of antibodies

3.1. *Merozoite neutralization*

Various neutralization tests have been developed to assay the biological activity of immune serum on the growth of *Babesia in vitro*. Bautista and Kreier [13] found antibodies prevented penetration of hamster erythrocytes by *B. microti*. Ristic and Levy [14] have also used the *B. bovis* merozoite neutralization test as an *in vitro* correlate of humoral immunity in infected cattle. When cell-free merozoites are pre-incubated with sera of recovered or immunized animals and then introduced into *in vitro* cultures [11], they fail to invade erythrocytes. In contrast, similar merozoites incubated in sera of susceptible non-immunized animals remain fully functional in their ability to invade erythrocytes and multiply *in vitro*.

The merozoite surface coat is known to elicit the production of antibodies that prevent erythrocyte invasion by parasites and facilitates their immune destruction by macrophages. Smith et al. [15] observed that antisera to antigens in *B. bovis* culture supernatant fluids react directly with the merozoite surface coat, causing thickening of the surface coat, aggregation, and lysis of merozoites.

Recent studies [15, 16, 17] have demonstrated that these parasite products are effective in inducing protective immunity to bovine babesiosis. Vaccinated cattle respond with a characteristically strong anamnestic humoral response to blood or tick-borne challenge exposures. Immunity induced by vaccination has been shown to persist for at least a 6-month period [17].

3.2. Antibody kinetics

Our research group at the University of Illinois has recently studied the kinetics of specific indirect fluorescent antibody (IFA) titers and total serum IgG and IgM levels in yearling Angus heifers vaccinated twice with culture-derived soluble *B. bovis* antigens and challenged wth live *Babesia* organisms [18]. Besides the usual increase in IFA responses pre-challenge, vaccinated animals demonstrated significant increases in mean serum IgG values soon after each injection with soluble *B. bovis* immunogen and following challange exposure (Fig. 1). Slight post-vaccination increases in serum IgM values were noticed with a marked increase seen 19 days post-challenge. Following challenge a decrease in total IgG (in the controls) and IgM (vaccinated and control animals) was noted, coinciding with the period of peak parasitemia.

Although the afore-mentioned is the first report of suppression of immunoglobulin levels in *B. bovis*-infected animals, others have reported immunosuppression to heterologous antigens in mice infected with *B. microti*. Purvis (19) found decreased antibody production to sheep erythrocytes in infected mice. Depression of IgM and IgG plaque-forming cells began 3 days after peak parasitemia and was maximal 4 days later. As in the above study, specific anti-babesial

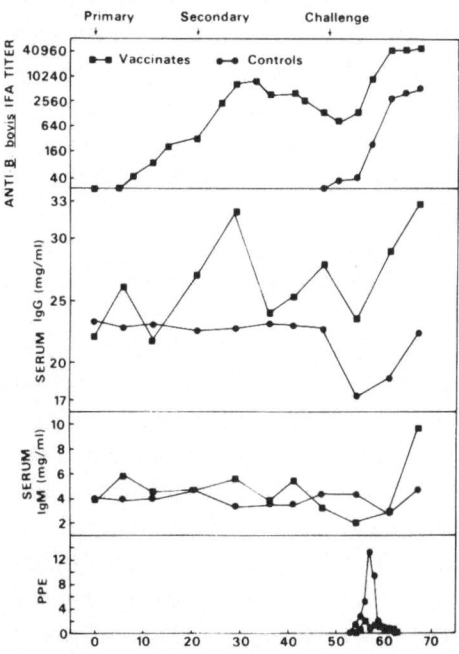

Figure 1. Anti-*B. bovis* IFA titers, total serum IgG and IgM concentrations, and percentage of parasitized erythrocytes (PPE) from animals vaccinated with culture-derived soluble *B. bovis* antigens and challenge exposed with live *Babesia* organisms. Values derived from nonvaccinated controls are also indicated.

antibody continued to rise throughout the infection period. Likewise, return to normal immune responsiveness was correlated with the gradual disappearance of parasites from the blood. Similarly, Gray [20] has observed an effect of *B. microti* on both primary and secondary responses to sheep erythrocytes with maximal depression associated with peak parasitemia. Cell-mediated immunity during *B. microti* infection, as manifested by skin graft injection, is not significantly altered, while macrophage phagocytic activity has been shown to be enhanced [21].

The immunosuppressive effects of *B. bovis* may have important implications on the transmission rate of the parasite in endemic areas. *Babesia bovis* has been known to cause a decrease in host immunity to its natural tick vector, *Boophilus microplus* [22]. A primary infection with *Babesia* at the time of first tick exposure prevents development of resistance to this tick, thereby enabling increased tick infestation. In an earlier study, Mahoney and Ross [23] found that the prevalence of *Babesia* was indeed related to vector density.

3.3. *Mechanisms of antibody responses*

The role of antibody-mediated immune responses to *Babesia* parasites is now well established, however the nature of these immunological mechanisms is still, to a great extent, speculative. A simplified schema for mechanisms of antibody responses to *Babesia* is proposed in Figure 2. Possible mechanisms for the antibody response are as follows: The *Babesia* organism possesses an array of surface coat antigens, each constructed of different antigenic determinants or epitopes which are either thymic-independent or thymic-dependent in nature. The thymic-independent determinants have an antigenic structure designed to stimulate B cells committed for IgM production. Immunoglobulin M functions as an opsonin and a potent agglutinating antibody. Thymic-dependent determinants induce IgG formation with the aid of helper T cells. The helper T cell interacts with specific B cells to produce IgG antibodies capable of opsonic, cytophilic and neutralizing activities. Memory cells of both B and T lineages are produced and will be responsible for the anamnestic response upon a second encounter with parasite antigens. Macrophages probably are necessary for antigen processing and for cooperation with B and T cells in the anti-parasite humoral response.

Although *Babesia* are capable of inducing copious amounts of specific antibody, certain suppressive effects may arise through immunologic mechanisms. Any of these mechanisms may be operative in *Babesia*-induced immunosuppression. Macrophages may be inherently defective in their ability to process antigen or may belong to the subpopulation of macrophages which secrete soluble suppressor factors capable of depressing humoral responses. Furthermore, parasites may activate nonspecific suppressor T cells and, in effect, suppress antibody responses to heterologous antigens. Lastly, parasite-induced mitogenic substances may stimulate polyclonal antibody responses unrelated to specific *Babe-*

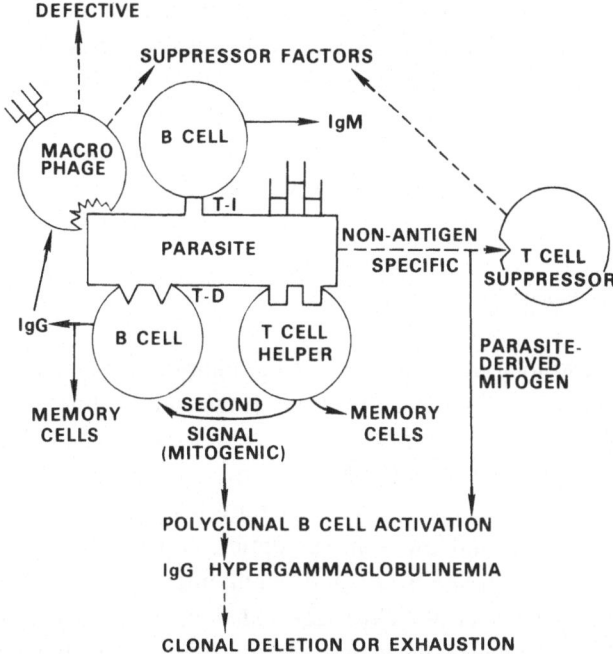

Figure 2. A proposed schema for the mechanism of the antibody response to *Babesia*. T-D=thymic-dependent; T-I=thymic-independent; broken line=suppressive effect.

sia immunogenicity. Benach et al. [6] recently observed that during acute human babesiosis responses to nonspecific mitogens are suppressed while levels of serum IgG and IgM increase significantly.

4. Role of cell-mediated immunity

4.1. *T Lymphocytes*

Since Clark and Allison [24] first reported that nude mice differed from intact mice in their ability to eliminate *B. microti* parasites, there has been little direct evidence of cell-mediated immune mechanisms in *Babesia* infection. However, Ruebush and Hanson (25, 26) have reported that lymph node and spleen cells from BALB/c mice infected with *B. microti* of human origin developed the ability to transfer adoptive immunity to naive mice. Results suggested that immunologic memory was modulated by the T lymphocyte. Furthermore, they found that resistance to and recovery from a primary *B. microti* infection is T cell-dependent with a concurrent depression in B cell function. Timms et al. [27] recently studied the lymphocyte response to *B. bovis* antigen in cattle vaccinated with live parasites or with culture-derived soluble antigens. Lymphocyte transformation assays indicated that the lymphocyte response to live vaccine was short-lived, a low positive stimulation index being recorded 10–18 days after vaccination. The response in cattle given culture-derived soluble antigens was very different. These animals showed positive stimulation indicies for an entire 6-month period, reaching a maximum after approximately 18 weeks.

4.2. *Natural killer cells*

Studies have also focused on the role of the natural killer (NK) cell in cellular immune responses to babesial infection. Eugui and Allison [28] found that differences in the susceptibility to *B. microti* infections among various mouse strains could be correlated with NK cell activity. Natural killer cell activity is known to be high in strains of mice which are resistant to *B. microti*, such as C57Bl and CBA mice, and low in the susceptible A strain. In the resistant strains there is also a rapid increase in size and cell number, which is still more marked during recovery. Irvin et al. [29] suggested that NK cells may be important mediators of functional splenic activity during *Babesia* infections of mice. Conversely, Wood and Clark [30] have shown that increased NK activity in the spleens and peritoneal cavities of *B. microti*-infected mice is not associated with protective host responses. The finding was also supported in studies with mice genetically deficient in NK cells. Therefore, it does seem that caution is warranted when we attempt to define the role of cell-mediated immune mechanisms in *Babesia* infection. Yet, it can be assumed from present concepts that specifically reactive T lymphocytes increase the supply of mononuclear phagocytes (and probably NK cells), direct them at filtration sites in the reticuloendothelial system, and stimulate them to increase metabolic activity.

5. Antigen characterization

Recent studies concerned with the immunochemical characterization of potential immunogens for bovine babesiosis have utilized *B. bovis* antigens derived from culture supernatant fluids [31, 32, 33, 34] and from lysates of parasitized erythrocytes [35, 36, 37]. In our laboratory, a critical development in the first isolation and identification of culture-derived soluble *B. bovis* antigens was the adaptation of *B. bovis* for growth in a heterologous rabbit erythrocyte-serum system using the MASP method [11]. This was important in that suboptimal reactivity was found when bovine antiserum was used in gel immunoprecipitation techniques. The rabbit-derived culture system also allowed for the production of antisera against an antigenic preparation relatively free of bovine serum contaminants.

Crossed immunoelectrophoretic (CIE) analysis [31] of supernatants from infected and uninfected cultures showed that at least three soluble antigens are produced *in vitro* (so-called antigens 1, 2 and 3). Antigen 1 has an electrophoretic mobility in the albumin range, whereas antigens 2 and 3 migrate to the alpha-1 region.

The estimated molecular weights for at least two of the antigens as determined by SDS-PAGE approximate 37,000–40,000 daltons [31]. Kahl et al. [33] have demonstrated that certain biosynthetically labeled protein antigens of culture-derived *B. bovis* parasites are strain-specific and correlate with the degree of virulence. At least one protein (molecular weight 43,000 daltons) was identified as being a dominant labeled antigen of an avirulent strain with potential protective capabilities.

Preliminary evidence derived from analytical polyacrylamide gel isoelectro-focusing experiments suggests that three soluble *B. bovis* antigens purified from culture supernatant fluid focus in the range of pI 5.0–5.5 (James, unpublished data). This range is consistent with that of known acidic protein antigens derived from detergent extracts of *B. bovis* organisms [33].

Preparative purification of culture-derived soluble antigens has been conducted by selective precipitation with ammonium sulfate and anion-exchange chromatography [32]. Parasite antigens could be demonstrated in fractions precipitated with 60–70% saturated ammonium sulfate. Additionally, fractionation of culture fluid in a stepwise gradient (0.1–0.4M Tris-HCl buffer pH 6.5) over diethylaminoethyl (DEAE) cellulose revealed that most of the soluble antigenic components were recovered in the fractions eluted with the 0.1M buffer.

To localize the culture-derived soluble *B. bovis* antigens as they exist within the infected erythrocyte, Montenegro-James et al. [34] utilized established procedures for the production of monospecific antibodies to individual antigens. Immunoprecipitates derived from CIE of *B. bovis* culture supernatant fluid against polyspecific anti-*B. bovis* serum were used to produce monospecific rabbit antibodies to individual *B. bovis* antigens. These antibodies were utilized in an immunofluorescence test to identify the location of the respective antigens in the infected erythrocyte. The study revealed that antigen 1 was bound to the erythrocyte membrane, antigen 2 was found in the cytoplasm of the infected erythrocyte, and antigen 3 was directly associated with the parasite (Fig. 3). Goodger et al. [38] have reported that membrane and stromal *Babesia* antigens (antigens 1 and 2) are fibrinogen-associated with the parasite-associated antigen (antigen 3) most probably a constituent of the merozoite surface coat. Very recently, Wright et al. [36] isolated a protective antigen by using monoclonal antibodies. Strong protective immunity was induced by an antigen which has a reported molecular weight of 44,000 daltons, confirming similar physicochemical data obtained by two other research groups (31, 33). Immunofluorescent staining patterns revealed that monoclonal antibodies to this antigen intensely stained

LOCATION OF THREE <u>BABESIA</u> <u>BOVIS</u> ANTIGENS IN INFECTED ERYTHROCYTE

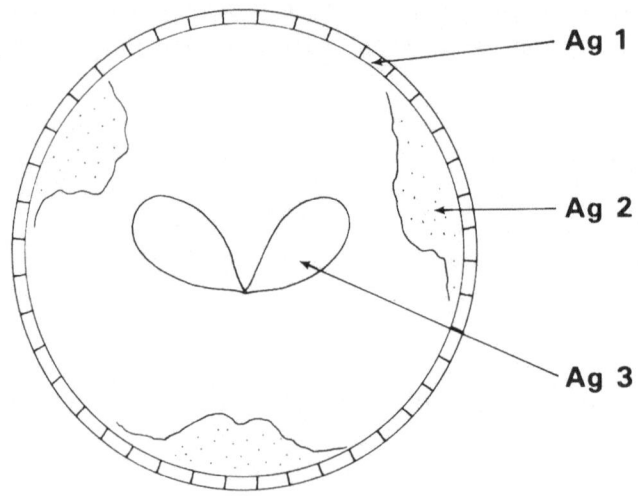

Figure 3. Diagram of the location of three *B. bovis* antigens in the infected erythrocyte. Parasite antigens indicated by arrows.

only the parasite. Probably, this antigen is identical to our so-called antigen 3.

6. Immunodiagnosis

Various innovative serodiagnostic techniques have been implemented to supplement the standard tests such as indirect immunofluorescence, complement fixation, and the indirect card and capillary agglutination tests. Most of the techniques have been designed to meet the requirements for field use, those being sensitivity and specificity with inherent simplicity of performance. Young and Purnell [39] have modified the micro ELISA for field serodiagnosis of *B. divergens* by utilizing dried blood samples as the antibody source. Barry et al. [40] also have described a micro ELISA method for the detection and measurement of antibodies to *B. bovis*. This was shown to be even more sensitive than the classical IFA test. Montenegro et al. [41] have used culture-derived soluble *B. bovis* antigens in the latex agglutination test for the serodiagnosis of *Babesia* species. Additionally, a highly specific and sensitive test developed to titer and rank anti-*B. bovis* antibody has been reported by Kahl and colleagues [42]. They developed a solid-phase radioimmunoassay using antigens from infected bovine erythrocytes. Logically, this test may best be employed as a prelude to other laboratory procedures.

7. Summary and conclusions

The role of antibody- and T cell-mediated immune responses to *Babesia* parasites is now well established, however the nature of these and other immunological effector mechanisms has been defined only recently. New knowledge obtained from the study of host defense mechanisms to babesial infections has elucidated specific and nonspecific, humoral and cellular aspects of resistance. The recovery from experimental *B. microti* infection in BALB/c mice has been shown to be T-lymphocytic dependent, particularly with regards to the modulation of immunologic memory. Depressed B cell function and normal T cell function are correlates of this infection. There are also indications that natural killer cell activity may be important in controlling *Babesia* infection.

Various nonspecific serum factors have been demonstrated to affect babesial growth *in vivo* and *in vitro*. Complement (C3) and the C3b receptor may facilitate *B. rodhaini* infection in the rat. *In vitro* cultivation of *B. bovis* in erythrocyte cultures demonstrated that blood from young animals contains a factor(s) responsible for their resistance to severe babesiosis.

Soluble antigens derived from cultures of *B. bovis* have been shown to be efficient immunogens for induction of protective immunity against bovine babesiosis. Immunochemical analysis of culture supernatants has demonstrated that at least three parasite antigens are released *in vitro*. Molecular weights of these culture-derived antigens range from 35,000–47,500 daltons.

New developments are also being made in serological tests designed for detection of anti-*Babesia* antibodies. Use of the micro ELISA test and solid-phase radioimmunoassay has provided more sensitivity in detecting changes in antibody titer.

Progress toward the understanding of protective anti-babesial immune responses and the antigens which induce them has proceeded at a credible rate since the last meeting on malaria and babesiosis in Mexico City. The identification of host protective antigens and their recent incorporation into monoclonal antibody systems have provided us with a solid foundation for future investigation. Continued study of protective immune mechanisms and ways by which they may be optimized are not only worthy research considerations but paramount in our efforts to resolve bovine babesiosis.

References

1. Jack RM, Ward PA: *Babesia rodhaini* interactions with complement: relationship to parasitic entry into red cells. J Immunol 124(4):1566–1573, 1980.
2. Jack RM, Ward PA: The role *in vivo* of C3 and the C3b receptor in babesial infection in the rat. J Immunol 124(4):1574–1578, 1980.
3. Ward PA, Jack RM: The entry process of *Babesia* merozoites into red cells. Am J Pathol 102:109–113, 1981.

4. Chapman WE, Ward PA: *Babesia rodhaini*: requirement of complement for penetration of human erythrocytes. Science 196:67–70, 1977.
5. Mahoney DF, Wright IG, Goodger BV: Changes in the haemolytic activity of serum complement during acute *Babesia bovis* infection in cattle. Z Parasitenkd 62:39–45, 1980.
6. Benach JL, Habicht GS, Hamburger MI: Immunoresponsiveness in acute babesiosis in humans. J Infect Dis 146(3):369–380, 1982.
7. Goodger BV, Wright IG, Mahoney DF: Changes in conglutinin, immunoconglutinin, complement C3 and fibronectin concentrations in cattle acutely infected with *Babesia bovis*. Aust J Exp Biol Med Sci 59(5):531–538, 1981.
8. Clark IA, Allison AC, Cox FEG: Protection of mice against *Babesia* and *Plasmodium* with BCG. Nature (London) 259:309–311, 1976.
9. Clark IA, Cox FEG, Allison AC: Protection of mice against *Babesia* spp. and *Plasmodium* spp. with killed *Corynebacterium parvum*. Parasitology 74:9–11, 1977.
10. Clark IA: Resistance to *Babesia* spp. and *Plasmodium* spp. in mice pretreated with an extract of *Coxiella burnetii*. Inf Immun 24(2):319–325, 1979.
11. Levy MG, Ristic M: *Babesia bovis*: continuous cultivation in a microaerophilous stationary phase culture. Science 207:1218–1220, 1980.
12. Levy MG, Clabaugh G, Ristic M: Age resistance in bovine babesiosis: role of blood factors in resistance to *Babesia bovis*. Inf Immun 37(3):1127–1131, 1982.
13. Bautista CR, Kreier JP: Effect of immune serum on the growth of *Babesia microti* in hamster erythrocytes in short-term culture. Inf Immun 25(1):470–472, 1979.
14. Ristic M, Levy MG: A new era of research toward solution of bovine babesiosis. In: Babesiosis, Ristic M, Kreier JP (eds), New York, Academic Press, 1981, p. 509–544.
15. Smith RD, James MA, Ristic M, Aikawa M, Vega CA: Bovine babesiosis: protection of cattle with culture-derived soluble *Babesia bovis* antigen. Science 212:335–338, 1981.
16. Kuttler KL, Levy MG, James MA, Ristic M: Efficacy of a nonviable culture-derived *Babesia bovis* vaccine. Amer J Vet Res 43(2):281–284, 1982.
17. Kuttler KL, Levy MG, Ristic M: Cell culture-derived *Babesia bovis* vaccine: sequential challenge exposure of protective immunity during 6-month postvaccination period. Amer J Vet Res 44(8):1456–1459, 1983.
18. James MA, Kuttler KL, Levy MG, Ristic M: Antibody kinetics in response to vaccination against *Babesia bovis*. Amer J Vet Res 42(11):1999–2001, 1981.
19. Purvis AC: Immunodepression in *Babesia microti* infections. Parasitology 75:197–205, 1977.
20. Gray GB: The effect of *Babesia microti* on the immune response of mice to sheep erythrocytes. Parasitology 77:xliv, 1978.
21. Purvis AC: Immunodepression in rodent piroplasmosis. *(Babesia microti)*. Parasitology 75:197–205, 1976.
22. Callow LL, Stewart NP: Immunosuppression by *Babesia bovis* against its tick vector, *Boophilus microplus*. Nature (London) 272:818–819, 1978.
23. Mahoney DF, Ross DR: Epizootiological factors in the control of bovine babesiosis. Aust Vet J 48:292–298, 1972.
24. Clark IA, Allison AC: *Babesia microti* and *Plasmodium berghei yoelii* infections in nude mice. Nature 252:328–329, 1974.
25. Ruebush MJ, Hanson WL: Transfer of immunity to *Babesia microti* of human origin using T lymphocytes in mice. Cell Immunol 52:255–265, 1980.
26. Ruebush MJ, Hanson WL: Thymus dependence of resistance to infection with *Babesia microti* of human origin in mice. Am J Trop Med Hyg 29(4):507–515, 1980.
27. Timms P, Stewart NP, Barry DN, Dalgliesh RJ: Nonliving *Babesia bovis* vaccines from culture. How good are they? Proc 2nd Intl Conf Mal Bab Annecy, France, Abstract 40, p. 109.
28. Eugui EM, Allison AC: Differences in susceptibility of various mouse strains to haemoprotozoan infections: possible correlation with natural killer activity. Parasite Immunol 2:277–292, 1980.

29. Irvin AD, Young ER, Osborn GD, Francis LMA: A comparison of *Babesia* infections in intact, surgically splenectomized, and congenitally asplenic (Dh/+) mice. Int J Parasitol 11(3):251–255, 1981.

30. Wood PR, Clark IA: Apparent irrelevance of NK cells to resolution of infections with *Babesia microti* and *Plasmodium vinckei petteri* in mice. Parasite Immunol 4:319–327, 1982.

31. James MA, Levy MG, Ristic M: Isolation and partial characterization of culture-derived soluble *Babesia bovis* antigens. Inf Immun 31(1):358–361, 1981.

32. Montenegro S: Studies of culture-derived soluble *Babesia bovis* antigens: purification, characterization and application in serodiagnosis. PhD thesis University of Illinois, Urbana-Champaign, Illinois.

33. Kahl LP, Anders RF, Rodwell BJ, Timms P, Mitchell GF: Variable and common antigens of *Babesia bovis* parasites differing in strain and virulence. J Immunol 129(4):1700–1705, 1982.

34. Montenegro-James S, James MA, Ristic M: Localization of culture-derived soluble *Babesia bovis* antigens in the infected erythrocyte. Vet Parasitol 13:311–316, 1983.

35. Mahoney DF, Wright IG, Goodger BV: Bovine babesiosis: the immunization of cattle with fractions of erythrocytes infected with *Babesia bovis* (syn. *B. argentina*). Vet Immunol Immunopathol 2:145–156, 1981.

36. Wright IG, White M, Tracey-Patte PD, Donaldson RA, Goodger BV, Waltisbuhl DJ, Mahoney DF: *Babesia bovis*: isolation of a protective antigen by using monoclonal antibodies. Inf Immun 41(1):244–250, 1983.

37. Goodger BV, Wright IG, Waltisbuhl DJ: The lysate from bovine erythrocytes infected with *Babesia bovis*. Z Parasitenkd 69:473–482, 1983.

38. Goodger BV, Wright IG, Mahoney DF, McKenna RV: *Babesia bovis (argentina)*: studies on the composition and location of antigen associated with infected erythrocytes. Int J Parasitol 10:33–36, 1980.

39. Young ER, Purnell RE: Evaluation of dried blood samples as a source of antibody in the micro ELISA test for *Babesia divergens*. Vet Rec 106:60–61, 1980.

40. Barry DN, Rodwell BJ, Timms P, McGregor W: A microplate enzyme immunoassay for detecting and measuring antibodies to *Babesia bovis* in cattle serum. Aust Vet J 59:136–140, 1982.

41. Montenegro S, James MA, Levy MG, Preston MD, Esparza H, Ristic M: Utilization of culture-derived soluble antigen in the latex agglutination test for bovine babesiosis and anaplasmosis. Vet Parasitol 8:291–297, 1981.

42. Kahl LP, Anders RF, Callow LL, Rodwell BJ, Mitchell GF: Development of a solid-phase radioimmunoassay for antibody to antigens of *Babesia bovis*-infected bovine erythrocytes. Int J Parasitol 12(2/3):103–109, 1982.

4. The red cell cytoskeleton and invasion by malaria parasites

ROBERT J.M. WILSON*, ANTON R. DLUZEWSKI,
KAVERI RANGACHARI AND WALTER B. GRATZER

* National Institute for Medical Research, Mill Hill, London NW7 1AA, UK, and Medical Research Council Cell Biophysics Unit, King's College, London WC2, UK.

Introduction

In recent years, considerable progress has been made in understanding how malaria parasites recognise and interact with the surface of human red cells. However, our knowledge of molecular events in the invasion process decreases as the parasite passes through the sequential stages of recognition, attachment, junction formation, and internalisation. The purposes of what follows in this review is to consider the later stages of invasion in the light of the increasingly detailed picture available of the organisation of the membrane skeleton of the red cell itself. Emphasis will be given to new information recently gathered from experimental work with red cell ghosts which are both amenable to cytoskeletal modification and susceptible to invasion.

1. The invasion process

Malaria parasites enter red cells by a complex process that is complete within tens of seconds. Direct observations and high resolution video analysis of living organisms [1, 2] have led to comprehensive descriptions of the morphological events involved. Transmission electron micrographs [3, 4] and freeze-fracture studies [5, 6] have revealed further important details. We know very little, however, about the fundamental steps which operate at the molecular level.

There are many data to indicate that the invasion of human red cells by merozoites of *Plasmodium falciparum* follows specific binding of parasite surface components to glycophorin, the major intrinsic sialoglycoprotein of the erythrocyte membrane. Three lines of evidence support this conclusion: red cells from subjects genetically devoid of glycophorin are resistant to invasion [7, 8, 9]; antibodies to certain epitopes of glycophorin A, such as the Wright b (Wr^b) antigen, inhibit invasion *in vitro* [10, 11]; liposomes containing purified glycophorin A compete with and inhibit invasion by merozoites *in vitro* [12, 13].

Ristic, M. et al. (eds.) *Malaria and babesiosis.*
© 1984, Martinus Nijhoff Publishers, Dordrecht/Boston/Lancaster.

The red cell membrane has a highly charged surface due to lipid phosphoryl groups and ionised side chains on proteins and glycoproteins. To what extent the overall charge determines the interaction with the merozoite is unclear. As normal red cells treated with trypsin have a greatly reduced susceptibility to invasion, despite enhanced accessibility of the Wr^b antigen, more than a single region of the glycophorin molecule seems to be involved [10]. The amount of sialic acid on the red cell surface appears to become critical only after more than half has been removed, but there is still some controversy as to whether a high charge density or only a high affinity ligand is required to generate sufficient binding energy. Friedman [see ref. 11] has claimed that the adsorption of serum orosomucoid increases the surface charge of erythrocytes treated with neuraminidase and restores susceptibility to invasion. It has also been found that the efficiency with which N-acetylglucosamine blocks invasion is greater, by a factor of 10^5, if the saccharide is first conjugated with a protein matrix such as bovine serum albumin [13].

A further level of biological complexity is reflected by the requirement that it is specifically the apical region of the merozoite which must be applied to the red cell membrane before invasion can eventuate. A favourable interaction between the surfaces of the merozoite and the potential host cell can thus be viewed as a prelude to initiation of invasion *per se*. In what appears to be an active process, the erythrocyte is deformed by the merozoite over an area of several μm^2 at the point of attack. An electron dense material, sometimes resolvable into short fibres, can be seen to extend from the apex of the parasite on to the red cell surface. Whether a membrane-reactive substance is released on triggering of receptors in the apical region of the parasite is still unknown. Membrane material is internalised by the red cell at the attachment point, and a localised thickening of the inner leaflet of the red cell bilayer forms a discrete junction zone where the host cell and merozoite surfaces are closely apposed (10 nm gap). Freeze-fracture studies show that the density of intramembrane particles (IMP) becomes much reduced in the P face of the red cell bilayer in the vicinity of the attachment site, and a ring of densely packed IMP surrounds the attachment point. These packed particles evidently correspond to the thickened inner leaflet observed at the junction zone in transmission electron micrographs. It is noteworthy that there does not seem to be any marked change in the distribution of IMP in the E face of the red cell membrane. At this stage of the invasion process, Dvorak et al. [1] observed that the deformed host cell temporarily resumes it normal contour, but with the merozoite attached by its apical prominence.

Encapsulation of the merozoite next ensues by the formation and internalisation of a parasitophorous vacuole. Because cytochalasin B treatment of merozoites blocks internalisation but not attachment [2] the intervention of some form of contractile mechanism is implied. During encapsulation, the apex of the merozoite remains attached to the invaginated red cell membrane by the small electron opaque deposit alluded to earlier. The junction zone separates from this point and forms a rim round the contour of the merozoite as it penetrates into the red cell. The parasite and host cell membranes are tightly bound only in the junction zone which forms a narrow annulus. This zone of tight binding might have several functions; it could be the site of a motile force to propel the merozoite into the cell; it may confine enzymatic or other processes within the incipient parasitophorous vacuole - the 'surface coat' of the merozoite becomes modified within the expanding vacuole and it is widely held that it becomes enzymatically degraded during invasion [14, 15]; a third conjecture is that membrane flows past the junction zone so that the parasite, anchored at its apical tip to the expanding vacuole, is pulled into the cell - this hypothesis requires that some mechanism maintains the junction zone in the region of membrane flow. In the final stages of invasion the junction zone coalesces at the posterior end of the merozoite and is eventually enclosed within the red cell as part of the parasitophorous vacuole membrane. Sealing of the red cell membrane to restore its continuity at the site of invasion completes the process.

2. The red cell membrane skeleton

An infrastructure of protein molecules called the membrane skeleton, or cytoskeleton, covers the cytosolic surface of the erythrocyte membrane [16, 17]. The discoid shape and elasticity of the cell depend on the cytoskeleton which is associated with the intrinsic membrane proteins and probably also with the phospholipid bilayer. On disruption of the cytoskeleton the membrane disintegrates into vesicles. The main components of the membrane skeleton are spectrin, ankyrin, band 4.1 and actin. The predominant protein is the large filamentous molecule known as spectrin that is densely packed over the membrane surface. The α and β subunits of spectrin (bands 1 and 2) associate laterally to form heterodimers. These interact by specific head-to-head association to produce rod-like tetramers, 1.1×10^5 per cell. Small proportions of higher oligomeric complexes of spectrin also exist *in situ* [18]. Spectrin has the capacity to bind F-actin. The actin present is in the form of short proto-filaments, connected by spectrin tetramers to form a lattice-like mesh [19]. The interaction between spectrin and actin depends on another globular protein, band 4.1 (M.Wt. 80,000) and this complex is responsible for the relatively low viscosity of erythrocyte suspensions under sheer-induced stress [20]. The cytoskeleton is linked to the membrane through ankyrin (band 2.1) which is not an intrinsic membrane protein. Ankyrin (M.Wt. 200,000) has a high affinity binding site for spectrin (10^{-8}M dissociation constant) and another for the cytosolic portion of band 3, the major transmembrane glycoprotein. Band 3 appears to be associated with the other major intrinsic membrane protein, glycophorin A [21]. This chain of interactions between spectrin and transmembrane glycoproteins neatly explains the observation that the introduction into ghosts of antibodies to spectrin can alter the

distribution of extracellular glycoprotein sites [22] and that, conversely, immobilisation of the externally orientated saccharide moieties facilitates cross-linking
of cytoskeletal proteins [23]. Band 3 is the predominant substance of the intramembrane particles seen by electron microscopy but only a minor proportion of
band 3 is associated with ankyrin.

The network of cytoskeletal proteins is attached to the membrane by non-
covalent bonds at many sites; not only through the spectrin-ankyrin complex, but
also apparently by way of interactions of band 4 with glycoproteins, and probably
an interaction of spectrin with the negatively charged phosphatidylserine in the
inner leaflet of the bilayer [17]. There is evidence [24] that maintenance of the
asymmetric distribution of phospholipids, particularly phosphotidylserine (PTS),
is dependent on spectrin, because oxidation of certain spectrin thiols leads to loss
of the phospholipid asymmetry. These interactions with the lipid bilayer appear
to provide an important stabilising force and contribute to the high deformability
modulus of red cells under shear-flow stress [20].

The stabilising effect of the cytoskeleton is such that it can adapt passively to
area changes in the intrinsic domain of the membrane, as reflected by echi-
nocytosis or stomatocytosis on intercalation of amphipathic drugs into one or
other membrane leaflet [25, 26]. Local rearrangements of extrinsic and intrinsinic
membrane proteins accompany the formation of protein-free areas of bilayer, or
'bare patches', in which exo- or endocytosis, vesiculation, or fusion can occur
[27]. Endocytosis is preceded by the clustering of IMP and the loss of spectrin in
the area of invagination[28]. This effect is readily induced in neonatal red cells
(predominantly a young population of cells) which can undergo spontaneous
endocytosis unlike mature red cells [29, 30]. The introduction of cross-links in the
cytoskeleton by antibodies to spectrin, blocks both fusion and endocytosis [31].
Stabilisation of erythrocyte shape can result, in converse manner, from non-
covalent linking by lectins of the external oligosaccharides of intrinsic membrane
glycoproteins[32]. Immobilisation of transmembrane proteins results in a loss of
motility of associated cytoskeletal components. There is evidence [54] that although most band (3) molecules are not attached to the membrane skeleton, their
lateral movement is impeded by the cytoskeletal network into the interstices of
which the cytoplasmic domains of the band 3 molecule are thought to penetrate.

In the presence of adenosine triphosphate (ATP) the β subunit of spectrin is
phosphorylated at four clustered sites by a cAMP-independent protein kinase
[33]. Dephosphorylation does not affect the stability of the membrane skeleton
[34] and, in contrast to earlier claims, it is by no means clear that shape changes of
erythrocytes are controlled directly by phosphorylation [35, 36]. However, pretreatment of red cell ghosts with alkaline phosphatase blocks endocytosis and
prevents the creation of spectrin-free areas. This raises the possibility that phosphorylation plays a role in endocytosis [28]. Other important physiological processes may also act through the membrane skeleton. Deformability of the cell, for
example, is affected by polyanions such as 2,3-diphosphoglycerate (2,3-DPG)

which destabilises the cytoskeleton [37, 38]. High concentrations of calcium cause extensive changes in the membrane by activating proteolytic and trans-glutaminase enzymes, as well as in other less drastic ways.

This survey has concentrated on defining the dynamic interdependence of cytoskeletal and transmembrane proteins, as well as the pathways by which external events can exert changes in the interior of the cell. As a greatly reduced number of IMP is common to both the parasitophorous vacuole and the endo-cytotic vesicle, we can postulate that uncoupling of the cytoskeleton from the site of invasion by an activity of the merozoite is accompanied by withdrawal of IMP and the formation of a bare patch of membrane within which the parasite becomes encapsulated.

3. Red cell ghosts

3.1. White ghosts and red ghosts

Most biochemical studies of the red cell membrane pertain to haemoglobin-free preparations obtained after hypotonic lysis and repeated washing, referred to as 'white' ghosts [39]. Although such membranes retain many of their biological properties, such as the capacity for glucose transport, some systems are altered, suggesting that structural perturbation has occurred [40]. From the observations of Miller and his colleagues [41], that merozoites of *P. knowlesi* attach to and then detach from white ghosts without inducing deformation, it can be inferred that the primary receptor site is retained but the structural changes required to trigger invasion or to labilize the red cell membrane, no longer take place.

We have reported [42] that resealed red ghosts prepared by hypotonic lysis by dialysis without separation of the membrane from the cytosol are susceptible to invasion by the malaria parasites *P. falciparum* and *P. knowlesi*. A similar observation has also been reported by Olson [43], using a different technique. According to Sprandel et al. [44], resealed ghosts prepared by dialysis at 70% haematocrit, retain, as expected, the original contents diluted to 70% of their starting concentration. Glucose transport is elevated but can still be inhibited by phloridzin as in intact cells. The influx of sodium ions is also considerably elevated but transport of metabolites such as L-phenylalanine and uric acid is identical to that in intact cells. Other comparisons between intact red cells and resealed ghosts revealed no differences in SDS-gel electrophoresis patterns following tryptic digestion [45], or of the sensitivity of band 3 to lactoperoxidase catalysed iodination [46]. On the other hand, some properties of the membrane do change if the ghosts are washed or depleted of cytosol by dilution prior to resealing [47, 65]. For one membrane-associated protein, band 4, it was concluded that signifi-cant dissociation occurred on dilution of the cytosol by a factor of ≥ 10. Bearing such limitations in mind, preparations of resealed red ghosts are nevertheless of interest to us because they are prone to invasion and offer a means of altering the internal milieu of the cell, and also of modifying specific cytoskeletal structures which might be involved in the invasion process.

3.2. *Cytoplasmic requirements for invasion*

Our studies on the invasion of resealed red ghosts with *P. falciparum* have shown a striking relation between the dilution of the cytosol upon hypotonic lysis and the retention of susceptibility to invasion [48]. Resealed ghosts prepared by dialysis at 70% haematocrit against 5 mM phosphate buffer, with no added solutes, were invaded only to about one-third the extent of intact red cells. The efficiency of invasion fell further as the haematocrit was reduced and reached zero at a haematocrit of about 30%. When lysis and resealing at reduced haematocrit were carried out in the presence of an undiluted haemolysate that had been prepared previously by repeated freezing and thawing of intact cells, the morphology of the resealed ghosts improved substantially (from 80% stomatocytes to 90% dis-cocytes) but there was still only a small increase in the efficiency of invasion [49].

Of the many cytoplasmic constituents whose loss or dilution might change the membrane properties appreciably, ATP seems to be of primary importance. When cells are lysed in the presence of 6 mM ATP and resealed in iso-osmotic buffer, susceptibility to invasion rises to a level comparable to that of control cells [50]. We now routinely add 1 mM Mg.ATP to both the lysis and the resealing buffers to obtain a similar effect [48]. The addition of ATP leads to retention of susceptibility to invasion down to much lower haematocrit as well as increased efficiency of invasion at high haematocrit, depending on the metabolic state of the cells. With decreasing concentrations of added ATP, susceptibility to invasion remains almost constant until a sharp drop almost to zero occurs below 10 μM ATP. The endogenous level of ATP, which varies in different preparations, governs to some extent the enhancing effect of added ATP and an inverse relationship has been demonstrated [48].

A limitation in our experimental system that complicates study of the role of ATP, is that we add mature schizonts rather than free merozoites to resealed ghosts, so there is always a lag of several hours before invasion occurs. Consequently, the concentration of ATP at the time of invasion cannot be expected to be the same as when the parasites and ghosts were first mixed together. Furthermore, the culture medium contains glucose so that ATP will be synthesised in the cytoplasm of resealed ghosts. Indeed we have observed that upon addition of AMP or ADP, rather than ATP, during the preparation of ghosts, ATP is synthesised in the maturation period required by the schizonts and susceptibility to invasion is largely retained [48].

Our preliminary report of the enhancing effect of ATP on invasion [50] was at variance with the study of Olson [43], but a subsequent paper by Olson and Kilejian [51] resolved this discrepancy which was ascribed to adverse experimental conditions. The beneficial effect of ATP shown by these studies is also consistent with the correlation between intracellular ATP concentration and parasitaemia levels *in vivo*, described previously by Brewer and Powell [52].

3.2.1. *The role of adenosine triphosphate (ATP) in invasion*
Some progress has been made towards identifying the site of action of ATP in promoting invasion. One possibility we considered was that ATP is required to maintain ion gradients across the host cell membrane. Ca^{2+} ions are of particular interest since they influence deformability of the membrane [53]. We found, however, that the introduction of 0.5-1 mM EGTA, an ion that cannot pass through the membrane, had little effect on the invasion of resealed ghosts, even though a reduction in the cytoplasmic concentration of Ca^{2+} from 0.1 μM to ~5 nM could be anticipated. To test for an effect of elevated concentrations of Ca^{2+} ions, such as would occur if reduced levels of ATP prevented efficient pumping of calcium out of the host cell, we utilised the vanadate ion. Vanadate is rapidly transported across the membrane and was introduced into intact red cells by equilibration with the medium. Invasion was not significantly inhibited (Fig. 1), though the concentration of vanadate was well above the level required to prevent active transport of calcium (20 μM).

It is believed, as already indicated, that ATP acting as a polyanion can influence

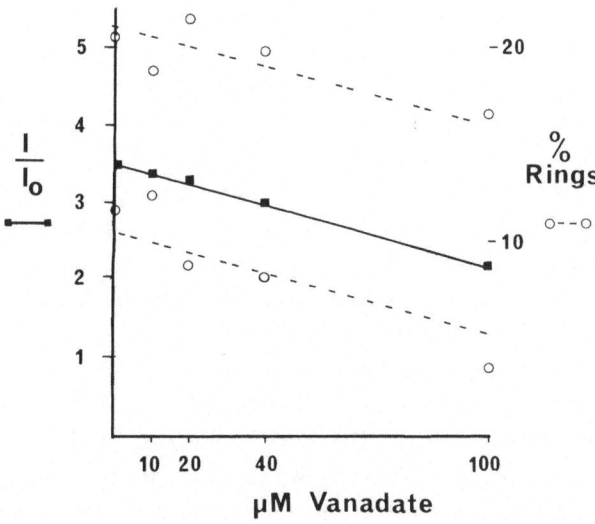

Figure 1. Susceptibility of intact human red cells to invasion by *P. falciparum* following equilibration of the cells in medium containing vanadate (10–100 μM). The mean invasion ratio (I/Io) is shown for two experiments (○———○) at different levels of parasitaemia.

the properties of the red cell membrane by a quite different non-enzymatic electrostatic mechanism. Sheetz and his coworkers [54] interpreted the increased lateral mobility of transmembrane proteins by physiological concentrations of polyanions such as ATP and 2,3-DPG as a loosening of the cohesion between the membrane and the cytoskeletal network. To test for such an effect on invasion, we introduced a non-hydrolysable analogue of ATP, namely, adenylyl-im-idodiphosphate (AMP.PNP) into resealed red ghosts [48]. This analogue did not prevent loss of susceptibility of the ghosts to parasite invasion. On the other hand, partial restoration of susceptibility resulted when the hydrolysable analogue of ATP, adenosine-5'-0-(3-thio-triphosphate) wad added. These results exclude a non-specific requirement for ATP in invasion. That ATP is required for phos-phoryl turnover in the phospholipids of the bilayer itself can also be excluded on the grounds that the esterase involved in this process is highly dependent on calcium ions [55] and we have found little effect on malarial invasion by the elevation or removal of Ca^{2+}.

We infer from these considerations that ATP is required as a phosphoryl source for kinases involved in the phosphoryl turnover of membrane-associated pro-teins. In support of this conclusion, we have demonstrated that the invasion of both red cell ghosts and intact cells is markedly reduced if they are loaded with high concentrations ($\geqslant 1$ mM) of adenosine [48], a powerful inhibitor of protein kinase activity [56]. We cannot yet indicate whether the turnover of phosphoryl groups is linked to the cAMP-dependent kinase that acts on ankyrin, the spectrin attachment protein, or to the cAMP-independent kinase that has the smaller subunit of spectrin as its main substrate. It also remains to be determined whether a threshold level of ATP is essential in the cytoplasm at the time of invasion or whether the role of ATP is in preconditioning the membrane. Another possibility is that ATP is required for a contractile process such as has been postulated for lectin-induced endocytosis [30].

3.2.2. *The role of other cytoplasmic constituents in invasion*
ATP is not the only cytoplasmic constituent that we have found to enhance invasion efficiency. The addition of physiological concentrations of 2,3-DPG (1–5mM) has a large stimulatory effect over and above the maximum produced by ATP (Table 1). The basis for this enhancement remains to be established. That still other unidentified cytoplasmic constituents are involved in invasion is indi-cated by the finding that neither ATP nor 2,3-DPG on their own are able to restore susceptibility to invasion when the haematocrit is reduced below a critical level during hypotonic lysis. As is shown in separate experiments in Fig. 2 and Table 1, resealed ghosts largely lose their ability to support invasion when prepared at an haematocrit of 1:16 (6%) or below, in the presence of 1 mM ATP, but the addition of fresh haemolysate allows substantial retention of suscep-tibility. Preliminary indications (Table 1) are that haemolysates which have been stripped of low molecular weight constituents, retain their ability to prevent the

Table 1. The invasion by P. falciparum of resealed ghosts loaded with ATP, 2,3-DPG or haemolysate

Cell type	Fluid in dialysis bag						Duplicate cultures[d]		X%
	Isoosmotic buffer	Hypoosmotic buffer with additives							
		ATP (1 mM)	DPG (1 mM)	Haemolysate					
				Fresh	Stripped	Aged[c]			
Untreated	−	−	−	−	−	−	4.1	3.8	100
Intact	+	−	−	−	−	−	3.2	3.0	79
Resealed ghost[a]	−	+	−	−	−	−	4.4	4.4	110
Resealed ghost[b]	−	+	−	−	−	−	0.8	0.6	17
ditto	−	+	−	+	−	−	1.9	1.9	48
ditto	−	+	−	−	+	−	2.1	1.6	48
ditto	−	+	−	−	−	+	1.0	0.6	20
ditto	−	+	+	+	−	−	3.1	3.0	79
ditto	−	+	+	−	+	−	3.3	3.4	86
ditto	−	+	+	−	−	+	0.8	0.6	18

[a] prepared at haematocrit of 1:1 (50%)
[b] prepared at haematocrit of 1:16 (6%)
[c] stored at 4°C for 18 hours
[d] Fold increase of parasites following invasion

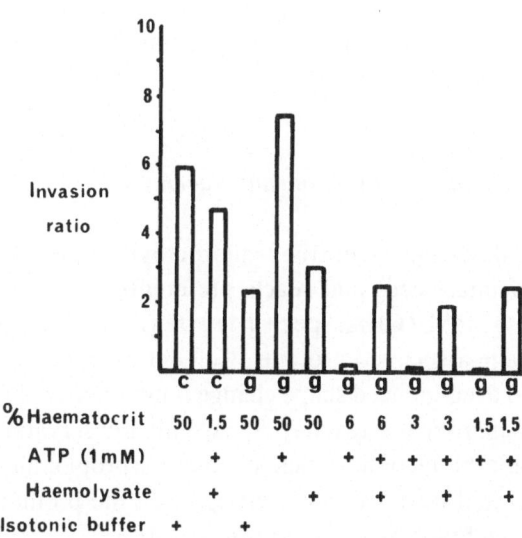

Figure 2. Resealed ghosts (g) lose their ability to support invasion when prepared at an haematocrit of 6% or less, even in the presence of 1 mM ATP. The inclusion of fresh haemolysate allows substantial retention of susceptibility. The invasion of intact cells (c) dialysed against isotonic buffer is shown for comparison.

loss of susceptibility to ghosts prepared at low haematocrit. By contrast, haemolysates stored at 4°C for 18 hours lose this capacity. Work is in progress in our laboratory to identify other active intracellular components revealed by these manipulations of resealed red ghosts.

4. Endocytosis, deformability and invasion

Immature red cells are believed to have spectrin-free areas within which clustering of receptors and endocytosis can occur [30]. By contrast, the binding of antibodies or lectins to mature erythrocytes does not induce redistribution of transmembrane proteins or endocytosis, i.e. the intrinsic membrane proteins of mature erythrocytes are relatively immobile compared to those of most other types of cell [29]. Nevertheless, mature erythrocytes do have the ability to form endocytotic vacuoles after exposure to certain membrane-active drugs or after loading with Mg.ATP during hypotonic lysis. At least two steps are required in endocytosis [57]. The first process is temperature dependent and requires Mg.ATP. The second involves a fluidizing or loosening of the structure as is brought about in the preparation of white ghosts washed in EDTA or by the introduction of amphipathic cationic drugs like primaquine. That endocytosis in mature erythrocytes requires a loosening of the membrane structure bears on our hypothesis concerning invasion by malaria parasites: the release of transmembrane proteins for lateral movement at the site of invasion is associated with a localized retraction or dissociation of the membrane skeleton. Tests of this concept, by the introduction of chemical or immunochemical cross-links into the cytoskeleton, will now be described.

4.1. *Chemical modification with permeant reagents*

The trifunctional alkylating agent tris(2-chloroethyl) amine (TCEA) penetrates the membrane of intact cells and reacts preferentially with spectrin [58]. At concentrations of 1-2 mM TCEA, spectrin is extensively cross-linked though not the other membrane-associated proteins. Cell deformability is slightly reduced and metabolic and drug-induced shape change is inhibited. An 80% inhibition of invasion by *P. falciparum* also results [59]. A similar observation has been made with the permeable bifunctional reagent, dithiobispropionimidate [60]. Reactivity again is directed towards amino groups with the promotion of extensive cross-linking of membrane-associated proteins [61].

A more limited degree of cross-linking results from exposure of red cells to the membrane-permeant oxidising agent, diamide. At low concentrations, this agent oxidises thiol groups capable of forming disulphide bridges between different spectrin chains [62]. Gel electrophoresis (Fig. 3) shows in accordance with earlier

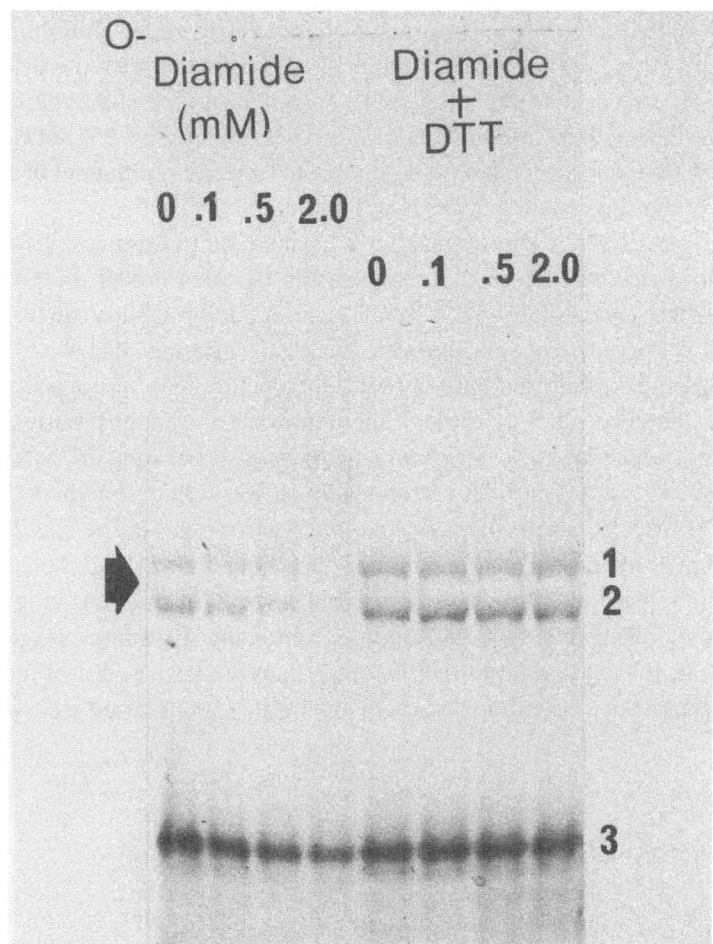

Figure 3. Exposure of intact red cells to diamide at concentrations ≤ 2 mM produces a limited degree of cross-linking of membrane-associated proteins that is essentially confined to spectrin. High molecular weight aggregates of spectrin (arrow) were separated on SDS–acrylamide agarose gel by electrophoresis according to Smith and Palek (1982).

work that intrinsic membrane proteins are not cross-linked up to concentrations of 2 mM diamide, though at higher concentrations there is a progressive accumulation of cross-linked spectrin and also of other membrane-associated proteins [63]. Cells treated with 0.5 to 2 mM diamide are much less susceptible to invasion by *P. falciparum in vitro*, an effect that can be reversed substantially by the reducing agent dithiothreitol [60]. At 5 mM diamide, irreversible effects were found.

4.1.2. *Chemical modification with impermeant reagents*

It must be supposed that any extensive chemical modifications of membrane

76

proteins would interfere with the process of malarial invasion. Thus inhibition of invasion by *P. falciparum* occurs if the cells are pretreated with the disulphonic stilbene, H₂DIDS, at a pH >8.6 [59]. As other surface components of the membrane besides band 3 are labelled under these conditions, it is not clear what modification renders the cells less susceptible to invasion. Treatment of cells with H₂DIDS at a more physiological pH did not inhibit invasion.

Erythrocytes have a low permeability to aliphatic polyamines. Erythrocyte ghosts, however, which have been resealed in the presence of the polyamine, spermine, become less deformable [64]. The loss of deformability can be detected at 10 μM spermine, the usual physiological concentration, but according to a mechanical index, deformability is reduced to below 50% of normal at 5 mM spermine. The two other physiologically important polyamines, putrescine and spermidine, which have shorter chain length and lower charge, are considerably less potent. This difference between polyamines was reflected in their effects on invasion of resealed ghosts by *P. falciparum in vitro* (Fig. 4). The loss of susceptibility to invasion in spermine-containing ghosts qualitatively paralleled the loss of membrane deformability over a range of 0.1 to 5 mM spermine (Fig. 5).

Loss of deformability of resealed ghosts containing spermine was inferred by Ballas et al. [64] to be due to factors other than the trivial ones of membrane damage caused by proteolysis, or cross-linking by Ca²⁺-induced transglutamin-

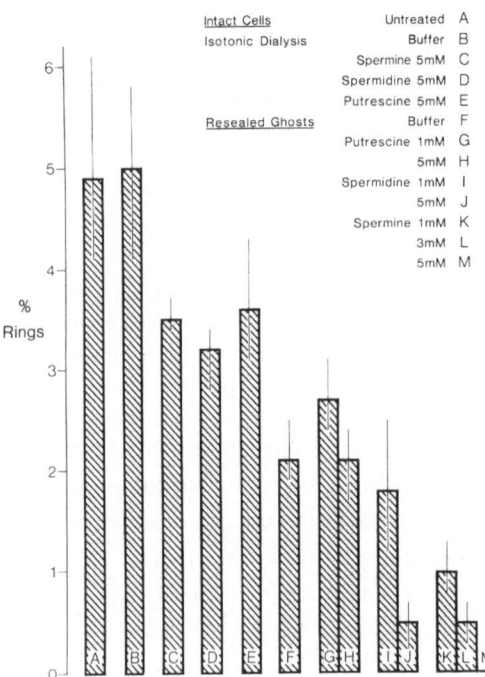

Figure 4. The susceptibility to invasion of intact cells or resealed red ghosts exposed to polyamines-putrescine, spermidine, and spermine. Each bar represents the mean of triplicate cultures.

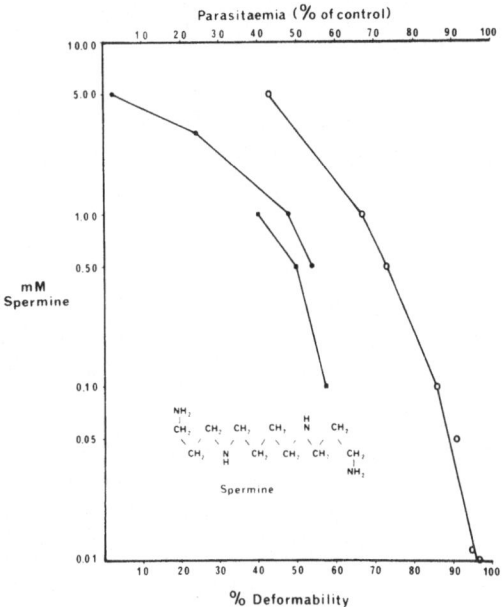

Figure 5. Titration of the inhibitory effect of spermine on the invasion of resealed red ghosts (●———●,two experiments) in comparison with the loss of membrane deformability (○———○, modified from Ballas et al. [64]).

ase. As the effect of polyamines is not mimicked by divalent cations such as Ca^{2+} or Mg^{2+}, it was suggested that an appropriately sized charged molecule, rather than a charge effect *per se,* was responsible for stabilisation of the resealed ghost membrane. Evidence that spermine increases the cohesion of the cytoskeletal network, in contrast to polyphosphates, is that at an intracellular concentration of <1 mM, spermine decreases the translational mobility of fluoresceinated membrane glycoproteins such as band 3 and glycophorin [54]. Microviscosity measurements revealed no change in the state of membrane lipids in spermine-treated ghosts so it may be inferred that polyamines affect the physical state of the cytoskeletal network.

4.2. *Temperature-induced protein aggregation*

The influence of temperature on red cell deformability also leads to the conclusion that membrane proteins rather than lipids determine red cell deformability characteristics under physiological conditions. Normal erythrocytes undergo fragmentation without haemolysis after brief incubation at 49°C. Diamide (1 mM) reduces the critical temperature of fragmentation to 47°C, an effect that is reversible with dithiothreitol, indicating that disulphide bonds may be involved [66]. The unfolding and cross-linking of spectrin bands 1 and 2 in normal erythro-

78

cytes corresponds to a narrow thermal transition (Tm) central at 50°C, whereas the Tm for bands 2.1, 4.1 and 4.2 is at 53°C [67]. The Tm for band 3 varies from 54°C to 67°C, depending on the ionic conditions and the interactions with other membrane proteins. The Tm of spectrin isolated from pyropoikilocytes is at 44°C, corresponding to a critical temperature of fragmentation of 45°C. Red cells heated to between 48°C and 50°C also exhibit a dramatic increase in their deformability under shear stress [68]. Upon cooling to 37°C, however, the elasticity and fluidity of the cells is decreased. As spectrin undergoes a transition at 49°C, losing nearly 30% of its helical content and becoming aggregated, there can be little doubt that its structural integrity plays a central role in red cell deformability.

The susceptibility of red cells to invasion by *P. falciparum in vitro* also shows a marked decrease following brief heating to between 48° and 50°C (Fig. 6). Heating between 37° and 48°C results in only a small loss of susceptibility. The interesting finding [69] that ovalocytic erythrocytes from Melanesians are both resistant to invasion by *P. falciparum* and have an elevated thermal deformation temperature (51°C) has yet to be explained; the Tm of spectrin in this heritable condition is normal [see Anders in ref.11]. Further experimental work is also indicated by the apparently normal susceptibility to invasion by *P. falciparum* of red cells from patients with hereditary spherocytosis [70]. The deformability of these cells is again reduced and in some cases the cytoskeletal defect involves an increased affinity between band 4.1 and the spectrin-actin complex [71].

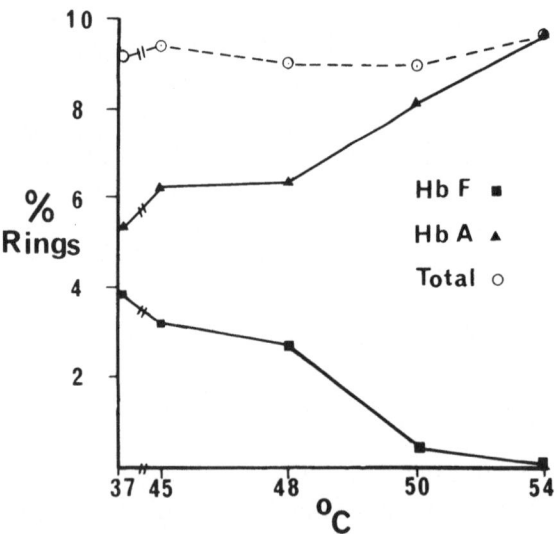

Figure 6. Loss of susceptibility to invasion of red cells heated to between 48° and 50°C. Cord blood cells recognisable by their content of fetal haemaglobin (HbF) were heated at various temperatures for five minutes and then mixed with an equal number of adult red cells (HbA) containing mature schizonts of *P. falciparum*. Following invasion the percentage of young ring-stage parasites in each cell type was compared.

4.2.1. *Immunochemical cross-links*

Evidence has been advanced that hypotonic lysis of erythrocytes produces a single hole in the membrane which can vary in radius from 0.7 to 14 nm, depending on the ionic strength, temperature and pH [72]. We have investigated resealed ghosts prepared by our procedure in the presence of a range of membrane-impermeant macromolecular solutes including albumin, immunoglobulin G (IgG) and Dextran 2000 [49]. The results are consistent with the observations of Lieber and Steck [73] in that Blue Dextran with a Stokes radius of some tens of nm is excluded from the unsealed ghosts, whereas albumin and IgG readily penetrate.

Both we [60] and Olson and Kilejian [51] have taken advantage of this system to introduce antibodies into the red cell cytoplasm; it seems likely that reactions with divalent antibodies may provide the least disruptive means of cross-linking the cytoskeletal complex and preventing it from undergoing topological rearrangement during invasion by *P. falciparum*. In both reports it was found that the inclusion of divalent rabbit anti-spectrin antibodies in resealed ghosts markedly reduced invasion whereas F(ab)[l] fragments did not. Partial restoration of the bifunctionality of F(ab)[l] fragments by the addition of goat anti-rabbit IgG, prior to resealing the ghosts, substantially restored the inhibitory effect [60]. This result indicates that it is the effect of bridging spectrin molecules *per se* that inhibits invasion.

Before drawing conclusions from these results, it is worth recalling that cross-linking of spectrin can alter the translational mobility of intrinsic membrane proteins [22] as well as reduce the deformability of the cell [74]. It has been suggested by Olson and Kilejian [51] that cross-linking of spectrin by antibodies incorporated into resealed ghosts might produce an unfavourable arrangement of the protein receptors on the erythrocyte surface and thus prevent interaction with the merozoite. This seems to us a rather unlikely explanation for inhibition of invasion because erythrocytes metabolically depleted under aerobic conditions also lose their susceptibility to invasion and have high molecular weight aggregates of spectrin and actin, but retain the usual random distribution of IMP [75]. It follows that loss of susceptibility to invasion can occur without gross alteration in the disposition of integral membrane proteins. Under the conditions of our experiments it appears that neither antibodies nor reagents like diamide introduce so many bridges into the cytoskeletal network as to present a continuously bonded barrier to the parasite. Rather, these bifunctional agents introduce a limited degree of cross-linking that prevents a rearrangement of the cytoskeleton required in the invasion process.

Conclusion

Reversible lysis of human red cells at high haematocrit gives rise to resealed ghosts which partially retain their susceptibility to invasion by *P. falciparum*. Addition of Mg.ATP during the lysis procedure, to maintain a concentration of about 1 mM, fully restores susceptibility and there is a direct correlation between the concentration of intracellular ATP at the time of resealing and the extent of subsequent invasion. The function of ATP in promoting invasion is probably not related to the maintenance of cation gradients but almost certainly involves the phosphorylation of membrane proteins. The evidence for this is that a non-hydrolysable analogue of ATP, adenylyl-imidodiphosphate (AMP.PNP) does not replace ATP. Furthermore, inhibition of phosphorylation by adenosine, introduced into cells or ghosts at high concentration, causes significant inhibition of invasion. These results suggest that ATP is required to maintain the turnover of phosphoryl groups of membrane-associated proteins such as spectrin. Dilution of the red cell cytosol during lysis by more than a critical factor of about ten, impairs susceptibility to invasion, even when a high concentration of ATP is maintained. The addition of 2,3-DPG and undiluted haemolysate has a favourable effect on invasion but does not restore the susceptibility of the ghost to invasion after dilution of the haemolysate. The additional essential constituent(s) in the cytoplasm has not yet been identified. The physical state of spectrin in the host cell is implicated in the finely regulated interactions between the components of the membrane skeleton, the intrinsic membrane proteins, and the lipid bilayer. The strong inhibition of invasion induced by limited reversible, cross-linking of spectrin, by chemical or immunochemical means, implies that rearrangement of the membrane cytoskeletal proteins plays an essential part in the invasion process.

Acknowledgements

This work was supported in part by the UNDP/World Bank/WHO Special Programme for Research and Training in Tropical Diseases.

References

1. Dvorak JA, Miller LH, Whitehouse WE, Shiroishi T: Invasion of erythrocytes by malaria merozoites. Science 187:748–750, 1975.
2. Miller LH, Aikawa M, Johnson JG, Shiroishi T: Interaction between cytochalasin B-treated malarial parasites and erythrocytes. Attachment and junction formation. J Exp Med 149:172–184, 1979.
3. Bannister LH: The invasion of red cells by *Plasmodium*. In: Parasite invasion. Taylor AER, Muller R (eds): Oxford, Blackwell Scientific Publications 1977, p 25–55.
4. Aikawa M, Miller LH, Johnson J, Rabbege J: Erythrocyte entry by malaria parasites. A moving junction between erythrocyte and parasite. J Cell Biol 77:72–82, 1978.
5. McLaren DJ, Bannister LH, Trigg PI, Butcher GA: Freeze-fracture studies on the interaction between the malaria parasite and the host erythrocyte in *Plasmodium knowlesi* infections. Parasitology 79:125–139, 1979.

6. Aikawa M, Miller LH, Rabbege JR, Epstein N: Freeze-fracture study on the erythrocyte membrane during malarial parasite invasion. J Cell Biol 91:55–62, 1981.

7. Miller LH, Haynes JD, McAuliffe FM, Shiroishi T, Durocher JR, McGinniss MH: Evidence for differences in erythrocyte surface receptors for the malarial parasites *Plasmodium falciparum* and *Plasmodium knowlesi*. J. Exp Med 146:277–282, 1977.

8. Pasvol G, Wainscoat JS, Weatherall DJ: Erythrocytes deficient in glycophorin A resist infection by the malarial parasite, *Plasmodium falciparum*. Nature (London) 297:64–66, 1982.

9. Facer CA: Erythrocyte sialoglycoproteins and *Plasmodium falciparum* invasion. Trans R Soc Trop Med Hyg 77:524–530, 1983.

10. Pasvol G, Jungery M, Weatherall DJ, Parsons SF, Anstee DJ: Glycophorin as a possible receptor for *Plasmodium falciparum*. The Lancet 2:947–950, 1982.

11. Pasvol G, Jungery M: Glycophorins and red cell invasion by *Plasmodium falciparum*. In: *Malaria and the red cell*. Evered D, Whelam J (eds). London. Ciba Foundation Symposium 94. p.174–195. 1983.

12. Perkins M: Inhibitory effects of erythrocyte membrane proteins on the *in vitro* invasion of the human malarial parasite (*Plasmodium falciparum*) into its host cell. J Cell Biol 90:563–567, 1981.

13. Jungery M, Pasvol G, Newbold CI, Weatherall DJ: A lectin-like receptor is involved in invasion of erythrocytes by *Plasmodium falciparum*. Proc Nat Acad Sci USA 80:1018–1022, 1983.

14. Banyal HS, Misra GC, Gupta CM, Dutta GP: Involvement of malaria proteases in the interaction between the parasite and host erythrocyte in *Plasmodium knowlesi* infections. J Parasitol 67:623–626, 1981.

15. Boyle DB, March JC, Newbold CI, Brown KN: Parasite polypeptides lost during schizogony and erythrocyte invasion by the malaria parasites *Plasmodium chabaudi* and *Plasmodium knowlesi*. Mol Biochem Parasitol 7:9–18, 1983.

16. Gratzer WB: The red cell membrane and its cytoskeleton. Biochem J 198:1–8, 1981.

17. Haest CWM: Interactions between membrane skeleton proteins and the intrinsic domain of the erythrocyte membrane. Biochim Biophys Acta 694:331–352, 1982.

18. Marchesi VT: The red cell membrane skeleton: recent progress. Blood 61:1–11, 1983.

19. Ungewickell E, Bennett PM, Calvert R, Ohanian V, Gratzer WB: *In vitro* formation of a complex between cytoskeletal proteins of the human erythrocyte. Nature 280:811–814, 1979

20. Cohen CM, Korsgren G: Band 4.1 vauses spectrin-actin gels to become thixiotropic. Biochem Biophys Res Commun 97:1429–1435, 1980.

21. Nigg EA, Bron C, Giradet M, Cherry RJ: Band 3-glycophorin A association in erythrocyte membranes, demonstrated by combining protein diffusion measurements with antibody-mediated cross-linking. Biochemistry 19:1887–1893, 1980.

22. Nicolson GL, Painter RG: Anionic sites of human erythrocyte membranes II. Antispectrin-induced transmembrane aggregation of the binding sites for positively charged colloidal particles. J Cell Biol 59:398–405, 1973.

23. Ji TH, Nicolson GL: Lectin binding and perturbation of the outer surface of the cell membrane induces a transmembrane organizational alteration at the inner surface. Proc Nat Acad Sci USA 71:2212–2216, 1974.

24. Haest CWM, Plasa G, Kamp D, Deuticke B: Spectrin as a stabilizer of the phospholipid asymmetry in the human erythrocyte membrane. Biochim Biophys Acta 509:21–32, 1978.

25. Mohandas N, Greenquist AC, Shohet SB: Bilayer balance and regulation of red cell shape changes. J Supramolec Struct 9:453–458, 1978.

26. Haest CWM, Plasa G, Deuticke B: Selective removal of lipids from the inner membrane layer of human erythrocytes without hemolysis. Consequences for bilayer stability and cell shape. Biochim Biophys Acta 649:701–708, 1981.

27. Schrier SL, Hardy B, Bensch KG: Endocytosis in erythrocytes and their ghosts. In: Normal and abnormal red cell membranes. Lux SE, Marchesi VT, Fox CF (eds): New York. A R Liss Inc 1978. p 437–449.

28. Hardy B, Bensch KG, Schrier SL: Spectrin rearrangement early in erythrocyte ghost endocytosis. J Cell Biol 82:654–663, 1979.

29. Schekman R, Singer SJ: Clustering and endocytosis of membrane receptors can be induced in mature erythrocytes of neonatal but not adult humans. Proc Nat Acad Sci USA 73:4075–4079, 1976.

30. Tokuyasu KT, Schekman R, Singer SJ: Domains of receptor mobility and endocytosis in the membranes of neonatal human erythrocytes and reticulocytes are deficient in spectrin. J Cell Biol 80:481–486, 1979.

31. Hardy B, Schrier SL: The role of spectrin in erythrocyte ghost endocytosis. Biochem Biophys Res Commun 81:1152–1161, 1978.

32. Anderson RA, Lovrien R: Erythrocyte membrane sidedness in lectin control of the Ca^{2+}-A23187-mediated diskocyte-echinocyte conversion. Nature (London) 292:158–161, 1981.

33. Harris HW jr, Lux SE: Comparison of the phosphorylation of human erythrocyte spectrin in the intact red cell and in various cell-free systems. J Biol Chem 255:11512–11520, 1980.

34. Liu Sh-Ch, Palek J: Spectrin tetramer-dimer equilibrium and the stability of erythrocyte membrane skeletons. Nature (London) 285:586–588 (1980).

35. Anderson JM, Tyler JM: State of spectrin phosphorylation does not affect erythrocyte shape or spectrin binding to erythrocyte membranes. J Biol Chem 255:1259–1265, 1980.

36. Patel VP, Fairbanks G: Spectrin phosphorylation and shape change of human erythrocyte ghosts. J Cell Biol. 88:430–440, 1981.

37. Conway R, Tao M: Effects of 2,3-diphosphoglyceric acid on the human erythrocyte membrane phosphorylation system. J Biol Chem. 256:11932–11938, 1981.

38. Sheetz MP, Casaly J: 2,3-diphosphoglycerate and ATP dissociate erythrocyte membrane skeletons. J Biol Chem 255:9955–9960, 1980.

39. Dodge JT, Mitchell C, Hanahan DJ: The preparation and chemical characterization of haemoglobin-free ghosts of human erythrocytes. Arch Biochem Biophys 100:119–130, 1963.

40. Mawby WJ, Findlay JBC: Some transport properties of resealed washed human erythrocyte membranes. Biochem J 172:605–611, 1978.

41. Miller LH Hypothesis on the mechanism of erythrocyte invasion by malaria merozoites. Bull WHO 55:157–162, 1977.

42. Dluzewski AR, Rangachari K, Wilson RJM, Gratzer WB: Entry of malaria parasites into resealed ghosts of human and simian erythrocytes. Brit J Haematol 49:97–101, 1981.

43. Olson JA: In vitro studies of malarial parasites using resealed ghosts of human erythrocytes. In: The Red Cell: Fifth Ann Arbor Conference. New York. AR Liss Inc. 1981. p.537–555.

44. Sprandel U, Hubbard AR, Chalmers RA: Membrane transport in resealed haemoglobin-containing human erythrocyte ghosts prepared by dialysis procedure. Biochem Biophys Res Commun 91:79–85, 1979.

45. Triplett RB, Carraway KL: Proteolytic digestion of erythrocytes, resealed ghosts and isolated membranes. Biochemistry 11:2897–2903, 1972.

46. Boxer DH, Jenkins RE, Tanner MJA: The organization of the major protein of the human erythrocyte membrane. Biochem J 137:531–534, 1974.

47. Staros JV, Haley BE, Richards FM: Human erythrocytes and resealed ghosts. A comparison of membrane topology. J Biol Chem 249:5004–5007, 1974.

48. Dluzewski AR, Rangachari K, Wilson RJM, Gratzer WB: A cytoplasmic requirement of red cells for invasion by malarial parasites. Mol Biochem Parasitol 9:145–160, 1983.

49. Dluzewski AR, Rangachari K, Wilson RMJ, Gratzer WB: Properties of red cell ghost preparations susceptible to invasion by malaria parasites. Parasitology 87:429–438, 1983.

50. Dluzewski AR, Rangachari K, Wilson RJM, Gratzer WB: The effect of ATP on the entry of malaria parasites into resealed ghosts of human erythrocytes. J Protozool 29:636, 1982.

51. Olson JA, Kilejian A: Involvement of spectrin and ATP in infection of resealed erythrocyte ghosts by the human malarial parasite, *Plasmodium falciparum*. J Cell Biol 95:757–762, 1982.

52. Brewer GJ, Powell RD: A study of the relationship between the content of adenosine triphosph-

ate in human red cells and the course of *falciparum* malaria: A new system that may confer protection against malaria. Proc Nat Acad Sci USA 54:741–745, 1965.

53. LaCelle PL, Weed RI: The contribution of normal and pathologic erythrocytes to blood rheology. Progr Hematol 7:1–31, 1971.

54. Schindler M, Koppel DE, Sheetz MP: Modulation of membrane protein lateral mobility by polyphosphates and polyamines. Proc Nat Acad Sci USA 77:1457–1461, 1980.

55. Downes CP, Michell EH: The control by Ca²⁻ of the polyphosphoinositide phosphodiesters in the Ca²⁺ pump ATPase in human erythrocytes. Biochem J 202:53–58, 1982.

56. Fairbanks G, Patel VP, Dino JE: Biochemistry of ATP-dependent red cell membrane shape changes. Scand J Clin Lab Invest 41:Suppl 156 139–144, 1981.

57. Penniston JT, Vaughan L, Nakamura M: Endocytosis in erythrocytes and ghosts: occurrence at 0°C after ATP preincubation. Arch Biochem Biophys 198:339–348, 1979.

58. Wildenauer DB, Reuther H, Remien J: Reactions of the alkylating agent (2-chloroethyl)-amine with the erythrocyte membrane. Biochim Biophys Acta 603:101–116, 1980.

59. Breuer WV, Ginsburg H, Cabantchik ZI: An assay of malaria parasite invasion into human erythrocytes. The effects of chemical and enzymatic modification of erythrocyte membrane components. Biochim Biophys Acta 755:263–271, 1983.

60. Dluzewski AR, Rangachari K, Gratzer WB, Wilson RJM: Inhibition of malarial invasion of red cells by chemical and immunochemical linking of spectrin molecules. Brit J Haematol 55:629–637, 1983.

61. Wang K, Richards FM: An approach to nearest neighbour analysis of membrane proteins. Application to the human erythrocyte membrane of a method employing cleavable cross-linkages. J Biol Chem 249:8005–8018, 1974.

62. Haest CWM, Plasa G, Kamp D, Deuticke B: Spectrin as a stabilizer of the phospholipid asymmetry in the human erythrocyte membrane. Biochim Biophys Acta 509:21–32, 1978.

63. Smith DK, Palek J: Modulation of lateral mobility of band 3 in the red cell membrane by oxidative cross-linking of spectrin. Nature (London) 297:424–425, 1982.

64. Ballas SK, Mohandas N, Marton LJ, Shohet SB: Stabilization of erythrocyte membranes by polyamines. Proc Nat Acad Sci USA 80:1942–1946, 1983.

65. Sauberman N, Snyder ML: Contribution of whole cell and cytoplasmic polypeptides to apparent red cell membrane alterations. Biochim Biophys Acta 602:323–330, 1980.

66. Zarkowsky HS: Membrane-active agents and heat-induced erythrocyte fragmentation. Brit J Haematol 50:361–365, 1982.

67. Lysko KA, Carlson R, Taverna R, Snow J, Brandts JF: Protein involvement in structural transitions of erythrocyte ghosts. Use of thermal gel analysis to detect protein aggregation. Biochemistry 20:5570–5576, 1981.

68. Williamson JR, Shanahan MO, Hochmuth RM: The influence of temperature on red cell deformability. Blood 46:611–624, 1975.

69. Kidson C, Lamont G, Saul A, Nurse GT: Ovalocytic erythrocytes from Melanesians are resistant to invasion by malaria parasites in culture. Proc Nat Acad Sci USA 78:5829–5832, 1981.

70. Koeweiden E, Ponnudurai T, Meuwissen JHETh: *In vitro* observations on hereditary spherocytosis and malaria. Trans R Soc Trop Med Hyg 73:589–590, 1979.

71. Sawyer WH, Hill JS, Howlett GJ, Wiley JS: Hereditary spherocytosis of man. Defective cytoskeletal interactions in the erythrocyte membrane. Biochem. J. 211:349–356, 1983.

72. Lieber MR, Steck TL: Dynamics of the holes in human erythrocyte membrane ghosts. J Biol Chem 257:11660–11666, 1982.

73. Lieber MR, Steck TL: A description of the holes in human erythrocyte membrane ghosts. J Biol Chem 257:11651–11659, 1982.

74. Nakashima K, Beutler E: Effect of anti-spectrin antibody and ATP on deformability of resealed erythrocyte membranes. Proc Nat Acad Sci USA 75:3823–3825.

75. Lux SE, John KM, Ukena TE: Diminished spectrin extraction from ATP-depleted human erythrocytes. J Clin Invest 61:815–827, 1978.

5. Pathogenesis of babesiosis

I. KAKOMA and M. RISTIC

College of Veterinary Medicine, University of Illinois, Urbana, Illinois 61801, USA.

1. Influence of host-parasite relationship on the pathogenesis of babesiosis

1.1. *Host range and specificity of the babesias*

Recent clinical and epidemiological observations demonstrate an unstable host-parasite interplay in babesiosis. This is particularly illustrated by increased incidences of infectivity of various *Babesia* spp. for human beings [1, 2, 3, 4, 5, 6]. Many of these organisms which are now of public health importance were originally considered to be host specific as implied by the nomenclature (e.g., *B. canis, B. bovis, B. equi*). Since the original identification of *Babesia* spp. as pathogens, virtually all domestic, wild animals and man have been shown to be susceptible to one or more species of *Babesia* [7, 8, 9, 10, 11]. Table 1 illustrates the host range of Babesias but it must be appreciated that the flexible host-parasite relationship will dictate frequent revision of this table.

1.2. *Factors predisposing to immunologic imbalance in babesiosis with special reference to human babesiosis*

It has been postulated that for every clinical case of animal babesiosis, there are hundreds of latent cases [11, 12, 13, 14]. Epidemiologic studies in human populations in Nantucket Island [4, 12, 15, 16], in Mexico [3], and in Nigeria [17] are lending credence to this theory. Surprisingly, there are no confirmed clinical cases of human babesiosis in the tropics; all have been in the temperate zones. It is possible that cross-immunity between Babesia species and other protozoa diseases endemic in many tropical regions prevents clinical infection. Thus, individuals resident in regions where malaria is endemic might be partially or completely immune to *Babesia* infections. This hypothesis should be rigourously tested by cross-immunization studies in laboratory animals and increased seroepidemiologic surveillance on babesiosis in Africa, Asia and South America, similar to

Ristic, M. et al. (eds.) *Malaria and babesiosis.*
© 1984, Martinus Nijhoff Publishers, Dordrecht/Boston/Lancaster.

Table 1. Examples of the wide host range for babesia species.

Major host	Babesia spp.	Infectivity for man
Bovidae	B. argentina	?
	B. berbera	?
	B. bigemina	?
	B. bovis	yes [4]
	B. divergens	yes [5]
	B. major	?
Cat	B. felis	?
Dog	B. canis	?
	B. gibsoni	?
	B. vogeli	?
Goat	B. motasi	?
	B. ovis	?
	B. taylori	?
Horse	B. cabali	?
	B. equi	yes [6]
Pig	B. perronciti	?
	B. trantimanni	?
Sheep	B. foliata	?
	B. motasi	?
	B. ovis	?
Rodents	B. microti	yes [7, 8, 9, 10]

those accomplished in Mexico [3] and Nigeria [17].

Clearly the immune status of the host plays a major role in susceptibility to babesiosis since splenectomy, irradiation, or treatment with antilymphocytic serum enhances susceptibility to various Babesias [18, 19, 20, 21].

The human *B. microti* cases illustrate the role of the immune status in that most of the patients manifesting clinical signs were over 50 years of age [4, 12]. Further, some of the patients were presumably immunosuppressed by corticosteriod therapy received prior to the development of *Babesia* infection but interestingly, not all the *B. microti* victims in the Nantucket study were splenectomized [4]. However, all previous cases from Europe which were due to bovine or equine *Babesia* occurred in splenectomized individuals [5, 6, 11]. Thus, immunologic compromise associated with splenectomy, hormonal, genetic or metabolic influences are important determinants in the susceptibility to, and pathogenesis of, *Babesia* infections.

2. Pathogenetic pathways in babesiosis

2.1. *General characteristics*

The classical work of Wright and his associates highlighted the involvement of the coagulatory system, complement cascade, reticuloendothelial system and other physiological systems [22, 23, 24] in the pathogenesis of babesiosis. Pathogenesis of babesiosis commences at the initial contact between the tick-born parasite and the mammalian erythrocyte. Indentation of the erythrocyte precedes penetration of the host cell by the parasite. As soon as it penetrates, the parasite begins to enlarge and multiply. The offspring are eventually released into the plasma to invade other susceptible erythrocytes. In some babesia infections, soluble plasma antigens are demonstrable in the circulation [25, 26, 27, 28]. These antigens are immunogenic [29, 30], and similar antigens have been demonstrated in *in vitro* cultures thereby providing prospects for vaccination [31].

The pathogenesis of babesiosis can be discussed from the standpoint of primary effects on the erythrocytes, and plasma and the secondary effects which follow dissemination into the reticuloendothelial system and other vital organs of the mammalian host of intact Babesia or products. The differences between the two proposed pathways are summarized in table 2. This discussion will be restricted to pathogenesis of babesiosis since the immunology and pathology of babesiosis are detailed elsewhere (see chapters 3 and 7).

2.2. *Proposed categories of the pathogenesis of babesiosis*

2.2.1. *The primary pathway – (antibody independent)*
This pathway does not involve any demonstrable participation of antibody and specific antigen. Classical examples include *B. bovis* infection in which the pathogenesis is characterized by massive release of pharmacologically active mediators [22, 23]. Simultaneously, soon after infection is initiated, parasites accumulate locally in the micro-circulation of the dermis [32, 33]. Infection then triggers release of kinins and other vasoactive substances that produce vasodilation, circulatory collapse, coma and death [23, 24]. This syndrome is the basis for canine and bovine 'cerebral' babesiosis caused by *B. canis* and *B. bovis,* respectively [34, 35, 36, 37] and also the babesiosis caused by *B. caballi* infection of horses [38].

A common feature of the infection caused by *Babesia* species in which the primary-type pathway predominates is the occurance of severe clinical effects at relatively low parasitemias. This is in contrast to infection by *B. bigemina, B. equi, B. gibsoni* in which high parasitemias occur before severe clinical manifestations [22]. The critical difference between the two major groups of organisms is the relative predeliction of the parasitized erythrocytes of the primary type infection to adhere to microcirculatory endothelium and thus to accumulate in blood capillaries. This characteristic is largely under splenic control in the case of *B. bovis* as described elsewhere in this publication and is an important factor in the attenuation of *B. bovis* strains for vaccine development (see chapter 7).

The vascular alterations in *B. bovis* precede development of high parasitemia and severe hemolysis [33] indicating that parasite load and destruction of erythrocytes are not a key factor in pathogenesis. In contrast the pathogenesis of *B. bigemina* coincides with severe parasitemia. Indeed, proteases extracted from *B. bovis* parasites can induce the shock syndrome indistinguishable from infection with the parasite. The effects appear to be mediated through esteraseactivated plasma kallikrein and generation of fibrinogenlike products and complexes from plasma. This hypothesis has been tested both *in vitro* and *in vivo* and the explanation seems scientifically correct [33]. It also appears that the protease content of *Babesia* strains might be linked to their relative virulence. These same proteases have been shown to cleave kinins from kininogen and to activate kallikrein and Hageman factor [23, 33].

Although the actual role of vasoactive amines in the pathogenesis of babesiosis is not known, it has been demonstrated that histamine and 5-hydroxy-tryptamine levels are high in the blood of *Babesia*-infected cattle and might reach even higher levels in the target areas of the microcirculation where their effects are exerted [39].

The disease produced by the primary pathway is further compounded by disturbances in the coaggulation cascade in *B. caballi* and *B. bovis* infections [23]. Both free fibrin, fibrinogen-fibrin complexes, and cryoprecipitates are demonstrable in the plasma of animals with the infection. A disseminated intravascular coagulation-like syndrome (DIC) characterized by massive fibrin deposition has also been described in *B. bovis* infected cattle [40]. According to Dalgliesh et al. [40], this DIC syndrome leads to reticuloendothelial blockade. The condition is potentiated by immunosuppression, including splenectomy.

The last component of the primary pathway is erythrocyte destruction. This partially explains the anemia frequently seen in most cases of babesiosis. A major effect is parasite load leading to erythrocyte rupture as the parasites exit [24]. In infections by some species of *Babesia* (e.g., *B. bigemina*), the parasitemias may be as high as 25–40%, and be associated with massive changes in the osmotic fragility of the entire erythrocyte population including uninfected erythrocytes – a phenomenon implying that there is a soluble mediator released by the parasite which attaches to and destabilizes normal erythrocytes. No data is yet available to explain this phenomenon. In infections caused by other *Babesias* (e.g., *B. bovis*), osmotic fragility occurs at very low parasitemias. Surprisingly, in these infections unparasitized erythrocytes are also more fragile than infected ones. This occurs when parasitemias may be as low as 1% or less. Up to 33% of the erythrocyte population may be destroyed within 48 hours and efforts to demonstrate lytic enzymes have proved negative [33]. Fragility of red blood cells is not typical of all babesia infections and varies according to species. During *B. canis* infection, for example, there may not be any significant alteration in osmotic fragility whereas in bovine babesiosis increased fragility is a common feature [24, 33].

2.2.2. *The secondary pathway in the pathogenesis of babesiosis*

Babesia infection induces specific and nonspecific effects which contribute to the pathogenesis of the disease, particularly in the acute phase of infection. These changes are thus classically associated with *Babesia* species that induce high parasitemia, such as *B. bigemina, B. canis* and *B. rhodhaini* [39]. One of the earliest events in babesiosis is macrophage activation. This activation leads to production and release of mediators such as tissue thromboplastin, kininforming enzymes, pyrogens, prostaglandins, macrophage migration inhibition factor [39]. Complement activation and possibly endotoxin release [33] associated with leucopenia and thrombocytopenia also may occur. The evidence for babesial associated endotoxin is largely circumstantial and indirect and is based on the observation that *B. rhodhaini* infected mice have increased susceptibility to endotoxin-induced shock due to *E. coli* lipopolysaccharide [39]. A similar effect has been observed in bovine babesiosis caused by both *B. bovis* and *B. bigemina*. The authors of this paper demonstrated that administration of low doses of LPS to parasitemic calves potentiated the clinical and hematologic changes due to *B. bovis* and *B. bigemina* infection.

During infection of rats with *B. rhodhaini* [41] there is a decrease in complement components. In rats it was demonstrated that the hypocomplementaemia coincided with formation of immune complexes containing *B. rhodhaini* specific antigen. Antibody was demonstrable in the plasma and also in eluates from glomeruli of acutely infected rats. The authors also later reported that C3 depletion prolonged the prepatent period of *B. rhodhaini* infection and thus they inferred that C3b was essential for the penetration phase of the parasite as it invaded the erythrocyte [42, 43]. Subsequent observations, however, have since shown that C3 was not required for the invasion of the erythrocyte by *B. rhodhaini* [44] or *B. bovis* [45].

The role of C3 in the initial encounter and interaction between the host erythocyte and *Babesia* organisms remains controversial. Nevertheless, complement plays an important nonspecific role in the pathogenesis of babesiosis during the acute phase of the disease. Thus, hypocomplementaemia in bovine babesiosis aggravated the clinical picture since it occurs at a critical time for the host [46]. The authors suggested that C3a and C5a are important anaphylatoxins in *B. bovis* infections. Levels of serum carboxypeptidase B, bradykinin and kallidin decreased during acute *B. bovis* infection [33, 39]. Such changes were always associated with infection by virulent *B. bovis* organisms only, thus emphasizing the pathogenic role of complement-mediated process.

The activation of complement is closely linked with the free serum babesial antigens which have been demonstrated in plasma of horses, dogs and rats [13, 14,

25, 26], in the acute phase of *Babesia* infection. The presence of complexes of the serum antigen and specific antibody during the severe phase of the infection provides further evidence of the possible pathogenetic role of immune complexes in babesiosis [41].

A major component of the pathogenesis of babesiosis is anemia. The demonstration of erythrophagocytosis and the presence of cold-active agglutinins for autologous and homologous red-blood cells in animals with acute *B. rhodhaini* infection [47] suggests auto-immunity. It has been suggested that the auto-antibodies are partly responsible for the anemia and glomerulonephritis in animals with *B. rhodhaini* infections. The role of auto-immunity in babesiosis needs further investigation.

3. Conclusion

The pathogenesis of *Babesia* infections can be categorized into two major pathways: (1) A primary pathway occurring early in infection when parasitemia is low, and in which the effects are through largely non-specific mechanisms mediated through vasoactive substances that interact with the coaggulatory and complement cascades leading to circulatory collapse and blockade of the reticuloendothelial system. This pathway can occur in the presence of very low parasitemias and is therefore largely independent of parasite load. A major factor in the primary pathway is the enigmatic increase in osmotic fragility of the erythrocyte population; (2) the secondary pathway which depends on parasite load and the

Table 2. Comparison of the primary and secondar pathways of the pathogenesis of babesiosis

	Primary	Secondary
1. Dependence on parasite load	−	+
2. Requirement of specific antigen	±	+
3. Requirement for specific antibody	−	+
4. Involvement of specific immune complexes	−	+
5. Coaggulatory disturbance	+	+
6. Involvement of complement & 1K	+ via Hageman factor	+
7. Involvement of autoimmunity	−	+ (circumstantial evidence on rodent model)
8. Involvement of an endotoxin	+?	+
9. Major effects	V as o diatation circulatory collapse/Anoxic and endotoxic shock	Intravascular hemolysis-Anemia glomerulon lymphocytopenia Thrombocytopenia circulatory collapse & shock.

associated presence of soluble plasma antigen, specific antibody, immune complexes, and fibrin-fibrinogen complexes. This pathway triggers cell-mediated immunity and activation of the macrophage system and induces indiscriminate phagocytosis of normal and infected erythrocytes. Immune complexes, complement and auto-immunity are incriminated in this pathway on the basis of largely circumstantial evidence.

This discussion has highlighted the need for systematic studies of pathogenesis of babesiosis. Such studies are required if we are to understand the disturbance of the host which occurs during babesial infection. Such understanding is necessary, not only in the control of animal babesiosis, but also for control of the escalating numbers of human babesiosis cases. It is suggested that immunologic, hormonal, metabolic and genetic factors are important modulating factors in the clinical manifestation of human and animal babesiosis.

The paucity of documented cases of human babesiosis in the tropics where animal babesiosis is hyperendemic suggests that infections have either been missed or that other protozoal infections interfere in the clinical expression of babesiosis. This warrants more attention for epidemiologic research in the tropics. If, in fact, people exposed to other protozoal diseases (especially malaria) are resistant to babesiosis, this information would be particularly useful in interpreting clinical data on candidate protozoal vaccines.

References

1. Skrabo Z and Deanovic Z: Piroplasmosis in man. Report on a case. Doc Med Geog Trop 9:11–16, 1957.
2. Lykins JC, Ristic M, Weisiger M and Huxsoll DL: *Babesia microti*: Pathogenesis of parasite of human origin in the hamster. Exp Parasit 37:388–397, 1975.
3. Osorno BM, Vega C, Rish CM, Robels C and Ibarra S: Isolation of *Babesia* spp. from asymptomatic human beings. Vet Parasit 2:111–120, 1976.
4. Ruebash TK: Human Babesiosis in North America. Trans R Soc Trop Med & Hyg 74:149–152, 1980.
5. Entrican JH, Williams H, Cook IA, Lancaster WM, Clark JD: Joiner LP and Lewis D: Babesiosis in man: report of a case from Scotland with observations on the infective strain. J Infect 1:227–234, 1979.
6. Lewis D and Young ER: The transmission of a human strain of *Babesia divergens* by *Ixodes ricinus* ticks. J Parasit 66:359–360, 1980.
7. Purnell RE: Babesiosis in various hosts. In: *Babesiosis*. M Ristic and JP Kreier (eds). Academic Press, Inc., New York, NY p. 25–63, 1981.
8. Babes V: Sur l'hemoglobinuria bacterine de boeufs. CR Acad Sci (Paris) 107:692–700, 1888.
9. Mahoney DF: Babesiosis of domestic animals. In: *Parasitic Protozoa*. JP Kreiner (ed). Academic Press, Inc., New York, NY 1977. p. 1–52, 1977.
10. Smith T and Kilbourne FL: Investigation into the nature, causation and prevention of Texas and Southern Cattle Fever. In: Eighth and ninth Ann. Reports of Animal Industry for 1891 and 1892. Dept. of Agriculture, Washington, DC p. 177–304.
11. Ristic M and Lewis GE: *Babesia* in man wild laboratory-adapted mammals. In: Parasitic Protozoa Vol IV. JP Kreiner (ed). Academic Press, Inc., New York, NY. 1977, p. 53–76.

92

12. Ristic M and Healey GR: Babesiosis. In: Parasitic Zoonosis – I. JH Steel and P Arambulo (eds). CRC Press, Cleveland, Ohio. 1980, p. 151–165.

13. Ristic M: Babesiosis. In: Bovine Medicine and Surgery. W.J. Gibbons, E.J. Calcott and J.F. Smithers (eds). American Veterinary Publications, Wheaton, Illinois. 1970, p. 355–369.

14. Ristic M: Babesiosis. In: Equine Medicine and Surgery. E.J. Calcott and J.F. Smitheors (eds). American Veterinary Publications, Wheaton, IL. 1972, p. 137–144.

15. Healey GR, Spielman A and Gleason NN: Human Babesiosis reservoir of infection on Nantucket Island. Science 192:479–480, 1976.

16. Spielman A, Clifford CM, Piesman J, Corwin MD: Human Babesiosis on Nantucket Island, USA: description of the vector, *Ixodes (Ixodes) damni n. sp. (Acarina ixodidae)*. J Med Ent 15:218–234, 1979.

17. Leeflang P, Oomen JM, Zwart D and Meuwissen JH: The prevalence of *Babesia* antibodies in Nigerians. Int J Parasit 6:159–161, 1976.

18. Jansen BC: The parasiticidal effect of aureomycin (Lederle) on *Babesia equi* (Laveran, 1899) in splenectomized donkeys. Onderst J Vet Res 26:175–182, 1953.

19. Lohr KF: Susceptibility of non-splenectomized and splenectomized sahiwal cattle to experimental *Babesia bigemina* infection. Zentrabl Vet Med 20:52–56, 1973.

20. Irvin AD, Omwooyo P and Ledger MA: Comparison of the effects of irriation and splenectomy on *Babesia rhodhaini* infection in mice. Int J Parasitol 3:773–781, 1973.

21. Wolf RE: Effects of anti-lymphocyte serum and splenectomy on resistance to *Babesia microti* infection in hamsters. Clin Immunol and Immunopath 2:381–394, 1974.

22. Wright IG and Goodger BV: Acute *Babesiosis bigemina* infection: changes in coaggulation and kallidrein parameters. Z Parasitenkol 53:63–73, 1977.

23. Wright IG: The kallikrein-kinin system and its role in the hypotensive shock syndrome of animals infected with haemoprotozoan parasites: *Babesia, Plasmodium* and *Trypanosoma*. Gen Pharmacol 10:319–325, 1979.

24. Wright IG: Osmotic fragility of erythrocytes in acute *Babesia argentina* and *Babesia bigemina* infections in splenectomized *Bos taurus* calves. Res Vet Sci 15:299–305, 1973.

25. Sibinovic KH, Ristic M, Sibinovic S and Phillips TN: Equine babesiosis: isolation and characterization of a blood serum antigen from acutely infected horses. Am J Vet Res 26:153–247, 1965.

26. Sibinovic S, Sibinovic KH, Ristic M and Cox HW: Physical and serological properties of antigen prepared from erythrocytes of horses with acute babesiosis. J Prozool 13:551–553, 1966.

27. Mahoney DF: Circulating antigens in cattle infected with *Babesia bigemina* or *B. argentina*. Nature (London) 211:422, 1966.

28. Mahoney DF and Goodger BV: The isolation of *Babesia* parasites and their products from blood. In: *Babesiosis*. M Ristic and JP Kreier (eds). Academic Press, Inc., New York, NY. 1981, p. 323–335.

29. Sibinovic KH, Sibinovic S, Ristic M and Cox HW: Immunogenic properties of *Babesia* serum antigens. J Parasitol 53:1121–1129, 1967.

30. Mahoney DF and Goodger BV: *Babesia argentina*: Immunogenicity of plasma from infected animals. Exp Parasit 32:71–85, 1972.

31. Ristic M, Smith RD and Kakoma I: Characterization of *Babesia* antigens derived from cell cultures and ticks. In: *Babesiosis*. M Ristic and JP Kreier (eds). Academic Press, Inc., New York, NY. 1981, p. 337–380.

32. Hoyte HMD: Differential diagnosis of *Babesia argentina* and *B. bigemina* infections in cattle using thin blood smears and brain smears. Aust Vet J 47:248–251, 1971.

33. Wright IG: Biochemical characteristics of *Babesia* and physiochemical reactions in the host. In: *Babesiosis*. M Ristic and JP Kreier (eds). Academic Press, Inc., New York, NY. 1981, p. 171–205.

34. Malherbe WD: Clinico-pathological studies of *Babesia canis* infection in dogs. I. The influence of the infection on bromosulphalein retention in the flood. JS Afr Vet Med Assoc 36:25–30, 1965.

35. Maegraith BG, Giles HM and Devakul K: Pathological Processes in *Babesia canis* infections. Z Parasitenmed Parasitol 8:485–514, 1957.

36. Callow LL and Johnston LAY: *Babesia* species in brains of clinically normal cattle and their detection by a brain smear technique. Aust Vet J 39:25–31, 1963.

37. Callow LL and McGavin MD: Cerebral babesiosis due to *Babesia argentina*. Aust Vet J 39:15–21, 1963.

38. Malherbe WD: The manifestations and diagnosis of *Babesia* infections. Ann NY Acad Sci 64:128–133, 1956.

39. Wright IG: Biogenic amine levels in acute *Babesia bovis* infected cattle. Vet Parasitol 4:393–398, 1978.

40. Dalgliesh RJ, Dimmock CK, Hill MWM and Mellors LT: *Babesia argentina*: disseminated intravascular coaggulation in acute infections in splenectomized calves. Exp Parasitol 40.

41. Annable CR and Ward PA: Immunopathology of the renal complications of babesiosis. J Immunol 112:1–8, 1974.

42. Jack RM and Ward PA: The role *in vivo* of C3 and C3b receptor in *Babesia* infections in the rat. J Immunol 124:1574–1578, 1980.

43. Chapman WE and Ward PA: *Babesia rhodhaini*: requirement of complement for penetration of human red erythrocytes. Science 169:67–70, 1977.

44. Seinen W, Stegman T and Kuil H: Complement does play a role in promoting *Babesia rhodhaini* infections in Balb/c mice. Z Parasitenkd 68:249–257, 1982.

45. Kakoma I, Levy MG and Ristic M: Lack of complement participation in the *in vitro* infectivity of erythrocytes by *B. bovis*. Manuscript in Preparation. 1984.

46. Mahoney DF, Wright IG and Goodger BV: Changes in the haemolytic activity of serum complement during acute *Babesia bovis* infection in cattle. Z Parasitenkd 64:39–45, 1980.

47. Schroeder WF, Cox HW and Ristic M: Anaemia, parasitaemia, erythrophagocytosis and haemagglutinins in *Babesia rhodhaini* infection. Ann Trop Med Parasitol 60:31–38, 1966.

6. Research towards vaccination against malaria; an update

CARTER L. DIGGS

Division of Communicable Disease and Immunology, Walter Reed Army Institute of Research. Washington, DC 20307.

1. Introduction

A total change in the complexion of the malaria vaccine problem has taken place since this author last commented in print on this topic [1]. At that time the discussion centered around an evaluation of the feasibility of vaccine development utilizing currently available culture and insect rearing technology (for production of blood stage and sporozoite vaccines respectively), and it was concluded that, at best, such efforts would be tedious, fraught with dangers, and generally inadequate. It was suggested, with some reticence, that the theoretical alternative of production of antigen through recombinant DNA technology should be investigated. It was further concluded that a prerequisite to this approach was considerable advancement in the immunochemical characterization of the plasmodial antigens.

In the slightly more than four years since the above mentioned discussion, there has been a veritable explosion of information both on the immunochemistry of plasmodia and on progress in the utilization of recombinant DNA methods to address the malaria problem. There is now almost universal consensus that most probably, malaria vaccines will ultimately be produced either by nonplasmodial cells into which the relevant genes have been inserted or by direct synthesis of the antigens using non-living chemical systems.

The purpose of this overview will be to highlight the major milestones over the last four years and to attempt to project where the emphasis will lie in the next period. Most of the progress made has been towards an understanding of the antigens involved, and these comments will reflect this fact. At the present time, it appears likely that a sporozoite vaccine will be developed first. Therefore, the literature on this subject will be presented first. Blood stage antigen characterization is currently in an extremely active phase, but there are many more alternatives with respect to the most likely avenues to yield useful results with this vaccine than with the sporozoite vaccine. Research on blood stage vaccine will be covered second. Finally, the gamete antigen approach, only mentioned briefly

Ristic, M. et al. (eds.) *Malaria and babesiosis.*
© 1984, Martinus Nijhoff Publishers, Dordrecht/Boston/Lancaster.

four years ago, has developed remarkably, and can be considered a serious possibility for practical implementation.

2. Sporozoite vaccine

Progress in sporozoite immunochemistry was heralded by the development of a monoclonal antibody against *Plasmodium berghei* which produced circumsporozoite precipitates, neutralized sporozoite infectivity, and reacted with a M_r-44,000 antigen that could be labeled by iodination of intact sporozoites [2]. As little as ten micrograms of the monoclonal antibody passively transferred into a mouse was effective in preventing infection on subsequent challenge [3]. The antigen could be labeled metabolially. It was designated as Pb44, and two additional antigens were demonstrated which reacted with the same monoclonal antibody [4]. These are of somewhat higher molecular weight and are designated as Pb52 and Pb54 respectively. Pulse chase experiments indicate that Pb52 is an intracellular precursor of Pb44.

Subsequent studies have demonstrated that these findings are valid for other malaria parasites. Monoclonal antibodies were developed against *P. knowlesi* sporozoites which identified antigens designated Pk52, Pk50 and Pk42 which are analogous in function to those discovered for *P. berghei* in that the smaller of the three is a surface antigen whereas the others are intracellular and neutralization of sporozoite infectivity can be effected by the antibody or its FAb fragment [5]. Monoclonal antibodies have also been developed against analogous circumsporozoite (CS) antigens of *P. falciparum* and *P. vivax* which have been designated as Pf67, Pf58, Pv51 and Pv45. The results of experiments to evaluate the sporozoite neutralizing activity of these monoclonal antibodies in chimpanzees indicate that they reduce infectivity of the sporozoites in each of the two species.

Studies on the structure of these sporozoite antigens using two dimensional electrophoretic analyses or HPLC analyses of tryptic digests indicate striking homology among them [7]. Furthermore, some of the monoclonal antibodies cross react with proteins derived from sporozoites of several species. Specifically, antibody against *P. knowlesi* reacts with both *P. cyanomolgi* and *P. falciparum* and an antibody against a *P. yoelii* nigeriensis antigen reacts with a *P. berghei* antigen and in this case neutralizes infectivity.

The most exciting development in print at the time of this writing regarding sporozoite antigens is the cloning and expression in *E. coli* of a gene coding for *P. knowlesi* sporozoite surface antigen [8]. Messenger RNA was prepared from *P. knowlesi* infected mosquitoes and a cDNA library constructed and inserted into the plasmid pBR322. When *E. coli* was transformed with these plasmids, colonies were detected by immunoassay which expressed antigen reactive with a monoclonal antibody to the *P. knowlesi* sporozoite antien. Preliminary information suggesting the occurrence of a repeated peptide segment within the surface antigen protein was obtained through DNA sequence data and through the fact that two molecules of the same monoclonal antibody apparently reacted with two sites on an antigen molecule in the sandwich immunoassay. Intensive efforts are currently being made to exploit these findings to devise a synthetic vaccine against human malaria. Theoretically, once the peptide sequence of the relevant epitope is known it can be produced either by microorganisms into which the gene has been inserted or by direct synthesis. The immunogenicity of such a synthetic molecule would be a function of a large number of variables, among which is its size. Extensive studies will still be needed to determine the best method of producing a sporozoite vaccine. Nevertheless, there is good reason to be very optimistic that a practical vaccine can be devised in the near future.

3. Blood stage vaccine

A number of possibilities exist for the development of malaria vaccine directed against blood stage parasites. None of these developments are as advanced as is the approach based on the circumsporozoite protein. However, compelling arguments for continued vigorous exploration on the feasibility of blood stage vaccines exist. A long recognized limitation of sporozoite vaccines is the all or none quality of the immunity induced. Unless the immunity is of such intensity as to completely prevent infection, unmodified disease due to the resulting blood stage parasites will result. Immunization against blood stage antigens, while providing total immunity only in exceptional cases, results in a much less severe course of infection on challenge. A blood stage vaccine would thus have the advantage of preserving life, although not preventing infection, in those individuals in which there was less than optmal immunity.

The many possibilities for blood stage vaccine development fall into two categories; those in which the target of the immune response is the free merozoite and those in which the target is the infected erythrocyte. Only fragmentory information on the antigens involved in the various antiparasitic phenomena which might lead to vaccine development is available. Nevertheless, striking advances in the immunochemistry of blood stage plasmodia have been made in these last four years. Immunochemical studies, combined with studies to assess the antiparasitic effects in *in vitro* culture have provided much information. Furthermore, it is possible through the use of synchronized cultures and appropriately timed experimentation to deduce the probable cellular target, merozoite as opposed to infected erythrocyte, of antibody or other mediator.

Antibody mediated immunity against merozoites is perhaps the most studied immune reaction. A variety of immune sera from rhesus monkeys immune to *P. knowlesi* and from owl monkeys or humans immune to *P. falciparum* contain antibodies which react with the merozoite surface and cause agglutination of these cells at the time of their release from schizonts. Penetration of erythrocytes by merozoites in such agglutinated masses is impeded although not totally prevented [9, 10, 11].

Monoclonal antibodies have been produced against *P. knowlesi* [12], *P. yoelii* [13] and *P. falciparum* [14] which react with high molecular weight proteins ranging from M_r-195,000 to M_r-250,000. These are major antigens of the schizont and merozoite as determined through immunoprecipitation experiments utilizing immune sera [14, 15]. Antibody which agglutinates merozoites by cross-linking surface coat may provide an immunoprophylactic methodology, but many sera exist which precipitate large amounts of what appear to be these antigens, but which have no growth inhibitory activity. Furthermore, there is some evidence that inhibition of growth through agglutination is a strain specific phenomenon [15]. Further work is needed to elucidate these questions.

Other antigens may serve as targets of antibodies which impede the penetration of erythrocytes by released merozoites. A prominent example is the M_r-140,000 antigen of *P. knowlesi* [16]. Monoclonal antibodies directed against this antigen are highly protective [17] although they do not agglutinate merozoites.

A theoretical but as yet unrealized possibility for development of anti-merozoite vaccine is the utilization of the erythrocyte receptor on merozoites as an immunogen; presumably antibodies which react with this receptor would block penetration of erythrocytes by merozoites. It seems clear that glycophorin is important in the binding of merozoites to erythrocytes, and lectin-like proteins of M_r-140,000, 70,000 and 35,000 reactive with glycophorin have been identified on the merozoite surface [18]. Further developments in this area will be of great interest.

Collaboration of phagocytic cells with antibody to phagocytize merozoites and thus prevent infection of erythrocytes has been reported [19]. There is evidence that this reaction may be due to antibodies which are cytophilic for monocytes [20]. These findings point out the necessity for continued study of effector mechanisms which may be more effective than the simple agglutination which appears to be operative in most cases of antibody mediated antimerozoite immunity.

In addition to immunity directed against the merozoite as target, there are several instances in which the immune system exerts an influence on intracellular parasites. Studies by a number of workers have clearly indicated the presence of antigenic determinants on the surfaces of infected erythrocytes [21, 22]. Such antigens are associated, at least in part, with the knobs on the surfaces of erythrocytes infected by mature *P. falciparum*. They are also associated with the binding of the infected erythrocytes to endothelial cells providing a putative mechanism of escape for the parasites from destruction in the spleen [23]. The development of an *in vitro* assay for the binding of infected erythrocytes to endothelial cells has made possible the testing of immune sera for ability to block this interaction. Blockade is presumably due to the presence of antibodies reactive with the determinants on the infected erythrocytes which react with the endothelial cell surface [23]. Since endothelial binding has been suggested to be necessary for optimal parasite growth and pathogenicity, such blockade, induced through prior artificial immunization with the appropriate antigens, is an attractive strategy for the development of a vaccine.

Opsonization of infected erythrocytes by immune serum with subsequent phagocytosis by monocytes is a further possible immune effector mechanism which has been demonstrated *in vitro* and which might be operative in an immunized individual [24].

In addition to antibody mediated effector mechanisms, nonantibody mediated mechanisms also play a role in immunity against malaria. A series of observations ranging from the demonstration of B cell independent immunity in avian [25] and rodent [26] malarias to the recent demonstration of toxicity of tumor necrosis factor for *P. falciparum* [27] make this clear. Whether or not it is feasible to devise strategies for the production of nonantibody mediators toxic to malaria parasites as a part of the response to artificial immunization remains to be seen. However, these phenomena need to be considered in the overall approach to vaccine development.

In the final analysis, when sufficient data have been accumulated, it might be advisable to design vaccines which include more than one of the antigens and systems described in this brief survey. For example, a polyvalent vaccine which induced antibodies which not only interfered with erythrocyte reinvasion but blocked endothelial adherence would clearly have a synergistic inhibitory effect on the development of parasitemia.

It is clear from the foregoing discussion that much research, especially along the lines of identification of the pertinent antigens, must be performed before good choices can be made with respect to candidate antigens for vaccine development. An exciting recent development which will undoubtedly accelerate this work is the first demonstration of expression of *P. falciparum* blood stage antigens in *E. coli* [28]. Five percent of bacterial clones isolated after infection with an ampicillin-resistant bacteriophage into which *P. falciparum* cDNA had been inserted expressed peptides reactive with antibody from human immune sera. Analysis of these antigens with respect to their possible relevance to functional immunity is eagerly awaited.

4. Gamete vaccines

The development of our understanding of vaccination against gametes has been impressive over the last four years. At the time of the previous review [1], only *P. gallinaceum* and *P. knowlesi* had been investigated. Currently, monoclonal antibodies are available which block infectivity of *P. falciparum* gametes for mosquitoes [29]. The antigens reactive with these monoclonal antibodies have been identified as three proteins with $M_r = 155,000$, $59,000$ and $53,000$. These are antigenically related and present in both male and female gametes. In principle, there is no reason why appropriate peptides cannot be identified which could serve as synthetic vaccines to induce antibodies reactive with these materials.

5. Summary and conclusions

Progress in research on all three types of malaria vaccines has been truly impressive during this four year period. It would appear that the information necessary for the design of a vaccine against sporozoites and gametes will be available soon, perhaps within a year. Use of this information, which will utilize an amino acid sequence for the genetic development of a practical immunogen, will require great effort. In the case of blood stage vaccination, emphasis must remain for the immediate future on extensive immunochemical characterization of the pertinent antigens.

The question of a decision point at which a selection between vaccines can be made deserves discussion. All approaches to vaccination against malaria have advantages and disadvantages. Clearly a gamete vaccine, for example, even if it were capable of blocking transmission entirely over a period of time would not provide the immediate protection needed in many situations. The disadvantage of a sporozoite vaccine, namely its all or none quality, has already been discussed. In the light of current knowledge then, it would appear that the optimal vaccine would be polyvalent; it would prevent infections by malaria parasites in a large percentage of cases by virtue of its sporozoite antigen constituent; it would limit morbidity by virtue of antigens which induce immunity to the blood stages which are responsible for the signs and symptoms of disease; and it would limit transmission in the community by virtue of gamete antigen constituents. Needless to say, any one of these constituents of the optimal polyvalent vaccine will be welcomed as soon as it appears.

Acknowledgement

Alice Boarman is gratefully acknowledged for her superb assistance in preparing the manuscript.

References

1. Diggs CL: Prospects for development of vaccines against *Plasmodium falciparum* infection. In: Malaria, Vol. 3, JP Kreier, Ed. Academic Press, New York, pp 229–315, 1980.
2. Yoshida N, Nussenzweig R, Potocnjak P, Nussenzweig V, Aikawa M: Hybridoma produces

protective antibodies directed against the sporozoite stage of malaria parasite. Science 207:71–73, 1980.

3. Potocnjak P, Yoshida N, Nussenzweig R, Nussenzweig V: Monovalent fragments (Fab) of monoclonal antibodies to a sporozoite surface antigen (Pb44) protect mice against malarial infection. J Exp Med 151:1504–1513, 1980.

4. Yoshida N, Potocnjak P, Nussenzweig V, Nussenzweig R: Biosynthesis of Pb44, the protective antigen of sporozoites of *Plasmodium berghei.* . J Exp Med 154:1225–1236, 1981.

5. Cochrane AH, Santoro F, Nussenzweig V, Gwadz RW, Nussenzweig R: Monoclonal antibodies identify the protective antigens of sporozoites of *Plasmodium knowlesi*. Proc Natl Acad Sci 79:5651–5655, 1982.

6. Nardin EH, Nussenzweig V, Nussenzweig RS, Collins WE, Harinasuta KT, Tapchaisri P, Chomcharn Y: Circumsporozoite Proteins of human malaria parasites *Plasmodium falciparum* and *Plasmodium vivax*. J Exp Med 156:20–30, 1982.

7. Santoro F, Cochrane AH, Nussenzweig V, Nardin E, Nussenzweig RS, Gwadz RW, Ferreira A: Structural similarities among the protective antigens of sporozoites from different species of malaria parasites. J Biol Chem 258(5):3341–3345, 1983.

8. Ellis J, Ozaki LS, Gwads RW, Cochrane AH, Nussenzweig V, Nussenzweig RS, Godson GN: Cloning and expression in *E. coli* of the malarial sporozoite surface antigen gene from *Plasmodium knowlesi*. Nature 302:536–538, 1983.

9. Miller LH, Aikawa M, Dvorak JA: Malaria *(Plasmodium knowlesi)* merozoites: immunity and the surface coat. J Immunol 114(4):1237–1242, 1975.

10. Chulay JD, Aikawa M, Diggs C, Haynes JD. Inhibitory effects of immune monkey serum on synchronized *Plasmodium falciparum* Cultures. Am J Trop Med Hyg 30(1):12–19, 1981.

11. Vernes A, Haynes JD, Tapchaisri P, Williams JL, Dutoit E, Diggs CL: *Plasmodium falciparum* strain-specific human antibody inhibits merozoite invasion of erythrocytes. Am J Trop Med Hyg 33(2):197–203, 1984.

12. Epstein N, Miller LH, Kaushel DC, Udeinya IJ, Rener J, Howard RJ, Asofsky R, Aikawa M, Hess RL: Monoclonal antibodies against a specific surface determinant on malarial *(Plasmodium knowlesi)* merozoites block erythrocyte invasion. J Immunol 127(1):212–217, 1981.

13. Freeman RR, Trejdosiewicz AJ, Cross GAM: Protective monoclonal antibodies recognizing stage-specific merozoite antigens of a rodent malarial parasite. Nature 284:366.

14. Holder A, Freeman RR: Biosynthesis and Processing of a *Plasmodium falciparum* schizont antigen recognized by immune serum and a monoclonal antibody. J Exp Med 156:1528–1538, 1982.

15. Brown GV, Ander RF, Knowles G: Differential effect of immunoglobulin on the *in vitro* growth of several isolates of *Plasmodium falciparum*. Infect Immun 39(3):1228–1235.

16. Hudson DE, Miller LH, Richard RL, David PH, Alving CR, Gitler C: The malaria merozoite surface: a 140,000 M.W. protein antigenically unrelated to other surface components on *Plasmodium knowlesi* merozoites. J Immunol 130(6):2886–2890, 1983.

17. Miller LH, David PH, Hudson DE, Hadley TJ, Richards RL, Aikawa M: Monoclonal antibodies inhibit malaria invasion of RBCs. J Immunol 132(1):438–442, 1984.

18. Jungery M, Boyle D, Patel T, Weatherall DJ: Lectin-like polypeptides of *P. falciparum* bind to red cell sialoglycoproteins. Nature 301:704–705, 1983.

19. Khusmith S, Druilhe P: Cooperation between antibodies and monocytes that inhibit *in vitro* proliferation of *Plasmodium falciparum*. Infect Immun 41(1):219–223, 1983.

20. Khusmith S, Druilhe P: Specific arming of monocytes by cytophilic IgG promotes *Plasmodium falciparum* merozoite ingestion. Trans R Soc Trop Med Hyg 76:423–424.

21. Kilejian A: Characterisation of a protein correlated with the production of knob-like protrusions on membranes of erythrocytes infected with *Plasmodium falciparum*. Proc Natl Acad Sci USA 76(9):4650–4653, 1979.

22. Langreth SG, Reese RT: Antigenicity of the infected erythrocyte and merozoite surfaces in

falciparum malaria. J Exp Med 150:1241–1254, 1979.

23. Udeinya IJ, Schmidt JA, Aikawa M, Miller LH, Green I: *Falciparum* malaria-infected erythrocytes specifically bind to cultured human endothelial cells. Science 213:212–214, 1981.

24. Celada A, Cruchaudl A, Perrin LH: Opsonic activity of human immune serum on *in vitro* phagocytosis of *Plasmodium falciparum* infected red blood cells by monocytes. Clin Exp Immunol 47:635–644, 1982.

25. Rank RG, Weidanz WP: Nonsterilizing immunity in Avian malaria: an antibody-independent phenomenon (39186). Proc Soc Exp Biol Med 151:57–259, 1976.

26. Roberts DW, Weidanz WP: T cell immunity in the B-Cell deficient mouse. Am J Trop Med Hyg 28:1–3, 1979.

27. Haidaris CG, Haynes JD, Meltzer MS, Allison AC: Serum containing tumor necrosis factor is cytotoxic for the human malaria parasite *Plasmodium falciparum*. Infect Immun 42:385–393, 1983.

28. Kemp DJ, Coppel RL, Cowman AF, Saint RB, Brown GV, Anders RF: Expression of *Plasmodium falciparum* blood-stage antigens in *Escherichia coli:* Detection with antibodies from immune humans. Proc Natl Acad Sci 80:3787–3791, 1983.

29. Rener J, Graves PM, Carter R, Williams JL, Burkot TR: Identification of target antigens of malaria transmission blocking monoclonal antibodies on gametes of *Plasmodium falciparum*. J Exp Med. In press, 1983.

7. Research on babesiosis vaccines

MIODRAG RISTIC

Department of Pathobiology, College of Veterinary Medicine, University of Illinois. Urbana, Illinois 61801 USA.

1. Disease and causative agents

Babesiosis is a tick-transmitted disease of animals characterized by pyrexia, anemia, occasionally hemoglobinuria, and the presence of infecting protozoa in the host's erythrocytes[1]. Losses due to babesiosis may be higher than 50% when susceptible cattle are introduced into endemic areas of the disease. Animals which survive the acute phase of the disease remain carries of the agent for variable periods of time. Accordingly, two categories of infection are recognized being babesiosis and babesiasis. Babesiosis refers to the period when there is rapid growth and multiplication of the parasite and there are clinical signs of disease, while babesiasis encompasses the latent infections observed in animals which have recovered from the clinical disease and in newborn animals passively immunized via colostrum. Other occasionally used synonymous terminologies for babesiosis are: Texas cattle tick fever, prioplasmosis, tick fever, red water and tristesa.

Among 71 *Babesia* species known, 18 species cause disease in domestic animals including cattle, sheep, goats, horses, pigs, dogs and cats. Babesiosis also occurs in man and laboratory animals. Clinical signs observed in acute human babesiosis include: high fever, chills, headache and backache. Bovine, equine and rodent *Babesia* species were identified as the causative agents of human babesiosis [2].

Of the different diseases, bovine babesiosis caused by *Babesia bigemina, B. bovis* (synonymous with *B. argentina*), *B. divergens* and *B. major* is the most important economically. The disease caused by *B. bovis* is more severe and more difficult to control than that caused by the other species.

The tick is known to be a biologic vector of various *Babesia* and an earlier suggestion that a sexual phase exists in the vector was documented by recent electron-microscopic studies [3, 4]. *Babesia bigemina* and *B. bovis* are generally transmitted by *Boophilus* ticks, *B. divergens* by *Ixodes ricinus,* and *B. major* by *Haemaphysalis punctata*. More recently, the Hyaloma tick has been identified as a vector of a *Babesia* in Africa [5].

Ristic, M. et al. (eds.) *Malaria and babesiosis.*
© 1984, Martinus Nijhoff Publishers, Dordrecht/Boston/Lancaster.

With its wide geographic distribution, bovine babesiosis exerts a very important economic impact, particularly on livestock industries of developing countries and frequently presents a major obstacle to the establishment of more productive breeds of cattle in these regions. Reflecting the magnitude of the problem is the statement: 'Tickborne diseases are the cause of probably the most economically serious losses of ruminants in Southeastern Africa', made as a result of a recent study by the FAO of tick-borne diseases in that region [6]. Limited studies indicate that similar situations exist in Europe and other regions of Africa, Asia, South America and Australia where babesiosis is endemic. The only cattle producing regions free of babesiosis are the US, Canada, New Zealand, South Australia, and possibly areas of Northern Asia (Figure 1).

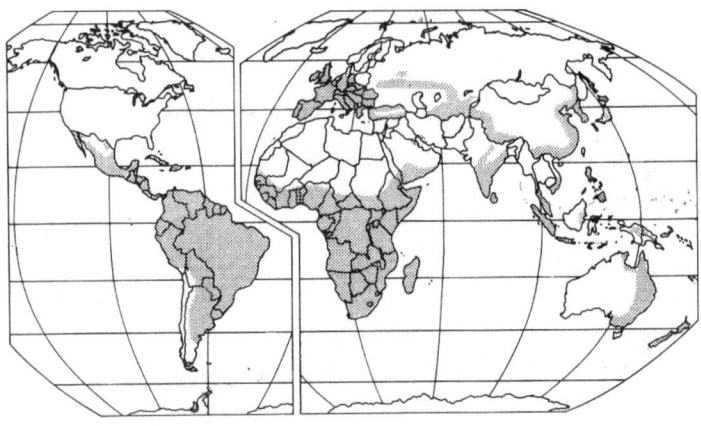

Figure 1.   The geographical distribution of bovine babesiosis.

2. Historical background

The term *Babesia* was adopted to honor a Rumanian scientist, Babes, who in 1888 first described the *Babesia* parasite in blood of African cattle showing hemoglobinuria [7]. The classic work of Smith and Kilbourne [8], which was underway in the United States at approximately the same time, signified the beginning of the scientific history of babesiosis. It is through this study that the tick was unequivocally identified for the first time as a vector of a protozoan agent, *B. bigemina*. For several decades thereafter, babesiosis caused by *B. bigemina*, was responsible for serious losses of cattle in the United States. These losses were estimated in millions of dollars and mortalities in excess of 50% were common. This serious situation prompted a proposal for eradication of the tick vector as a means of disease control. Hence, a national eradication program, backed by a multimillion dollar budget started in 1906, and was successfully completed during a four decade period (Figure 2).

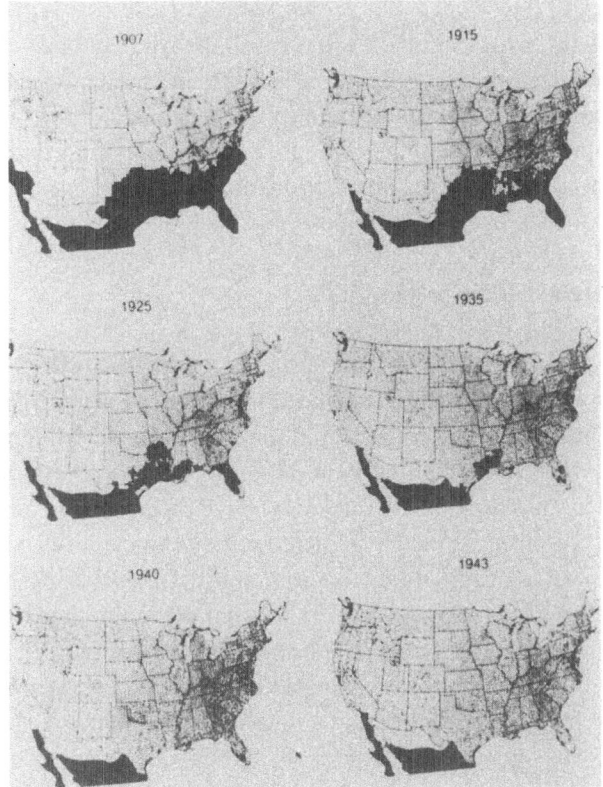

Figure 2. The progress of eradication of bovine babesiosis in the United States during the early part of the 20th century. Areas with babesiosis are marked in black.

On a global basis, the success of the United States in eliminating babesiosis by eradication of the vector remains an isolated but exemplary instance. Babesiosis persists as one of the most important diseases of cattle in all tropical and semitropical regions of the world between the 32nd parallel south and the 40th parallel nort of the equator. It is estimated today that half a billion cattle throughout the world may be endangered by the disease caused by one or more species of *Babesia*. This situation prompted research efforts in many parts of the world aimed at the development of control measures for babesiosis other than by vector eradication. In all these studies, infected cattle were the only source of *Babesia* and its antigens. There are a number of difficulties associated with the use of reagents derived from the living host. In most instances, the antigens were affected and degraded by immune and enzymatic machinery of the host, respectively. Furthermore, preparations were usually contaminated with host tissue constitutents, thus reducing their safety as routinely used immunogens.

A major breakthrough in babesiosis vaccine research was achieved by the development of cultural methods for continuous *in vitro* propagation of *Babesia bovis* [9, 10, 11].

This achievement, which signified a new era in the study of bovine babesiosis, has opened a vast horizon of possibilities for easier and more accurate studies of biophysical, immunochemical and immunogenic properties of the organism and for the development of modern and efficacious immunoprophylactic and serodiagnostic methods for the control of babesiosis [12].

3. Pathologic mechanisms of babesiosis

Many of the pathologic effects of babesiosis are the indirect effects of babesial multiplication in the host. Immune complex disease and associated glomerulone-phritis, anemia and thrombocytopenia have been described in rodent babesiosis caused by *B. rodhaini*. Circulating babesial antigens also appear to attach to parasitized and nonparasitized erythrocytes. The formation of immune complexes on the erythrocyte surface may increase the permeability and fragility of circulating erythrocytes. Formation of such complexes in the plasma may serve as a means of evasion of parasite destruction by immune antibodies.

During the exit of *B. bovis* and *B. bigemina* parasites from infected bovine erythrocytes, two or more parasite-associated proteolytic enzymes are released into the plasma. These enzymes and/or similar parasite metabolic products are believed to interact with blood components and are ultimately responsible for several of the pathologic signs and symptoms associated with bovine babesiosis, including icreased erythrocyte fragility, hypotensive shock, and disseminated intravascular coaggulation [13].

Preliminary experiments in our laboratory showed the enormous ability of *B. bigemina* to release massive quantities of proteases which are filtered into the blood plasma and by interaction with erythrocytes cause hemolysis and occasion-ally hemoglobinuria. Accordingly, anemia, which is caused by intravascular destruction of erythrocytes by escaping babesias and associated humoral prod-ucts, is the major pathologic manifestation of babesiosis caused by *B. bigemina*.

The pathologic effects caused by the small babesia *B. bovis* seem to be quite different from those induced by *B. bigemina*. This organism seems to be able to avoid splenic filtration by sequestration of infected erythrocytes in the small capillaries of the brain and other organs. Thus in infections with *B. bovis*, there is a poor correlation between parasitemia, anemia, and clinical manifestations. In the acute form of the disease parasitemia in peripheral blood may be 1 to 2%, while the parasite rate in blood of brain capillaries may exceed 90%. An earlier belief maintained that the coating of erythrocytes by soluble parasite antigens neutralized the normal surface charge of these cells, thus favoring autoagglutina-tion of erythrocytes in the capillaries. Recent studies produces striking evidence on the mechanisms by which *B. bovis* escapes splenic filtration by sequestering in the blood capillaries. These studies revealed that, similar to *Plasmodium falciparum*, *B. bovis* possesses the ability to induce changes in the membrane of the host erythrocytes [14, 15]. These changes, appearing in the form of electron dense spikes, seem to be specific antigens which find corresponding receptor sites on the endothelial cells of blood capillaries facilitating adhesion of the altered erythrocytes to the endothelium (Figure 3 - a, b, c). The resulting sequestration of erythrocytes in the narrow capillary passages impairs blood circulation in the vital organs such as the brain, bringing about anoxia and other clinico-pathologic manifestations. Such animals may develop rabies-like clinical signs and usually die before any appreciable parasitemia is manifested in the peripheral blood.

A method of bringing about a transitory attenuation of *B. bovis* by subjecting the organism to a series of rapid passages in splenectomized calves has been used in Australia as a means of producing a vaccine against babesiosis for nearly 20 years [16]. In order to study the underlying mechanism of the attenuation process we subjected tick-derived *B. bovis* to 20 consecutive blood passages in splenectomized calves. Studies of the parasite in infected animals and *in vitro* cultures [11] revealed that with each passage there was an increase in blood parasitemia level and that each increase was followed by a gradual shift of the parasite morphology from predominantly pyriform type to predominantly ring forms (Figure 4). Subsequent studies revealed that the selection from pyriform to ring form parasite type was due to the ability of the latter type to multiply at nearly twice the rate of the pyriform type. Finally, an electron microscopic examination of the parasite population at various passages showed that the majority of erythrocytes hosting low passage parasites (passages 1 to 4) possessed membrane knobs and that these structures were rarely, if at all, observed in parasitized erythrocytes beyond the 8th consecutive passage in splenectomized calves [15]. It could therefore be concluded that rapid passages in splenectomized calves abrogated the ability of the organism to escape splenic filtration thereby rendering it less virulent. When a knobless 'attenuated' parasite population was passed two times through intact (spleen *in situ*) cattle, a reversion to the knobbed virulent form occurred in a rather rapid fashion. Thus, the knobs appear to be a reversible specific 'marker' for the 'wild-type' *B. bovis*. Infection with the knobless type, however, confers complete protection to cattle against the virulent knobbed type.

4. Protective immunity

For many decades, the consensus of opinion was that induction of effective immunity against bovine babesiosis required exposure of the host to the live, preferably replicating, causative agents of this disease. A procedure for induction of protective immunity by infection and treatment, known as premunization, is the oldest known method. The subsequent carrier of chronic infection renders

108

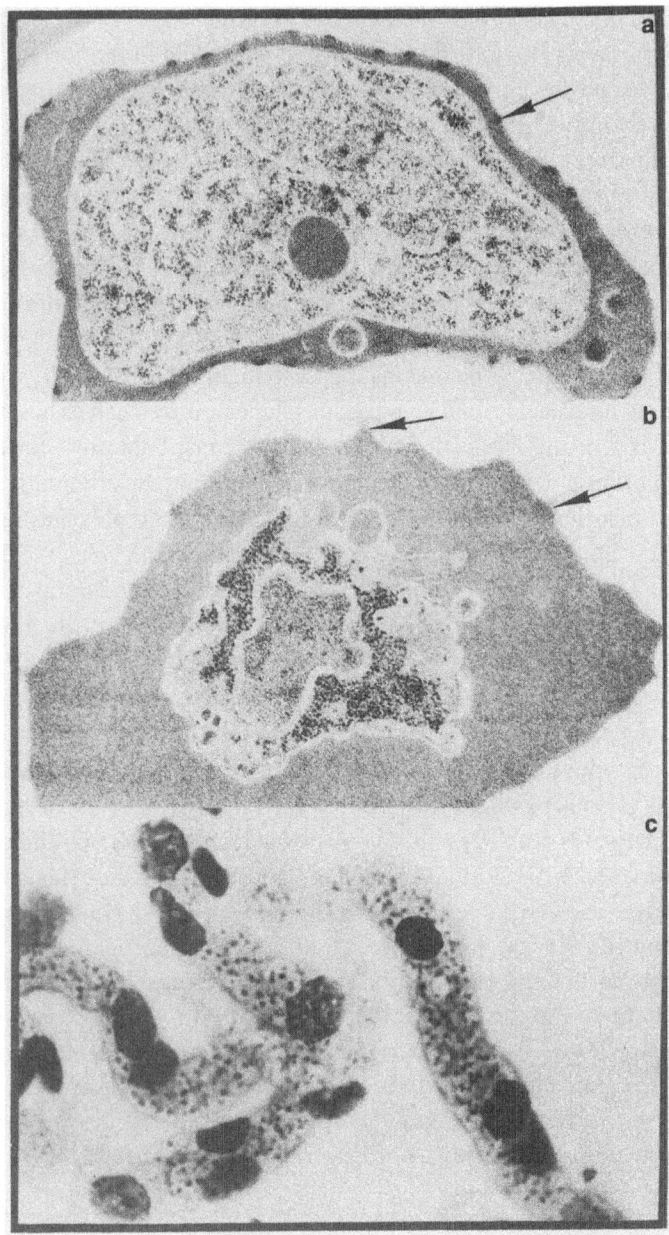

Figure 3. Electron micrographs of erythrocytes infected with *Plasmodium falciparum* (a) and *Babesia bovis* (b). Note knob-like structures in the membrane of *P. falciparum* infected erythrocyte and stellate-like protrusions in the erythrocyte infected with *B. bovis* (arrows) X-30,000. Bovine brain capillaries of an animal with acute infection caused by *B. bovis* (c). Note that these vessels are filled with sequestered erythrocytes most of which are infected. Giemsa stain × 1200. Electronmicrographs kindly provided by Dr. M. Aikawa, Institute of Pathology, Case Western Reserve University, Cleveland Ohio.

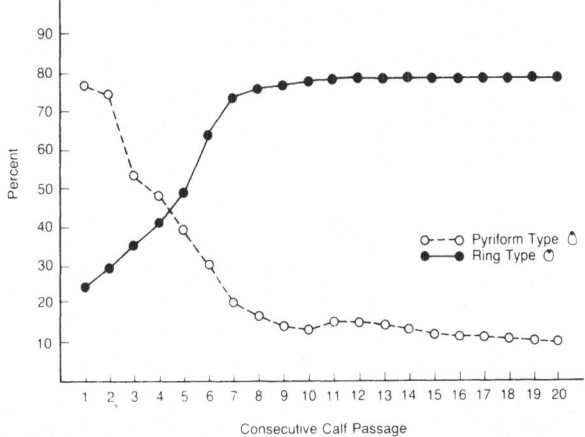

Figure 4. Attenuation of *Babesia bovis* by continuous frequent passages through splenectomized calves. Note a shift in parasite morphology from a typical pyriform type, which predominates in the low passage virulent population, to ring type, which represents the majority of parasites in the high passage 'attenuated' population (M. Filipov and M. Ristic, 1984).

cattle solidly immune to future homologous challenge. This procedure induces both humoral and cell mediated immune responses which jointly confer optimal protective immunity [17, 18].

Cattle immunization studies utilizing blood-derived non-living *Babesia* antigens and resistance to clinical infection after elimination of the agent from carrier animals by chemotherapy indicated that the sterile immunization approach was possible [19, 20, 21]. The duration of the infection prior to treatment seems to influence the level and duration of protective immunity, but these factors need to be studied further in order to understand their interrelationships. Further indications that sterile immunity occurs in babesiosis are derived from studies on passive transfer of immunity *via* serum and colostrum [22, 23, 24].

The development of a method for continuous *in vitro* propagation of *B. bovius* provided suitable means for the study of the antigens of that organism [25]. The studies thus far completed revealed that the major antigenic determinants associated with induction of protective immunity to *Babesia* are localized in the surface coat of the merozoites [12, 26]. The protective role of the merozoite surface coat antigens is further reflected by their apparent interaction with specific receptor sites on the surfaces of erythrocytes (Figure 5a-d). Merozoites deprived of the surface coat do not seem capable of attachment and penetration of erythrocytes.

Merozoite surface coat antigens may be obtained from the supernatant medium of *B. bovis* cultures. These antigens have been isolated and generally characterized as being proteinaceous moities, 30-40,000 molecular weight, degraded by papain and trypsin, stable at 60°C for 30 minutes, having fast electrophoretic mobility and isoelectric point at pH 5.0 - 5.5 [27].

Most of the information about the mechanisms of protection induced by antibodies to the merozoite surface coat was obtained by the use of the *in vitro*

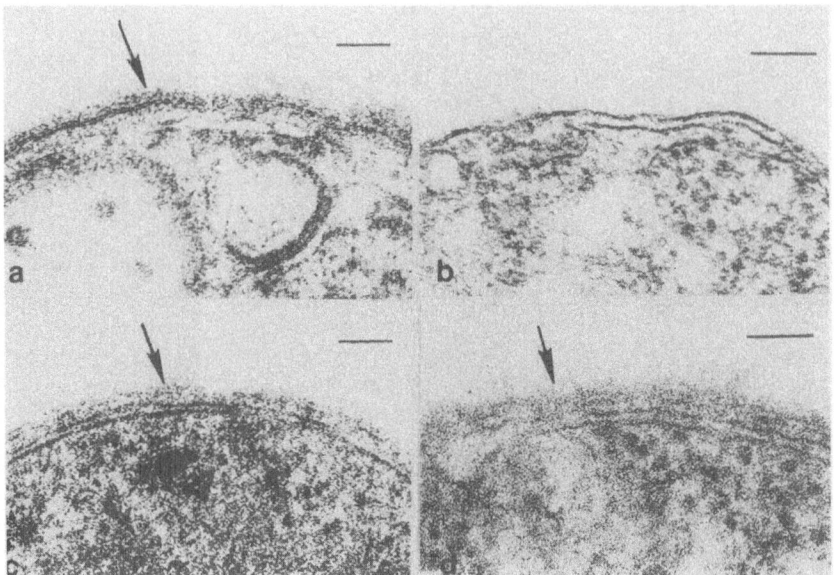

Figure 5. Electron micrographs demonstrating the effect of immune serum on *B. bovis* merozoite surface coat. Merozoite treated with the serum of an immune animal (a); merozoite treated with serum collected prior to vaccination with exoantigens (b); merozoite treated with antiserum collected at peak post-vaccination antibody titer (c) and merozoite incubated with serum of a vaccinated animal collected on the day of challenge (d). Note thickening of the surface coat in a, c, and d, and no such evidence in b, indicating specific interaction between the three sera and *B. bovis* merozoite surface coats.

merozoite serum neutralization test [12]. It was shown that antibodies to these antigens prevent attachment of extracellular babesia merozoites to erythrocytes. The opsonizing effect of those antibodies in collaboration with the phagocytic elements of the body present a powerful defense system which may be induced by immunization with culture-derived soluble merozoite surface coat antigens. Bases upon electron microscopic evidence, the interaction between these antibodies and the parasite may also bring about disruption and/or lysis of the organisms [28]. Finally, it was shown that immunization with soluble antigens induces formation of macrophage-bound cytophilic antibodies which seem to activate the phagocytic function of these cells and assists in immobilizing cell-free babesias on the surfaces of the macrophages (Figure 6a-d).

In a more recent study macrophage monolayers derived from *Babesia*-free cattle were exposed to soluble culture-derived *B. bovis* antigens. It was shown that these sensitized macrophages released a soluble factor capable of inhibiting *in vitro* growth of the organism [29]. Whether this factor inhibits the growth by direct action on the merozoites or by blocking erythrocyte surface receptors is the subject of future studies.

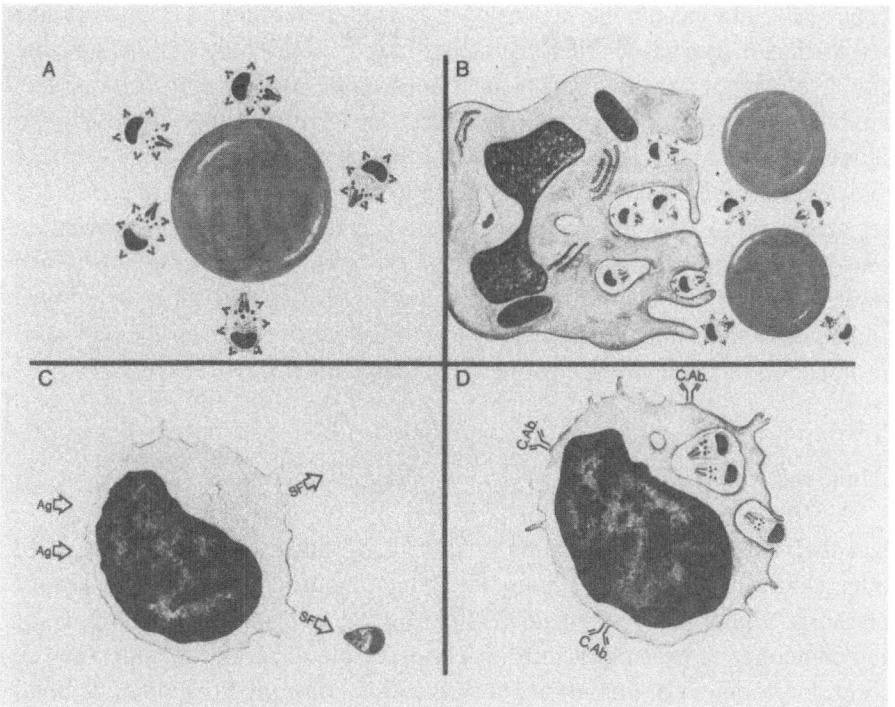

Figure 6. Proposed mechanism of protective immunity induced by soluble culture-derived exoan-tigens: Antibodies to these antigens may prevent attachment of cell-free merozoites to host cell erythrocytes (a) and induce opsinization of these parasites that triggers their removal by phagocytic activity (b). *In vitro* treatment of normal bovine blood macrophages with soluble exoantigens results in a release of a soluble factor (SF) by these cells which inhibits growth of *B. bovis* in cultures (c). Blood macrophage activity may be stimulated by a cytophilic antibody produced in response to vaccination with *B. bovis* exoantigens (d).

5. Antigenic variation

Babesia infections are frequently of long duration with the parasite surviving in the semi-immune host. Survival of the parasite may reflect its ability to evade the host's immune response by undergoing antigenic variation. Passage of the avi-rulent vaccine strain of *B. bovis* through either ticks, intact calves or intact calves, then ticks, resulted in development of two distinct protein antigens which were identified by two dimensional gel electrophoresis of biosynthetically labelled proteins and by immunoprecipitation [30, 31]. In contrast, passage through ticks of the virulent strain of the homologous *B. bovis* led to expression of another major acidic protein. These data suggest that various selection pressures are exerted in the tick and the vertebrate host on subpopulations in the hetero-geneous isolates (i.e., high passage attenuated strains) to produce the changes in protein antigen profiles of *B. bovis* [32].

The results of vaccination studies, however, using heterologous *B. bovis* strains suggest that a degree of cross protection may be achieved, thus minimizing possible effects of antigenic variation. Evidence of cross protection among certain, but not all, *B. bovis* strains·was recently documented using culture-derived soluble antigens as immunogens [32, 33]. It is suggested that the mechanism of cross immunity is based on priming of the host's immune system by antigens of the vaccine strain so that a secondary response against the heterologous strain occurred soon after challenge [34]. Based on various observations, some of which are described in this communication, it appears that soluble antigens derived from heterogeneous high passage *B. bovis* strains may be efficient immunogens for induction of immunity against heterologous challenge.

6. Immunization

Over the years various vaccination methods have been developed and studied under laboratory and field conditions as immunoprophylactic means against babesiosis. Generally, the antigens, either as live or inactivated organisms, or their components, were derived from ticks or the blood of infected animals. The recent development of methods for continuous *in vitro* propagation of *B. bovis* has provided the means for producing the first vaccine against an intra-erythrocytic parasite in a manner commonly used in the preparation of vaccines against viral and bacterial diseases. Various vaccination methods for bovine babesiosis using antigens derived from the blood of infected animals and from *in vitro* cultures are presented in table 1.

6.1. *Vaccines from infected ticks*

In view of the difficulty in adapting *Babesia* to growth in laboratory animals (*B. divergens* in mice is an exception) or tissue cultures, there has been a continuous effort to use tick stages of *Babesia* as potential immunogens [35, 36].

It was reported that sera from animals that had recovered from *B. bigemina* infections cross-reacted serologically with tick-derived vermicules of that organism [37]. In order to test the possible use of tick-derived vermicules as immunogens against bovine blood phase infections, we conducted several vaccination and challenge experiments. The vermicules derived from engorged *B. microplus* ticks were purified on a discontinuous Ficoll density gradient and then emulsified with Freund's complete adjuvant (FCA) and used to vaccinate four calves. The calves were inoculated with 1.9×10^7 vermicules divided into two doses given at 2-weeks intervals. Autofluorescence of vermicule preparations interfered with the interpretation of IFA tests when vermicular antigens were used. No significant cross-reactivity with blood-phase parasites was observed.

Table 1. Vaccination methods for bovine babesiosis: potentials and difficulties

Type of vaccine	Repro-ducibility	Commer-cial potential	Potential infection source	Possible reversion to virulence	Degree iso-immuni-zation	Protective efficacy
1. Live						
a. Premunization [1, 17]	Poor	No	Yes	Yes	Low	Good
b. Irradiated parasites [38, 39, 40, 41]	Poor	No	NI	NI	Low	Good
c. 'Attenuated' (passaged) [16]	Variable	No	Yes	Yes	Low	Good
2. Inactivated						
a. Corpuscular (whole organisms) [42]	Poor	No	None	None	High	Low
b. Solubilized antigens [44]	Poor	No	None	None	High	Low
c. Plasma soluble antigens [43, 46, 47]	Poor	No	None	None	Low	Low
d. Cell culture-derived soluble exoantigens [12, 25, 32, 50, 52, 53, 54, 55, 56]	Good	Yes	None	None	Low	Moderate

NI = No information

This negative finding is consistent with the negative IFA test results obtained when serum from naturally infected calves was tested against vermicular antigen. To further elucidate a possible relationship between tick-derived vermicules and larvae-derived infectious *B. bovis* forms, five calves were each inoculated with 1.7 $\times$ 10^7 vermicules and each challenged with 1,000 larvae eight weeks later. There was no detectable difference in the resulting infection in the animals in the control and immunized groups. The IFA test with blood-phase antigen became positive approximately 10 days post challenge. When vermicules were used as antigens in the IFA test, no difference could be demonstrated between sera from control and immunized calves, even after homologous challenge. Despite the failure to detect antibodies cross-reacting with blood and tick-stage parasites, 38% less (p 0.05) adult females dropped from the immunized calves than from the control calves.

This reduction was probably mediated by an immune response to tick antigens present in the vermicule preparations injected into these calves.

Even if an immune response and protection against tick-borne challenge could have been induced with one or more injections of vermicules, the large number of female ticks needed to produce that many vermicules under the conditions employed would make this approach to vaccination impractical.

6.2. Live vaccines from infected cattle

For many years the most widely used 'vaccination' method for babesiosis has been premunization. In this procedure susceptible cattle are intentionally infected and the insuing infection controlled by chemotherapy. The subsequent carrier or chronic infection rendered cattle solidly immune to later homologous challenge.

A degree of protection developed in cattle injected with irradiated *B. bovis, B. bigemina* or *B. major* infected erythrocytes [38, 39, 40, 41]. The cells were irradiated with a dose sufficient to prevent a parasitemia from developing after injection of the irradiated parasites. Where the irradiation dose only 'inactivated' or 'killed' the majority of the parasites, the calves were later strongly immune to challenge with viable parasites. Mild clinical reactions and parasitemia followed injection of the immunizing dose of the irradiated parasites. The immunizing efficiency of irradiated parasites may be related to the fact that even after irradiation, there is some residual metabolic activity retained by the organism. The many inherent difficulties with irradiated vaccines have prohibited their commercial usefulness.

Immunization of cattle against babesiosis caused by *B. bovis* using an 'avirulent' vaccine strain has sucessfully been practiced in Australia since 1965 [16]. A vaccinal strain is produced by rapid passage of *B. bovis*-infected blood through splenectomized calves. The organism appears safe for inoculation into animals with spleen *in situ*; however. subsequent inoculation of blood from vaccinated animals into susceptible cattle may induce clinical babesiosis. The mechanism involved in change of the virulence of the organism by passage through splenectomized calves has not yet been fully analyzed. Recent studies (see section on pathogenic mechanism of babesiosis) indicate that the phenomenon concerns a selection of more rapidly multiplying ring forms of *B. bovis* which lack the ability of sequestering in blood capillaries and thus are not able to avoid destruction by splenic filtration.

The disadvantage of establishing and maintaining bovine reservoirs of infection and the occasional adverse reactions caused by use of so-called 'attenuated' organisms has prompted many workers to investigate the usefulness of inactivated vaccines and the sterile immunity induced by such vaccines.

6.3. *Inactivated vaccines from infected cattle*

Initially all inactivated vaccines were composed of soluble and/or corpuscular babesia immunogens collected at the peak of parasitemia, subjected to limited purification, lyophilized or used fresh, and inoculated emulsified with an adjuvant. Ordinarily, more than one injection was recommended for each vaccination regime and there was usually a need for two or more such regimens a year.

Cattle have been partially protected against homologous and heterologous challenge by immunization with inactivated *B. bovis* or soluble antigens derived from erythrocytes and plasma of acutely infected cattle, respectively [42, 43]. Infected erythrocyte antigen was more effective than the plasma. Development of iso-blood group antibodies in vaccinated animals constituted one of several serious obstacles for wider use of the method. Other studies focused on isolation and use of solubilized *B. bovis* antigens as immunogens. At least two fractions were found to be immunogenic in splenectomized calves. One of these fractions appeared to have greater potential because of its lower contamination with bovine erythrocyte isoantigens [44]. More recently, a number of these antigens were isolated using monoclonal antibodies [45]. One of these antigens, fortified with Freund's Complete adjuvant, induced protective immunity in splenectomized calves against challenge two weeks following the second dose [45].

6.4. *Inactivated vaccines from cell cultures*

Culture-derived antigens used for immunization against bovine babesiosis caused by *B. bovis* are naturally released 'exoantigens' found in the supernatant culture medium. Our knowledge of these antigens dates some two decades back when we first observed their presence in the serum of several non-bovine animal species infected with *Babesia spp* [46, 47, 48]. During these studies an interrelationship between parasitemia levels, concentration of plasma antigens, and the level of antibodies to these antigens was established. There was a direct relationship between the levels of parasitemia and plasma antigens while an inverse relationship existed between these two elements and serum antibody levels (Figure 7). Recognizing the immunogenic potential of these antigens we initiated vaccination studies of dogs against infections caused by *B. canis* utilizing soluble antigens as immunogens. It is in the course of these studies that we, for the first time, recognized the protective nature of these antigens. However, while such potential was clearly in evidence, it was also recognized that the immunogenicity of soluble plasma-derived antigens was low, probably because of immune complex formation and enzymatic degradation.

The development of methods for *in vitro* propagation of *B. bovis* renewed our interest in soluble 'exoantigens' as immunogens against bovine babesiosis [9, 10, 11, 49]. Preliminary studies demonstrated that *in vitro* generated soluble babesia

116

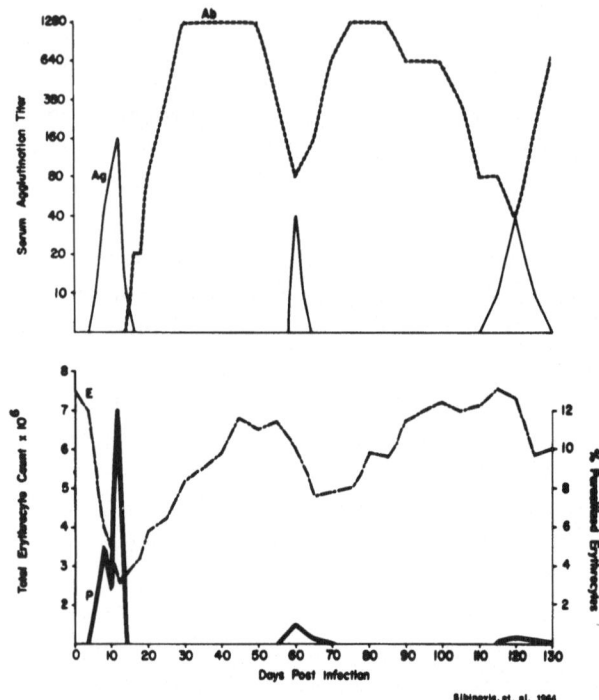

Figure 7. A diagram of parasitemia (P), soluble plasma antigens (Ag), and anti-babesia antibody titers (Ab) in a dog experimentally infected with *Babesia canis.* Note the direct relationship between the levels of parasitemia and plasma antigens and an inverse relationship between these two and serum antibody levels. It is apparent that in the presence of antibody excess, the levels of parasitemia and plasma antigens are suppressed, indicating the role of humoral antibody in protection against canine babesiosis.

antigens remained antigenically intact and immunogenically efficacious [12]. Initially the antigens used for production of *B. bovis* vaccines were derived from spinner flask cell cultures that produced an average of 3% parasitemia [9, 10].

In more recent studies, soluble *B. bovis* antigens were derived from the improved MASP cultures, which produced an average of 29% parasitemia [11, 50]. The antigens were concentrated approximately seven times by lyophilization, emulsified with a new saponin (Quil A) adjuvant and administered subcutaneously in two doses on days 1 and 21. Several small experiments were first conducted, each consisting of three to four cattle [12]. All inoculated animals showed a marked rise if IFA antibodies reaching a maximum titer of 1:20,000 at approximately 5-6 weeks after primary inoculation. The antibody titers persisted for 3-4 months and then subsided below detectable levels. Animals challenged at this time mounted a strong anamnestic antibody response that sometimes reached IFA titers as high as 1:327,680 at 24 days after challenge. Although contracting an infection due to challenge, vaccinated animals showed no detectable clinical or hematologic signs of the disease.

During the last two years, well controlled babesiosis vaccination experiments, using the culture-derived soluble antigen approach, were conducted in the United States, Mexico, Venezuela and Australia (Table 2). Evidence of protection against virulent *B. bovis* challenge using infected blood or ticks was demonstrated in all of these studies [32, 33, 51, 52, 53, 54, 55, 56, 57]. The challenge periods after vaccination varied from three weeks to six months. Depending on the study, both homologous and heterologous *B. bovis* challenges were used. Humoral immune responses to the vaccine antigen were demonstrated by the IFA, CF, and ELISA test systems [57]. In one instance where the cell-mediated immune response was measured by the lymphocyte transformation (LT) test, vaccinated animals showed positive stimulation indices for the entire six-month period, reaching a maximum index of 100 approximately 18 weeks after vaccination [32, 51]. Percent weight gain of vaccinated animals over controls ranged from 96 to 200 (Table 3).

In another study resulting from the collaborative research efforts between the scientists of the Institute Merieux of Lyon, France and those of our laboratory, a method for short-term *in vitro* cultivation of *B. canis,* the causative agent of canine babesiosis was developed [58]. This achievement was followed by the successful use of culture-derived soluble antigens as immunogens against infections with *B. canis* [59, 60]. Both laboratory and, most recently, completed field vaccination studies yielded satisfactory results indicating that the first commercially produced blood protozoan vaccine may be available in the near future (see chapter 9).

These initial successful developments in immunoprophylaxis against babesiosis must be followed by continuous basic studies in several areas in order to assure an optimal use of the system. It is obvious that the isolation and purification of

Table 2. Vaccination trials with culture-derived soluble B. bovis antigen

Location	No. Cattle	Days post vaccination and type of challenge	Results	Reference
USA — Beltsville	34	49, 131 and 178 Homologous-blood	Good*	Kuttler et al. [52, 53, 54]
USA — Urbana	28	30, 90 and 180 Homologous-blood	Good*	Levy & Ristic et al. [12]
Mexico - Mexico City	16	90 Homologous-tick	Good*	Smith et al. [55, 56]
Venezuela - Maracay	51	Homologous- and Hetrologous-blood	Satisfactory**	Montenegro-James et al. [33]
Australia - Brisbane	24	30 and 180 Heterologous-blood	Promising+	Timms et al. [32, 51]

* Mortalities among controls no need for treatment of vaccinates
** Morbidity among controls only
+ All controls and some vaccinates required treatment

protective antigens present in the culture medium may result in an amplification of both the degree and duration of protective immunity. Once physical and immunochemical characterization of these antigens is achieved, a more feasible means for their production would be by recombinant DNA or biochemical synthesis procedures. Other research should focus on the comparative examination of *B. bovis* and *B. canis* isolants from various geographic regions in order to delineate common and strain-specific immunodominant moeities of their merozoite surface coat antigens.

7. Conclusions

For many decades, the consensus of opinion was that induction of effective protective immunity against bovine babesiosis required prior exposure of the host to the live, preferably replicating, causative agents of this disease. A procedure for induction of protective immunity by infection and treatment, known as premunization, is the oldest known method. Safer immunization procedures have been developed subsequently by altering the virulence of the immunizing organism by rapid serial passages in splenectomized calves (*B. bovis)* and exposure of the infective blood to irradiation (*B. bovis* and *B. bigemina)*. The immune response to live immunogens includes both humoral and cell mediated (CMI) components. Cattle immunization studies utilizing blood-derived non-living babesia antigens and protection to clinical infection after elimination of the agent from carrier animals by chemotherpay indicated that the sterile immunization approach to vaccine development against babesiosis is possible.

A major breakthrough in babesiosis vaccine research was achieved by the development of methods for *in vitro* propagation of *B. bovis* and *B. canis* and by the discovery of abundant quantities of protective soluble exoantigens in the supernatant medium of these cultures. At least three such antigens with molecular weights in the range of 37,000 to 40,000 daltons have been identified in

Table 3. Immune response and weight gain in cattle vaccinated with culture-derived soluble *Babesia bovis* antigens

Post vaccination		Post challenge	
Immune response	Duration months	Immune reaction	% Weight gain of vaccinated over controls
IFA	4–5		
CF	2–3	Anamnestic	96–200
ELISA	4–6		
LT	6		

cultured *B. bovis*. These antigens were found to be effective immunogens useful for induction of protective immunity against infections caused by *B. bovis* and *B. canis*. The protective role of antibodies induced by soluble antigens was also demonstrated by means of the *in vitro* merozoite serum neutralization (MN) test. In addition, an *in vitro* interaction between soluble antigens and mononuclear phagocytes resulted in the production of soluble factors which inhibited growth and development of babesia parasites.

Various laboratory and field vaccination studies conducted in several regions of the world using culture-derived exoantigens of *B. bovis* and *B. canis* in combination with appropriate adjuvants yielded satisfactory results. These successful studies attest to the possibility that the first commerically produced blood protozoan vaccine may be available in the near future.

Some of the studies described in this communication have been made possible by a research grant from the Rockefeller Foundation, New York, NY.

8. References

1. Ristic Miodrag and Kreier JP: *Babesiosis*, Academic Press, Publishers, New York, NY, 1981.
2. Ristic Miodrag and Healy GR: Babesiosis. In: *Parasitic Zoonoses* (L. Jacobs, P. Arambulo, Eds.) CRC Press, Inc., Boca Raton, Florida, 1982, pp. 151–165.
3. Friedhoff KT: Morphologic Aspects of Babesia in the Tick. In: Babesiosis. M Ristic and JP Kreier, Eds. Academic Press, Publishers, New York, NY, 1981. pp. 143–169.
4. Rudzinskia MA: Morphologic Aspects of Host-Cell-Parasite Relationships in Babesiosis. In: Babesiosis. M Ristic and JP Kreier, Eds. Academic Press, Publishers, New York, NY 1981. pp. 87–141.
5. Gray JS, DeVos AJ: Studies on a bovine *Babesia* transmitted by *Hyalomma marginatum rufipes*. (Koch, 1844) Onderst J Vet Res 48:215–223, 1981.
6. Arnold RM, Asselbergs M: Tick borne diseases. World Animal Review 40:23–29, 1981.
7. Babes V: Sur l'Hemoglobinuria Bacterienne Du Boeuf. C.R. Bebd. Seances Adac Sci Paris 107:692–694, 1888.
8. Smith T and Kilbourne FL: Investigation into the Nature, Causation and Prevention of Texas or Southern Cattle Fever. US Department Agri Bur Anim Ind Bull *1*:1–301, 1893.
9. Erp EE, Gravely SM, Smith RD, Ristic M, Osorno BM and Carson CA: Growth of *Babesia bovis* in Bovine Erythrocyte Cultures. Am J Trop Med Hyg 27:1061–1064, 1978.
10. Erp EE, Smith RD, Ristic M and Osorno BM: Continuous *In vitro* Cultivation of *Babesia bovis*. Am J Vet Res 41:1141–1142, 1980.
11. Levy MG and Risic M: *Babesia bovis*: Continuous Cultivation in Microaerophilous Stationary Phase Culture. Science. 207 (No. 4426):1218–1220, 1980.
12. Ristic M and Levy MG: A New Era of Research Toward Solution of Bovine Babesiosis. In: Babesiosis. M Ristic and JP Kreier, Eds., Academic Press, Publishers, New York, NY 1981. pp. 509–544.
13. Wright IG: Biochemical Characteristics of Babesia and Physicochemical Reactions in the Host. In: Babesiosis. M Ristic and JP Kreier, Eds., Academic Press, Publishers, New York, NY, 1981. pp. 171–205.

120

14. Aikawa M, Rabbege J, Udeinya I and Miller LH: Electron microscopy of knobs in *P. falciparum*-infected erythrocytes. J Parasitology 62:435–437, 1983.

15. Aikawa M, Rabbege J, Ristic M and Miller LH: Structural Alterations of the Membrane of Erythrocytes Infected with *Babesia bovis*. In Press. J Trop Med and Hyg 1984.

16. Callow LT: Vaccination Against Bovine Babesiosis. Adv Exp Med Biol *93*:121–149, 1977.

17. Carson CA, Phillips RS: Immunologic responses of the vertebrate host to *Babesia*. In: Babesiosis. M Ristic and JP Kreier, Eds., Academic Press, New York, NY, 1981, pp. 411–443.

18. Goff WL, Wagner GG, Craig TM, Long RF: The bovine immune response to tick derived *Babesia bovis* infection: Serological studies of isolated immunoglobulins. Vet Parasit 11:109–120, 1982.

19. Mahoney DF and Wright EG: *Babesia argentina*. Immunization of Cattle with a Killed Antigen Against Infection with a Heterologous Strain. Vet Parasitol 2:273–282, 1976.

20. Kuttler KL, Johnson LW: Immunization of cattle with a *Babesia bigemia* antigen in Freund's complete adjuvant. Am J Vet Res 41:536–538, 1980.

21. Callow LL, McGregor W, Parker RJ, Dalgliesh RJ: Immunity of cattle to *Babesia bigemia* following its elimination from the host, with observations on antibody levels detected by indirect fluorescent antibody test. Austr Vet J 50:12–15, 1974.

22. Mahoney DG: Bovine Babesiosis: The passive immunization of calves against *Babesia argentina* with special reference to the role of complement fixing antibodies. Exp Parasit 20:119–124, 1967.

23. Weisman J, Goldman M, Mayer E, Pipano E: Passive transfer to newborn calves of maternal antibodies against *Babesia bigemina* and *Babesia berbera*. Refuah Vet *31*:108–113, 1974.

24. Dwivedi SK, Gautam OP: Experimental studies on passive immunization against *Babesia bigemina* infection in calves. Indian J Anim Sci 50:169–172, 1980.

25. Ristic M, Smith RD, Kakoma I: Characterization of Babesia Antigens Derived from Cell Cultures and Ticks. In: Babesiosis. M Ristic and JP Kreier, Eds., Academic Press, New York, NY 1982. pp. 337–380.

26. Montenegro-James S, James MA, Ristic M: Localization of culture-derived soluble *Babesia bovis* antigens in the infected erythrocytes. Vet Parasitology 13:311–316, 1983.

27. James MA, Levy MG and Ristic M: Isolation and Partial Characterization of Culture-derived Soluble *Babesia bovis* Antigens. Infec & Immun 31:358–361, 1981.

28. Ristic Miodrag: Babesiosis. In: Disease of Cattle in the Tropics. M Ristic and Ian McIntyre, Eds. Martinus Nijhoff Publishers, Hague, Netherlands, 1981. pp. 443–468.

29. Montealegre F, Levy MG, Ristic M: *In vitro* secretory activity of bovine blood mononuclear phagocytes and its effect on the growth of *Babesia bovis*. (Abstract). Proc 2nd Int Conf Malaria and Babesiosis, Sept. 18–22, 1983, Annecy, France, p. 7.

30. Kahl LP, Anders RF, Rodwell BJ, Timms P and Michell GF: Variable and Common Antigens of *Babesia bovis* Parasites Differing in Strain and Virulence. J Immunology, 129:1700–1705, 1982.

31. Kahl LP, Michell GF, Dalglish RH, Stewart NP, Rodwell BJ, Mellors LT, Timms P, Callow LL: *Babesia bovis*: Proteins of virulent and avirulent parasites passaged through ticks and splenectomized or intact calves. Exp Parasitology 56:222–236, 1983.

32. Timms P, Dalgliesh RJ, Barry DN, Dimmock CK, Rodwell BJ: *Babesia bovis*: Comparison of culture-derived parasites, non-living antigen and conventional vaccine in the protection of cattle against heterologous challenge. Austr Vet J 60:75–77, 1983.

33. Montenegro-James S, Leon E, Lopez R and Toro M: Heterologous Protection in Bovine Babesiosis Using a Culture-derived Vaccine. (Abstract). Proc 2nd Int Conf Malaria and Babesiosis, Sept 18–22, 1983, Annecy, France, p. 124.

34. Mahoney DF, Kerr JD, Goodger BV, Wright IG: The Immune Response of Cattle to *Babesia bovis* (syn. *B. argentina*). Studies on the Nature and Specificity of Protection. Int J Parasitol 9:297–306, 1979.

35. Mahoney DF, Mirre GB: *Babesia argentina*: The infection of splenectomized calves with extracts of larval ticks *(Boophilus microplus)*. Res Vet Sci 16:112–114, 1974.

36. Ronald NC, Cruz D: Transmission of *Babesia bovis*, using undifferentiated embryonic cells from *Boophilus microplus* tick eggs. Am J Vet Res 42:544–545, 1981.

37. Morzaria SP and Young AS: Identificaton of *Babesia bigemia* in the Tick Boophilus decoloratus by the Indirect Fluorescent Antibody Technique. Res Vet Sci 23:55–58, 1977.

38. Irvin AD, Brocklesby DW, Purnell RE: Radiation and isotopic techniques in the study and control of piroplasms of cattle: A review. Vet Parasit 5:17–28, 1979.

39. Wright IG, Mahoney DF, Mirre GB, Goodger BV, Kerr JD: The irradiation of *Babesia bovis*. II. The immunogenicity of irradiated blood parasites for intact cattle and splenectomized calves. Vet Immunol Immunopathol 3:591–601, 1982.

40. Wright IG, Mirre GB, Mahoney DF, Goodger BV: Failure of *Boophilus microplus* to transmit irradiated *Babesia bovis*. Res Vet Sci 34:124–125, 1983.

41. Purnell RE, Brocklesby DW, Stark AJ: Protection of Cattle against *Babesia* major by the Inoculation of Irradiated Piroplasms. Res Vet Sci 25:388–390, 1978.

42. Mahoney DF and Wright IG: *Babesia argentina:* Immunization of cattle with a killed antigen against infection with a heterologous strain. Vet Parasitology, 2:273–282, 1976.

43. Mahoney DF and Goodger BV: *Babesia argentina:* Immunogenicity of Plasma from Infected Animals. Exp Parasitol 32:71–85, 1972.

44. Mahoney DF, Wright IG and Goodger BV: Bovine babesiosis: The immunization of cattle with fractions of erythrocytes infected with *Babesia bovis* (syn. *B. argentina*). Vet Immun and Immunopath 2:145–156, 1981.

45. Wright IG, White M, Tracey-Patte PD, Donaldson RA, Goodger BV, Waltisbuhl DJ and Mahoney DF: *Babesia bovis*: Isolation of a protective antigen by using monoclonal antibodies. Inf and Immun 41:244–250, 1983.

46. Sibinovic KH: Immunogenic properties of purified antigens isolated from the serum of horses, dogs and rats with acute babesiosis. PhD Thesis, University of Illinois, Urbana, IL 61801, 1966.

47. Sibinovic KH, Sibinovic S, Ristic M and Cox HW: Immunogenic properties of babesial serum antigens. J Parasitol 53:1121–1129, 1967.

48. Sibinovic KH, Milar R, Ristic M and Cox HW: *In vivo* and *in vitro* effects of serum antigens of babesial infection and their antibodies on parasitized and normal erythrocytes. Ann Trop Med Parasitol 63:327–336, 1969.

49. Gravely SM, Smith RD, Erp EE, Conto, GJ, Aikawa M, Osorno MB and Ristic M: Bovine Babesiosis. Partial Purification and Characterization of Blood Culture-derived *Babesia bovis*. Int J Parasitol 9:591–598, 1979.

50. Levy MG, Clabaugh G, Ristic M: Age Resistance in Bovine Babesiosis: Role of blood factors in resistance to *Babesia bovis*. Inf and Immun 37:1127–1131, 1982.

51. Timms P, Stewart NP, Barry DN, Dalgliesh RJ: Nonliving *Babesia bovis* vaccines from culture. How good are they? (Abstract). Proc 2nd Int Conf Malaria and Babesiosis, Sept. 18–22, 1983, Annecy, France, p. 109.

52. Kuttler KL, Levy MG, James MA, Ristic M: Efficacy of a nonviable culture derived *Babesia bovis* vaccine. Am J Vet Res 43:281–284, 1982.

53. Kuttler KL, Levy MG, Ristic M: Cell culture-derived *Babesia bovis* vaccine: Sequential challenge exposure of protective immunity during a 6 month postvaccination period. Am J Vet Res 44:1456–1459, 1983.

54. Kuttler KL, Levy MG, Ristic M: Efficacy of cell culture-derived soluble *Babesia bovis* vaccines in the prevention of acute babesiosis. (Abstract). Proc 2nd Int Conf Malaria and Babesiosis, Sept. 18–22, 1983, Annecy, France, p. 108.

55. Smith RD, Carpenter J, Cabrera A, Gravely SM, Erp EE, Osorno M, Ristic M: Bovine Babesiosis: Vaccination against tick-borne challenge exposure with culture-derived *Babesia bovis* immunogens. Am J Vet Res 40:1678–1682, 1979.

56. Smith RD, James MA, Ristic M, Aikawa M, Vega CA: Bovine Babesiosis: Protection of cattle with culture-derived soluble *Babesia bovis* antigen. Science 212:335–338, 1981.

57. James MA, Kuttler KL, Levy MG, Ristic M: Antibody kinetics in response to vaccination against *Babesia bovis*. Am J Vet Res 42:1999–2001, 1981.
58. Laurent N, Moreau Y, Levy MG, Ristic M: A vaccine against canine babesiosis using a soluble antigen derived from cell culture of *Babesia canis*. (Abstract). Proc 2nd Int Conf Malaria and Babesiosis, Sept. 18–22, 1983, Annecy, France, p. 106.
59. Moreau Y: Vaccines Antibabesiens: Les contraintes industrielles. (Abstract). Proc 2nd Int Conf Malaria and Babesiosis, Sept. 18–22, 1983, Annecy, France, p. 121.
60. Molinar E, James MA, Kakoma I, Holland CJ, Ristic M: Antigenic and immunogenic studies on cell culture-derived *Babesia canis*. Vet Parasit 10:29–40, 1982.

8. Planning for malaria vaccine development

PHILIP K. RUSSELL AND CARTER L. DIGGS

Walter Reed Army Institute of Research, Washington, DC 20307.

1. Introduction

Over the past several years many laboratories have been engaged in basic research aimed at providing the fundamental information essential to the development of malaria vaccines. Targeted funding by the WHO TDR program and government agencies of several countries has accelerated the progress of this research. Studies in malaria immunology, parasite biochemistry, and molecular biology have progressed to the point where initiation of vaccine development is on the horizon. The malaria research community has effectively taken advantage of the important developments in the field of monoclonal antibodies, protein biochemistry, and molecular biology and have developed a very impressive and important information base [1]. These exciting developments in malaria immunology have convinced even the skeptics that the development of malaria vaccines is feasible and inevitable. The development of the malaria vaccine, however, presents an immense challenge to the scientific community. The complexity of the development process for malaria vaccine will be far beyond any vaccine development undertaken in the past and it presents many theoretical and practical problems which have not yet been systematically addressed and for which solutions will be essential if vaccine development is to be successful. At this point in time, it is instructive and necessary to consider the tasks which now still lie ahead in this endeavor. As we move from the area of basic research to the problems of implementation of the knowledge which has accrued to develop a practical vaccine, it is necessary to conscientiously devise a management strategy which can most nearly optimally address the problems inherent in exploratory and advanced vaccine development.

To begin with, not one but three types of vaccines are envisioned and of course ultimately against the several species of parasites. The three types of vaccines that are proposed include (1) an antisporozoite vaccine, (2) a transmission blocking vaccine and (3) an antimerozoite or antiblood stage vaccine. Carrying out development efforts in each of these areas for only a single species if done simul-

Ristic, M. et al. (eds.) *Malaria and babesiosis.*
© 1984, Martinus Nijhoff Publishers, Dordrecht/Boston/Lancaster.

taneously will strain the scientific and financial resources available for the development process. For all of these vaccines, stage specific protein antigens thought to be relevant to protective immunity have been described. The basic work is far from complete and much more needs to be done, especially in the field of blood stage vaccines. Nonetheless, the optimists among us can foresee in the coming year or two sufficient basis for undertaking studies to prove the feasibility of obtaining some of the objectives involved in vaccine development. Our main points in this presentation are to outline some of the problems that are facing us, to suggest some of the critical areas where scientific information will be necessary, and to make a plea for the effective collaboration among scientists and vaccine developers that will be needed to assure success.

2. Potential options for production of malaria vaccines

The vaccine that will probably be ready for a development effort first is the antisporozoite vaccine. The feasibility of immunization against sporozoite antigens has been established by experiments in man. The truly great work done by the NYU group has established the circumsporozoite protein as the critical antigen involved in protective antisporozoite immunity. Cloning and sequencing of the amino acids of the relevant protein and the relevant epitopes of the protein is progressing rapidly and it seems reasonable to expect the information to be available for a development effort quite soon. In malaria in particular, but in vaccine development in general, we will in the future be faced with the prospect of developing a practical biological product from the genetic information specifying antigenic peptide structures. Clearly, in the near future the structure of peptides which are portions of the human circumsporozoite proteins and which react with neutralizing monoclonal antibodies will be available. This will happen not only for *Plasmodium falciparum* but for *P. vivax* and in the long run not only for sporozoites but for other stages of the malaria parasite which might be used for vaccine development. This fact immediately poises a series of options which must be dwelt with. Peptides can be produced by conventional solid phase synthesis, or by microorganisms in which the genetic information has been inserted to produce the peptides, or by insertion of the genetic information into a nonvirulent microorganism which expresses the antigen which can be used as a live vaccine. With each of these options, a whole series of decision points exists.

2.1. Vaccines based on synthetic peptides

The selection of the peptide to be used in a vaccine is a key question. When the relevant epitope is represented in a repetitious fashion such as is the case with *P. knowlesi* CS protein, the single unit is high on the list as the best candidate for an optimal peptide for use in vaccine development. However, even in this case, and certainly in cases where such repetition is not evident, the possibility needs to be considered that changes in the sequence can improve immunogenicity. This fact implies the existence of the need for a systematic examination of the influence of discrete amino acid changes on binding affinity and immunogenicity of candidate peptide. In addition to the precise sequence which might be optimal, a number of other parameters must also be systematically examined. These include molecular size; it is entirely conceivable that increasing or decreasing the molecular size of a peptide could also influence its binding affinity and/or immunogenicity aside from considerations of the carrier molecule which will be discussed below.

Whether or not single or multiple epitopes should be represented on the immunogen needs to be considered; if multiple, how many are optimal needs to be determined.

Should a straight chain peptide be employed? Or is it advantageous to configure the immunogen with loops, or as side chains on a backbone carrier.

The optimal carrier to be used is also an open question. Arguments for the use of vaccines currently in use such as tetanus or diphtheria toxoid are that these have a vast amount of data to support their immunogenicity and safety. On the other hand modification of these materials may result in properties which are not anticipated.

Theoretical considerations such as the ability of the carrier to bind to cell surfaces, need also to be considered. For example, the labile toxin B of E. coli has this property and might be an excellent candidate for the carrier for peptide immunogens.

The outer membrane protein of the meningococcus has been shown to enhance immunogenicity of several antigens when presented in complex with it. The possible usefulness of this material in peptide vaccines needs to be explored. Keyhole limpet hemocyanin, a potent immunogen, has been used as a carrier for the production of antibodies against a variety of haptens. Whereas its use in humans can be questioned on the grounds of the paucity of experience with the material in man and of its relatively poor characterization, it is being used and needs to be evaluated in detail.

The presentation of certain antigens with hydrophobic moieties within liposomes has resulted in enhanced immunogenicity. The generality of these findings needs to be clarified.

In all of these cases, the rules by which choices of a carrier are made for a given hapten to be used in vaccine development need to be established.

The peptide carrier configuration is another subject which presents multiple options to the vaccine developer. The number of peptide molecules per carrier molecule needs to be studied systematically to determine the optimal ratio. The linking reaction will also undoubtedly be critical to optimal immunogenicity. Secondary cross-linking of peptide to carrier through aldehyde treatment is another consideration which needs to be dealt with.

Finally, in the preparation of a vaccine starting with the use of peptides, decisions must be made with respect to what adjuvants, if any, should be used.

2.2. *Vaccines based on expressed gene product*

A whole variety of choices are also available if a gene product is utilized as the basis of a vaccine. For example, the entire circumsporozoite protein, essentially as it appears naturally on the surface of sporozoites could be used. Alternatively, immunogenic segments of the protein could be produced and used as a starting point for further manipulation to produce a vaccine. Finally, a fusion protein which contains sequences unrelated to the native protein but which might endow the molecule with certain advantages, such as enhancement of immunogenicity, might also be contemplated.

Once the optimal genetic material is in place, an optimal expression system for it must be developed. Purification of the product in a manner suitable for human use is a whole additional subject for which there are presently few guidelines and which must be worked out. The problem of lipopolysaccharide contamination of materials purified from *E. coli* systems must be addressed, and is one argument for the use of a nonbacterial system for gene expression.

If live vaccines which have been genetically manipulated to express antigen *in vitro* are contemplated, careful risk/benefit analysis must be carried out.

After a product has been prepared, its evaluation in terms of safety and efficacy must be accomplished. Again, there are few ground rules from which to proceed using antigens produced in this way.

3. Needs of a program for the development of a malaria vaccine

Certain essential elements should be deliberately put into place for the efficient development of malaria vaccines. First and foremost is a strong basic research component to continue advancing the frontiers of knowledge which can be exploited in technology development. It is still the creative thinking of individual investigators which is the driving force of development efforts.

A management system to direct the development aspects of the work must be deliberately constructed and put into place. This system must have cognizance of the various aspects of the program and of its life cylce as it moves from basic research, through exploratory and advanced development to approved product for human use.

As a part of the exploratory developmental system, there should be laboratories geared to the production of immunogens, whether this be through peptide synthesis or recombinant DNA technology, and there should also be a systematic program for testing of the wide variety of experimental immunogens which must be assessed to optimize a final product to be used in humans.

Pilot vaccine manufacturing will be necessary with its component parts which involve safety testing, standarization and potency testing. This must all be done within the context of the governmental regulations which apply to such activities. In the US, the Food and Drug Administration Office of Biologic Products is responsible for implementing good manufacturing practices covered under existing federal law, so that the pilot vaccine manufacturing facility must maintain close liaison with this office. At this stage, the decisions made in optimization of the candidate vaccines will meet the test of being evaluated by governmental bodies.

After satisfactory preliminary safety testing, standarization, and potency testing, safety testing in human volunteers is a necessary next step. This can probably proceed in a manner similar to that of other more conventional vaccines. A small number of humans will be immunized and observed for signs of adverse effects.

Efficacy testing in humans for these engineered vaccines can take two forms. *In vitro* correlates, such as for example the appearance of antibody in appropriate amounts and with the appropriate affinity for certain sporozoite proteins, will give much assurance that vaccines will be efficacious. It also will be necessary, however, to perform limited challenge experiments in humans to confirm this fact.

Field testing will be the final step in evaluation. This will require careful design based on the status of the recipient population. For example, in endemic areas, there are many individuals who might have malaria at the time of immunization. Possible adverse effects due to immune complex formation must be carefully considered. On the other hand, populations such as military personnel at risk can be volunteers for field testing prior to exposure, thus avoiding this complication. Thus, it seems likely that a series of field evaluations starting with the simplest models with be required.

In spite of the complexity of the issues, we are confident that the developmental efforts can succeed. But in order to do so they must be very well organized by the scientific community and the funding agencies. There will be an absolute necessity for extensive collaboration between basic scientists, that is malariologists, molecular biologists, chemists and immunologists, with those undertaking the vaccine development. Any development effort raises important scientific questions that must be answered by the basic research communty if the development efforts are to proceed appropriately. The collaboration between basic scientists and development groups will need to be very effective if vaccines of this complexity are to be developed. An important aspect of the development effort is the systematic comparative testing of the various options. This will certainly involve multiple laboratories and will require a well conceived and well designed plan if it is to succeed in a reasonable time period.

It is at this point that the management requirements for these development efforts need to be considered by all concerned. The scientific developrents to date are remarkable and exciting. However, they impose on us a responsibility to exploit them in the most careful way possible. To do this we must plan together and implement the plans in a concerted manner. Our response to this ancient global disease must be global as well.

References

1. Diggs CL: Research Towards Vaccination Against Malaria; An Update (This volume.)

9. Antibabesial vaccination using antigens from cell culture fluids: industrial requirements

Y. MOREAU AND N. LAURENT

Rhone-Merieux, Laboratoire IFFA, 254 rue Marcel Merieux, 69007 Lyon, France.

1. Introduction

For half a century, various live antibabesial vaccines have been widely used in Australia, South Africa, South America and the Middle East [1]. In 1979, at the First International Conference on Malaria and Babesiosis, the development of cultural methods for short-term and continuous *in vitro* propagation of *Babesia bovis* and *Babesia canis* was reported [2, 3, 4, 5]. Mahoney affirmed at the conference that 'The culture of Babesia in blood and in tick tissues is showing promise and has now progressed sufficiently to indicate that material from these sources may revolutionize the production of babesial vaccines in the foreseable future' [6]. Ristic emphasized the subject by saying 'This achievement which signified a new era in the study of bovine babesiosis, has opened a vast horizon of possibilities ... for development of modern and more effective immunoprophylactic and serodiagnostic methods for control of the disease' [7, 8].

According to the concept of 'premunition' persistence of solid immunity to babesiosis depends upon a maintenance of the live causative agent in the blood. On the other hand, protection in the absence of infection has been demonstrated by Callow [9]. More recently, soluble exoantigens derived from *in vitro* cultures of *B. bovis* and *B. canis* have been shown to be highly immunogenic for cattle and dogs, respectively [8, 10, 11, 12, 13, 14, 15]. In view of a vaccine potential of these culture-derived immunogens, it is now necessary to evaluate the requirements for their industrial development and project certain difficulties that may be associated with such an endeavor. Some aspects of this problem are considered in this paper.

2. Characteristics of an antibabesial vaccine

The vaccine should have certain characteristics to be useful. The vaccine, for example, should prevent or attenuate the clinical disease caused by the babesia in

Ristic, M. et al. (eds.) *Malaria and babesiosis.*
© 1984, Martinus Nijhoff Publishers, Dordrecht/Boston/Lancaster.

question, be effective under field conditions, require a small number of inoculations, and induce protection lasting for a minimum period of six months. In addition the vaccination must not cause the production of antibodies against blood group antigens of the host, nor be harmful to the host. Further, the vaccine must be suitable for parenteral administration to the animal, i.e., it should not be excessively irritating or allergenic. Finally, the vaccine should be stable on storage and be easy to administer in the field, and production costs should be low.

3. Development of antibabesial vaccines

The development of antibabesial vaccines in analogy to those against viral or bacterial infections involves a scientific aspect which requires an evaluation of feasibility. For this, knowledge of the pathogenesis of the disease is required and the vulnerable point of the parasite's life cycle must be determined so that the target of the vaccine, e.g., sporozoite or merozoite can be selected. Vaccine development also has a technological aspect. Techniques for production in large quantities must be developed. Quality must also be assured which means that the vaccine must be safe and potent.

Formulation of the product is also important. Antibabesial vaccines will, as all other biological products, be made by a general scheme of organization according to the master-seed lot system.

3.1. Master seed lot system

3.1.1. Master-seed parasite strain (MSP)
This strain is the ancestral strain, used throughout the production process. It must be homogenous and aliquotes of it must be bottled in separate and clearly identified vials. This strain is used not only for production of the vaccine but also as a challenge strain for potency tests in animals.

3.1.2. Seed lot
The seed parasite is grown from an aliquot of the master-seed parasite strain and is expanded by culture to yield the production-seed parasites. A batch of seed parasites is called the seed lot. It is an homogenous strain bottled in separate and identified vials which is used to inoculate cell-cultures or animals.

3.1.3. Batch
The batch is a large quantity of product produced in a single production run. It is a finished product and is bottled in a number of vials on the same day. Each batch has its own identification number.

3.2. *Practical considerations*

3.2.1. *Cryopreservation*
While there are several important practical aspects to the production process which must be considered, cryopreservation of the parasite is one of the most important. Classical procedures for cryopreservation using the cryopreservatives glycerine, DMSO, PVP or SORBITOL are satisfactory for preservation of *B. canis* strains [16].

3.2.2. *In vitro culture*
In vitro culture of *B. canis* requires fresh parasites from an animal as it is impossible at present to initiate cultures of *B. canis* directly from cryopreserved babesia. The cryopreserved parasites are revived by *in vivo* passage in splenectomized dogs. When parasitemia has reached a maximum level in the splenectomized dog, blood is collected and *in vitro* culture is started. Clean dogs must be maintained in tick-free isolation units as it is important not to contaminate the *B. canis* strain being used. Rhone-Merieux maintains a large kennel of big hunting dogs for *B. canis* research. These dogs are available as blood and/or serum donors (Figure 1).

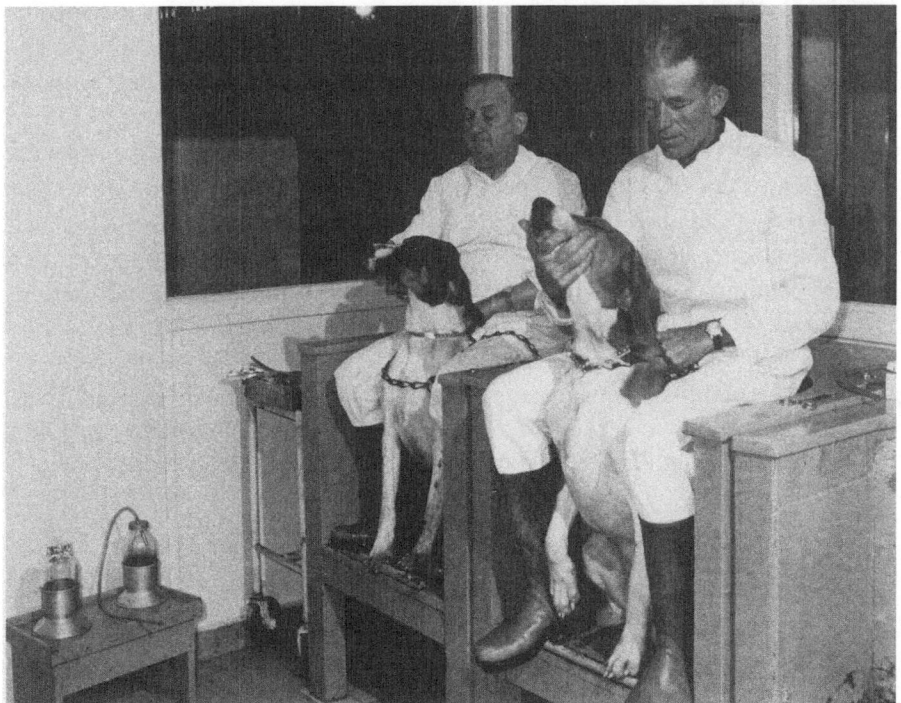

Figure 1. Experimental dogs with their handlers used for research in and production of canine babesiosis vaccine at the Rhone-Merieux Laboratories in Lyon, France.

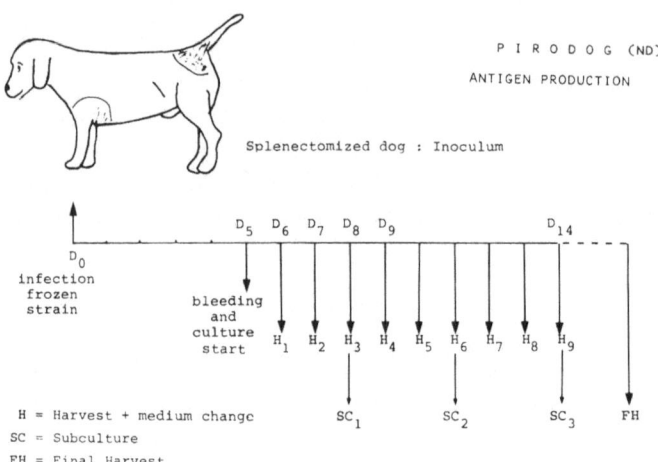

Figure 2. A scheme used for the production of *Babesia canis* 'Pirodog'* vaccine.
* Proposed commercial name for the canine babesiosis vaccine.

3.2.3. *Systemization of production of B. canis vaccine*

In order to produce a uniform product, a flow sheet for production is required
(Figure 2). Blood is collected from the dogs 4 or 5 days after infection with *B.
canis* by intravenous (IV) inoculation. This blood is used to initiate cultures. The
medium in these cultures is changed every 24 hours. Every three days, subcul-
tures using erythrocytes derived from babesia-free dogs are prepared. A final
harvest is made when parasitemia has decreased below 1% which usually occurs
after three weeks of continuous cultivation. Throughout the culture procedure
the supernatant fluids from the cultures are collected by centrifugation, purified
by filtration, and inactivated by formaline treatment. Finally, the supernatant
fluids containing soluble exoantigens are concentrated by ultrafiltration,
lyophilized, and stored frozen until needed. The final formulation of the vaccine
is made shortly before use. This formulation is accomplished by mixing equal
volumes of lyophilized antigens and a diluent which contains an adjuvant. Any
one of several adjuvants can be used. Saponin appears to be an effective adjuvant
for induction of immunity against plasmodia and babesia [8, 12, 15].

3.3. *Control of the vaccine*

A vaccine must be safe, and to determine this requires non-specific safety tests on
classical laboratory animals. Procedures are described by Holgate in the European Pharmacopea [17]. In addition, a specific safety test by use of a natural host,
e.g., the dog for *B. canis* and the cow for *B. bovis* is required. The test animals
must be observed for secondary effects including development of antibodies to
blood group antigens. The vaccine must be sterile. Appropriate tests for sterility

must be made. Sterility tests should include both for aerobic and anaerobic organisms. Finally, the vaccine must be potent. An indirect evaluation of vaccine potency is made by serological means using the IFA or ELISA tests [13].

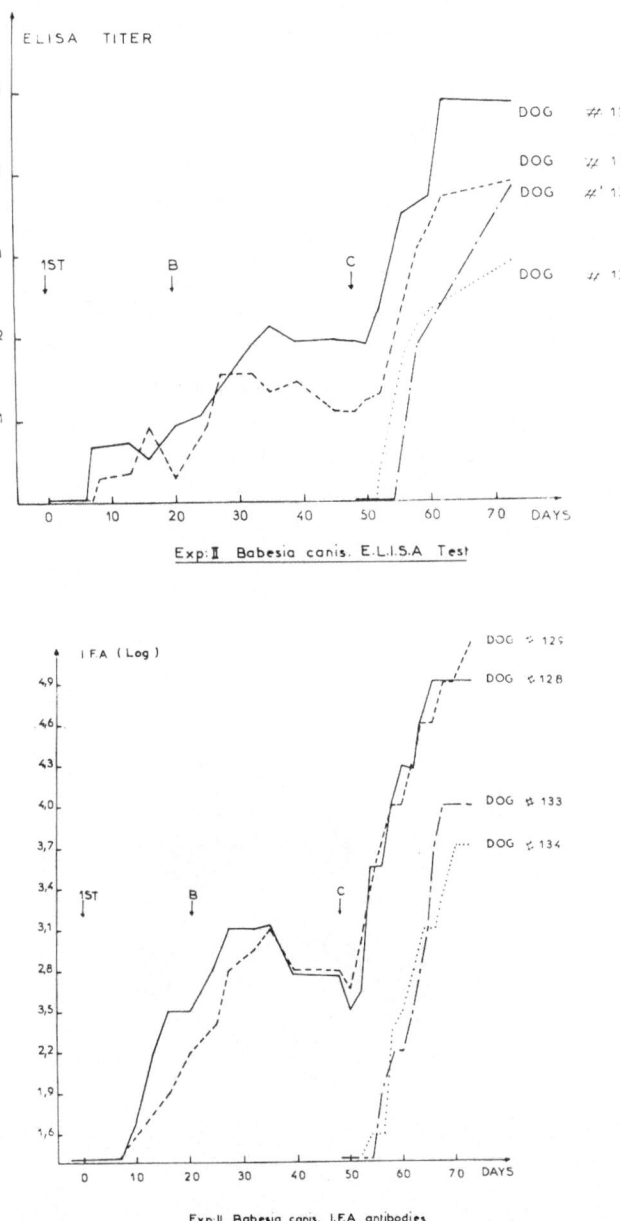

Figures 3 and 4. Immune responses in two vaccinated # 128 and 129 and two non-vaccinated dogs, # 133 and 134 measured by the ELISA (Figure 3) and IFA (Figure 4) tests. On challenge 50 days after the first vaccine dose only two non-vaccinated dogs developed clinical and hematologic responses typical of canine babesiosis. The two vaccinated animals remained clinically well.

134

3.4. *Protective immunity*

The examples of immune responses in two vaccinated dogs # 128 and 129 measured by the ELISA and IFA techniques are given in figures 3 and 4, respectively. These dogs received two vaccine doses within a period of three weeks. Prior to administration the vaccine was admixed with Saponin adjuvant (Quil-A, Superfos Export Company, Vedback, Denmark). The other two dogs, # 133 and 134 served as non-vaccinated controls. All four animals were challenged by intravenous administration of 1×10^7 virulent *B. canis* at 50 days after the first vaccine dose. Following challenge, a prompt anamnestic immune response was noted in the two vaccinated dogs which also failed to develop clinical signs of the disease. The two control dogs developed severe fever, anemia and parasitemia typical of canine babesiosis.

Following completion of a series of laboratory vaccination studies such as those described above, the efficacy of the vaccine was examined under field conditions in France. For this purpose eight regions known as being endemic for canine babesiosis have been selected (Figure 5). A total of 587 dogs (mainly German

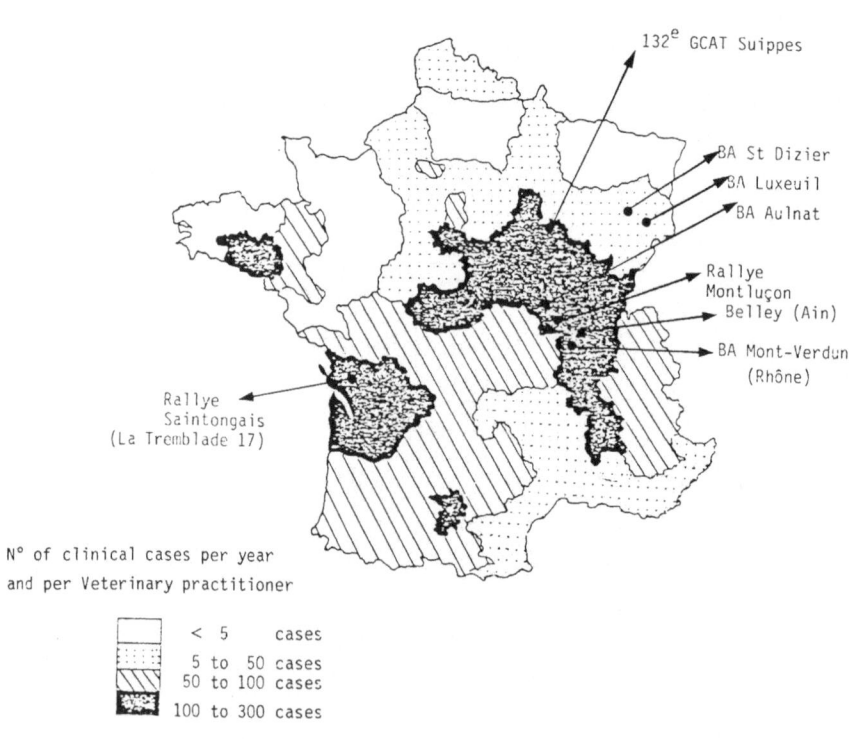

PIRODOG : FIELD CLINICAL TRIALS PLACES

Figure 5. Geographic distribution of canine babesiosis in France. Two principal areas are located on the Southeast coast (Bordeaux) and the east central part of the country, respectively.

Shepherd breed) with 167 vaccinated and 420 controls were used in the study. The distribution of each group of dogs for each of the eight regions is given in table 1.

The results of immune responses, measured by the ELISA technique for vaccinated dogs of the region Belley are given in table 2 and figures 6 and 7. Table 2 gives ELISA titers of individual vaccinated dogs during the examination periods of 35 days and nine months after vaccination. In the majority of dogs there was a good antibody titer conversion following vaccination. Figure 6 shows the pattern of ELISA antibody titer over a period of 9 months in reference to the initial titer at the time of vaccination. Figure 7 represents another version of data presented in figure 6 by providing a closer look into the pattern of titer conversion during individual post vaccination periods.

The numbers of clinical cases of babesiosis among vaccinated and control dogs in the region of Suippes are given in table 3. Among 314 control dogs there were 127 clinical cases of babesiosis as compared to six such cases among 40 vaccinated dogs representing the disease rate difference of 40.4% and 15%, respectively. Seasonal distribution of the disease among the two groups is presented in figure 8. It is evident that most cases occurred during the months of October and November.

These serologic and clinical data document immunogenic potency of the vaccine under both laboratory and field conditions. Accordingly, it is anticipated that the use of such vaccine in France and elsewhere should be useful for the prevention of canine babesiosis.

Table 1. Pirodog: Clinical cases vaccinated and non vaccinated dogs.

Experimental centers	Number		Clinical Cases		Dead	
	T	V	T	V	T	V
	T	V	T	V	T	V
1. Aulnat	4	7	1	0	/	0
2. Belley	0	20	/	0	/	0
3. Luxeuil	40	20	11	0	?	0
4. Mont-Verdun	7	13	0	0	0	0
5. Montluçon	0	17	/	0	/	0
6. Saint-Dizier	40	20	4 $(P^+ + P^-)$	0	0	0
7. Suippes	314	40	127 $(P^+ + P^-)$	6 $\begin{smallmatrix} 2P^+ \\ 4P^- \end{smallmatrix}$	14	0
8. La Tremblade	15	30	0	0	0	0

Observation:
T = Controls
V = Vaccinated
P^+ = Confirmed clinical cases (hematology)
P^- = Non confirmed hematological cases

Table 2. Pirodog: Center Nr. 2 Belley

	Elisa Log 10 Before vaccination	35 days After vaccination	9 months After vaccination	Clinical cases before vaccination	Clinical cases 9 months after vaccination
Waulna	0.50	2.21	0.50	No	No
Merlin	1.31	2.45	0.50	Yes (3)*	No
Milord	1.75	1.75	2.54	Yes (3)	No
Nefsky	0.50	2.23	1.00	Yes (2)	No
Finaud P.	0.50	2.03	2.01	No	No
Elsa	2.39	3.26	1.50	Yes (1)	No
Flora	0.50	1.71	–	No	No
Belle	0.50	2.26	0.50	No	No
Wolf	1.82	2.78	1.84	Yes (1)	No
Rack	1.14	2.67	1.91	Yes (1)	No
Roucky	1.34	2.48	1.00	Yes (1)	No
Junon	0.50	1.87	0.50	No	No
Nouchka	1.33	2.35	0.50	Yes (1)	No
Dick	0.50	1.97	1.00	No	No
Pataud	0.50	2.28	0.80	No	No
Finette	1.18	2.66	2.05	No	No
Nat	1.99	3.24	0.80	Yes (1)	No
Olaf	2.13	2.16	–	Yes (3)	No
Gamin	0.50	0.50	–	No	No
Finaud	1.23	2.18	–	No	No

* n° of relapses

3.5. *Economic aspects of immunization*

Marketing decisions may suggest that a compromise between performance and cost of the vaccine is required, but efficacy cannot be compromised excessively for economy. The product must produce strong immunity or it will soon be discarded and then not even be of value economically. The biologists must convince the marketing team that a weak product is not cheap at any cost.

4. Conclusion

In conclusion, there are three main phases in the industrial development of any antibabesial vaccine: (1) *Research phase:* here epidemiological surveys and analysis of existing models will be made. The type of vaccine to be developed is chosen. Living or killed, and sporozoite and merozoite vaccines are evaluated. In this phase trials with small volumes of vaccine are made. The conditions for production of antigens including media, temperature, gas and stability are evaluated.

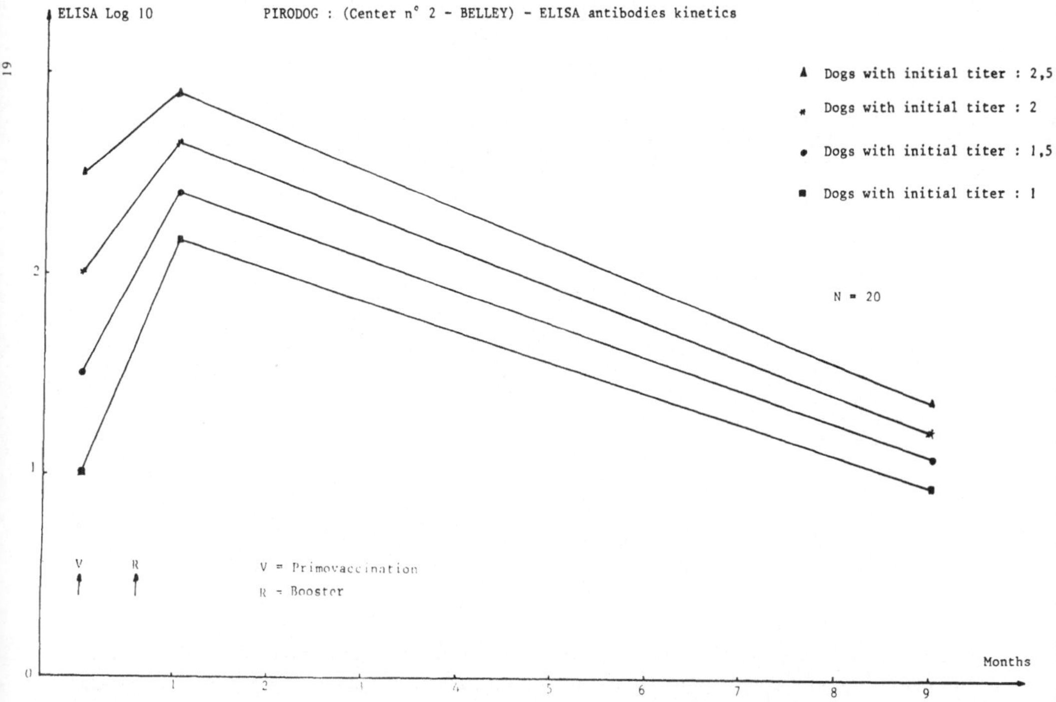

Figure 6. Field trial with *Babesia canis* vaccine in the region of Belley. The pattern of the ELISA antibody titer in vaccinated dogs over a period of 9 months is given.

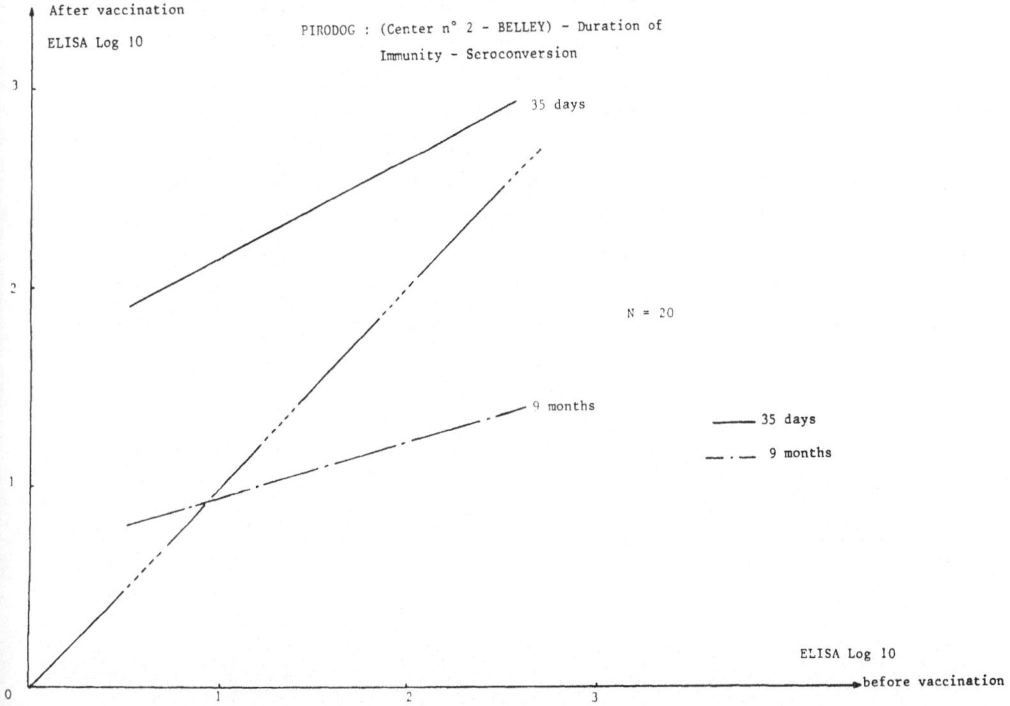

Figure 7. Field trial with *Babesia canis* vaccine in the region of Belley. A closer view of the pattern of titer conversion during individual post vaccination periods.

138

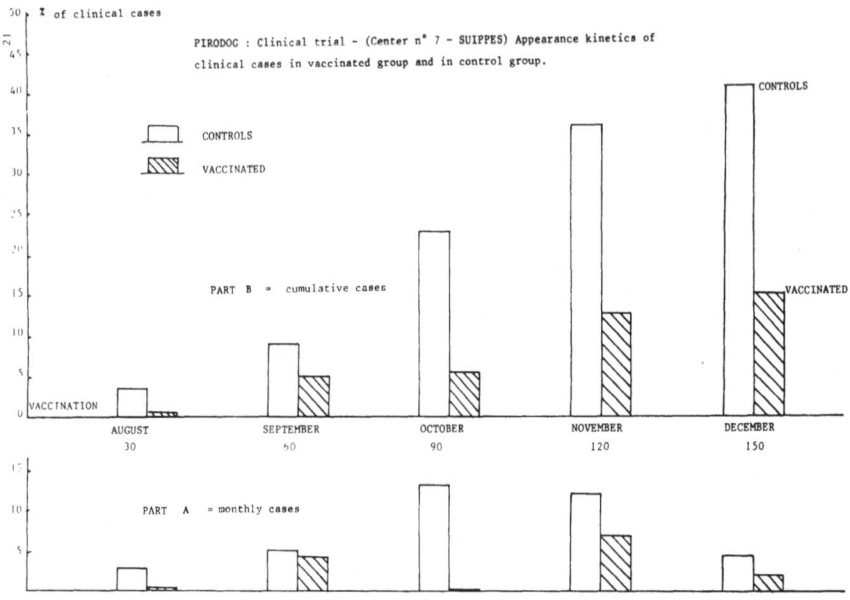

Figure 8. Field trial with *Babesia canis* vaccine in the region of Suippes with distribution of clinical cases in the vaccinated and control groups. It is indicated that most of the cases occurred during the months of October and November, reflecting seasonal disease manifestation.

The reproducibility of the technique is determined. Antigens and sera are used for serologic studies of the various batches of trial vaccines and experimental challenges are carried out. (2) *Pilot phase:* in the pilot phase the process is scaled up. The volumes of antigen produced are larger than in the research phase. Different types of materials for culture are evaluated in this phase; comparing cost and efficiency. This is crucial, because industrial cost evaluation is made from data collected in the pilot phase of development. In this phase, stability, safety, antibody kinetics, and immunity continue to be evaluated. These data are used in

Table 3. Pirodog: clinical trials (Center n° 7 - Suippes) Kinetics of appearance of clinical cases in vaccinated and control groups.

Clinical cases days after vaccination	Controls N = 314 dogs			Vaccinated N = 40 dogs		
	N° cases	%	Cumulative % cases	N° cases	%	Cumulative % cases
30	11	3.5	11	3.5 0	0	0	0
60	17	5.4	28	8.9 2	5	2	5
90	44	14	72	23 0	0	2	5
120	39	12.4	111	35.3 3	7.5	5	12.5
150	16	5.1	127	40.4 1	2.5	6	15

the preparation of the licensing dossier which must demonstrate to the licensing agencies that the producers of the vaccine have analytical, pharmacotoxicological, and clinical expertise and that the product is safe and effective. (3) *Industrialization phase:* if all is well, the decision to launch the product is taken. Industrialization of the process is a complex step. Raw materials must be purchased and systems for production and control of the vaccine on a commercial scale are developed. The product must be bottled and packaged in an attractive fashion and finally marketed.

At the present time, inactivated antigens prepared from *in vitro* culture supernatants of *Babesia canis* are in phase two of development. They have been demonstrated to be pure, safe, potent and efficacious by both laboratory and field trials. They will soon enter phase three, industrial production. Data is now being collected for submission to appropriate regulatory agencies. We can look forward to the availability of a vaccine against canine babesiosis based on antigens derived from cell culture fluids in the near future.

References

1. Mahoney DF: Immunization against blood-derived antigens of Babesia. In: Babesiosis. M Ristic and JP Kreier (eds.). Academic Press, Inc, New York, NY, 1981, p. 475–507.
2. Erp EE, Gravely SM, Smith RD, Ristic M, Osorno BM and Carson CA: Growth of *Babesia bovis* in bovine erythrocyte cultures. Am J Trop Med Hyg 27:1061–1064, 1978.
3. Erp EE, Smith RD, Ristic M and Osorno BM: Continuous *in vitro* cultivation of *Babesia bovis*. Am J Vet Res 41:1141–1142, 1980.
4. Levy MG and Ristic M: *Babesia bovis:* continuous cultivation in microaerophilous stationary phase culture. Science 207:1218–1220, 1980.
5. Moreau Y and Soula A: *Babesia canis.* La culture *in vitro* du parasite et son etude ultrastructurale. Bull Soc Sci Vet et Med Comparee - Lyon, 81 (5):255–261, 1979.
6. Mahoney DF: Prospects of an antibabesial vaccine. In: *Babesiosis.* M Ristic and JP Kreier (eds.). Academic Press Inc, New York, NY 1981, p. 555–562.
7. Ristic M: Comments on prospects for antibabesial vaccine. In: *Babesiosis.* M Ristic and JP Kreier (eds.) Academic Press Inc, New York, NY 1981, p. 563–566.
8. Ristic M and Levy MG: A new era of research toward solution of bovine babesiosis. In: Babesiosis. M Ristic and JP Kreier (eds.). Academic Press Inc, New York, NY 1981, p. 509–544.
9. Callow LL: Vaccination against bovine babesiosis. In: Immunity to Blood Parasites of Animals and Man. LH Miller, JA Pino, JJ McKelvey Jr (eds.). Pleanum Press, New York, NY 1977, p. 121–149.
10. Smith RD and Ristic M: Immunization against bovine babesiosis with culture derived antigens. In: *Babesiosis.* M Ristic and JP Kreier (eds.). Academic Press, Inc, New York, NY, 1981, p. 485–507.
11. Smith RD, James MA, Ristic M, Aikawa M, Vega CA: Bovine babesiosis: Protection of cattle with culture-derived soluble *Babesia bovis* antigen. Science 212:335–338, 1981.
12. Kuttler KL, Levy MG, Ristic M: Cell culture-derived *Babesia bovis* vaccine: Sequential challenge exposure of protective immunity during a 6-month post vaccination period. Am J Vet Res 44:1456–1459, 1983.
13. Laurent N, Moreau Y, Levy M and Ristic M: A vaccine against canine babesiosis using a soluble antigen derived from cell culture of *Babesia canis.* Vet Parasit. In Press, 1985.

14. Laurent N, Moreau Y, Levy MG, Ristic M: A vaccine against canine babesiosis using a soluble antigen derived from cell culture of *Babesia canis*. (Abstract). Proc 2nd Int Conf Malaria and Babesiosis, Sept. 18–22, 1983, Annecy, France, p. 106.

15. Molinar E, James MA, Kakoma I, Holland CJ, Ristic M: Antigenic and immunogenic studies on cell culture-derived *Babesia canis*. Vet Parasit *10*:29–40, 1982.

16. Joyner LP: The laboratory maintenance of tick borne protozoa. In: Isolation and maintenance of parasites *in vivo*. A Taylor and R Maller (eds.). Blackwell Scientific Publications, Oxford, England 1971, p. 1–37.

17. Holgate JA: European Pharmacopea, Counsil of Europe Paris, France 1980, p. v211–v225.

10. Recent developments in chemotherapy and drug resistance

WALLACE PETERS

Department of Medical Protozoology, London School of Hygiene and Tropical Medicine, Keppel Street, London WC1E 7HT, England.

1. Introduction

Resistance of human malaria parasites to drugs is of several types. It may be against: (1) compounds acting on pathways of folate metabolism, e.g., pyrimethamine, proguanil, sulphonamides, sulphones (these may affect all developmental stages); (2) compounds affecting haemoglobin metabolism of asexual intra-erythrocytic parasites, e.g. chloroquine and other 4-aminoquinolines; (3) compounds influencing asexual intraerythrocytic stages by mechanisms so far undetermined, e.g., quinine, mefloquine; (4) compounds influencing secondary hepatic stages (hypnozoites) and gametocytes, e.g., primaquine.

To date resistance of type 1 has been found in all species of human *Plasmodium* except *P. ovale*. *P. vivax* is commonly resistant to pyrimethamine and is inherently insensitive to sulphonamides and sulphones.

Resistance of types 2 and 3 has only been observed in *P. falciparum*. Scattered reports of chloroquine resistance in *P. vivax* have never been substantiated.

Type 4 resistance is only of importance in *P. vivax*. The level of resistance in the field is of a relatively low order and seldom prohibits the use of this compound for the radical cure of *P. vivax*, although in some areas, e.g., Papua New Guinea, high doses at the limit of tolerability may be required.

In practice problems arise mainly with *P. falciparum* since most strains resistant to type 2 compounds show concomitant resistance to type 1.

Some in addition are beginning to show resistance also to type 3. So far such strains of *P. falciparum* have retained their sensitivity to the gametocytocidal properties of primaquine.

2. Drug resistance in P. vivax, P. malariae and P. ovale

Plasmodium vivax is commonly transmitted in the same areas as *P. falciparum* particularly in Southeast Asia, the Western Pacific and in South America. This

Ristic, M. et al. (eds.) *Malaria and babesiosis.*
© 1984, Martinus Nijhoff Publishers, Dordrecht/Boston/Lancaster.

parasite is more localized on the African continent where *P. falciparum* causes over 90% of all infections, the rest being mainly *P. malariae* and *P. ovale*.

Resistance to pyrimethamine and proguanil is common in *P. vivax*. Consequently, these compounds cannot always be relied upon to provide prophylactic cover against this parasite. Pyrimethamine acts synergistically when given with sulphonamides (e.g., sulfadoxine), and possible with dapsone. This synergism does not appear to apply when the combinations are used against *P. vivax*, probably because this parasite is unresponsive to sulphonamides. As a result many infections break through the combination, suggesting that the parasites have become resistant to the pyrimethamine component.

Primaquine resistance in *P. vivax* implies the failure of normal doses to eliminate the intrahepatic hypnozoites, thus necessitating increased doses (e.g., 22.5 mg base daily for 14 days) to produce radical cure.

Resistance of *P. malariae* and *P. ovale* to antimalarial drugs does not appear to pose practical problems in clinical or field practice.

3. Spread of chloroquine resistance in P. falciparum

The geographical spread of chloroquine resistant *P. falciparum* with time may be assessed from figure 1. The first reports were in 1960 and 1961 [1]. The general pattern of spread appears to be exponential following the initial establishment of foci of resistant parasites [2]. First indications of resistance are the failure of chloroquine prophylaxis in nonimmunes and the failure of a standard therapeutic regimen to bring about radical cure of established infections. First resistant infections in a given geographical area may be of a low order (RI or RII) and are usually recognized in visitors or immigrants. Later on, RIII type resistance is seen [3]. At the same time RI and RII type responses start to appear in semi-immunes [4]. If *in vitro* sensitivity monitoring is carried out it will commonly be found at this stage that low level resistance is present in a significant proportion of the indigenous population, even before overt clinical resistance is seen. Finally the level, as well as extent of resistance in the indigenous population increase at an exponential rate until chloroquine becomes of little value as a radical curative drug.

4. Concomitant resistance of P. falciparum to other drugs

Since the earliest reports of chloroquine resistance in *P. falciparum* a variable pattern of concomitant resistance has been observed to drugs of quite different types (table 1).

Among the alternative drugs of which we have at least preliminary clinical experience (apart from the 4-aminoquinolines), the only ones to which con-

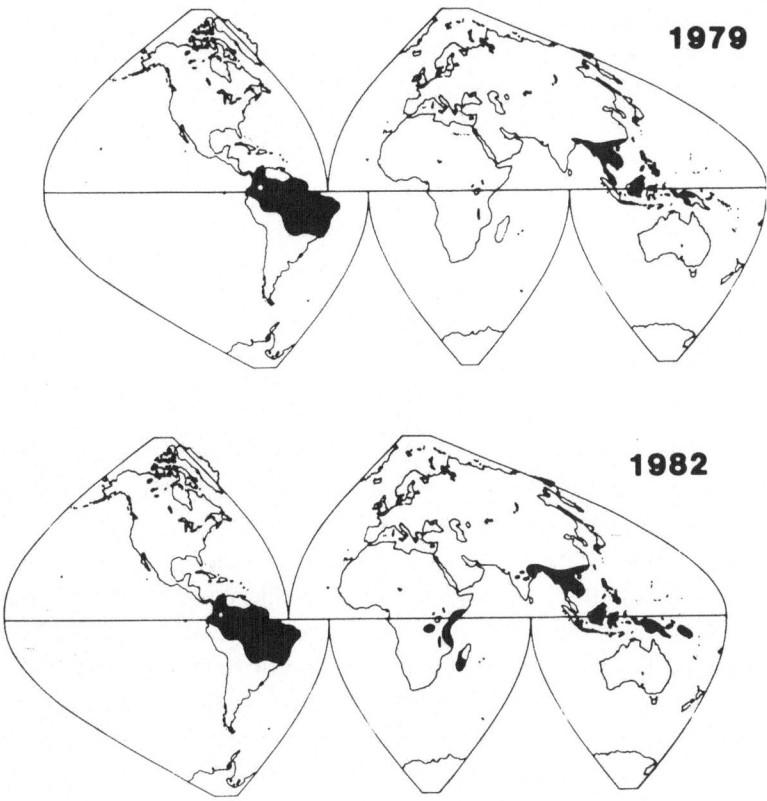

Figure 1. Distribution of chloroquine-resistant *P. falciparum* in 1979 and 1982.

comitant resistance seems not yet to have appeared are the tetracyclines, the artemisinine series, pyronaridine and hydroxypiperaquine. It is disturbing to note several indications, albeit preliminary and in isolated cases only, of poor responses to mefloquine in several localities [5]. This compound has, to date, only been employed officially in controlled clinical trials. The rapid appearance of concomitant resistance in chloroquine-resistant strains of *P. falciparum* underlines the need to 'protect' any new drugs that become available (see below). Quinine and tetracycline may be required for therapy if all else fails [6].

5. Mechanism of action of chloroquine and genetics of resistance

Current studies on the mode of action of chloroquine confirm earlier reports that this drug interferes in some manner with the digestion by the intraerythrocytic parasites of host cell haemoglobin. Exactly how this occurs, however, is not yet clear. The hypothesis that chloroquine binds with haematin, an intermediate breakdown product of haemoglobin, to form a highly haemolytic complex that

Table 1. Earliest reports of concomitant resistance to other drugs in chloroquine-resistant strains of *Plasmodium falciparum*

Compound	First reports Countries	Year
pyrimethamine	Venezuela	1961
proguanil	Thailand, Malaysia, Vietnam	1963
cycloguanil pamoate	Thailand, Malaysia	1965
pyrimethamine-dapsone	Cambodia	1968
pyrimethamine-sulfadoxine	Cambodia	1968
quinine	Brazil, Malaysia	1967
mefloquine	Thailand, Phillipines	1982

disrupts the host cell, does not satisfy all the known facts and other explanations are still being sought of the manner in which chloroquine kills the parasites.

This situation makes it difficult to explain how the malaria parasite becomes resistant to chloroquine. What can be shown is that erythrocytes containing chloroquine-resistant *P. falciparum* bind less chloroquine than do equivalent numbers containing chloroquine-sensitive organisms, an observation that was first made on the rodent parasite, *P. berghei.* In rodent malaria chloroquine resistance is a character that is inherited along classical Mendelian lines [7]. Resistant parasites appear to be dominant over sensitive ones. They also appear to be more readily infective to anopheline vectors that feed on chloroquine treated animals than are sensitive organisms. This observation has been confirmed in *P. falciparum* in Thailand [2]. Several investigators have commented on the relative vigour of chloroquine resistant *P. falciparum* when such lines are maintained *in vitro.* Chloroquine resistance appears to be associated, therefore, with several biological advantages as compared with sensitive parasites, perhaps thus explaining the rapidity with which the problem appears to spread in an endemic area once a focus is established.

6. New drugs in development

In figure 2 are shown several compounds that are in pre-clinical studies or clinical trial. One of the most promising of these is mefloquine (Figure 2A) which has been extensively studied in Southeast Asia, South America and tropical Africa [8]. Mefloquine should shortly be made available through national health authorities in areas where chloroquine and concomitant drug resistance make the treatment of falciparum malaria a practical problem at the present time. Test kits for monitoring the *in vitro* response of *P. falciparum* to mefloquine are available from WHO [9]. Another compound that has received extensive clinical trial in the People's Republic of China is artemisinine (Qinghaosu) (Figure 2C) [10]. Both

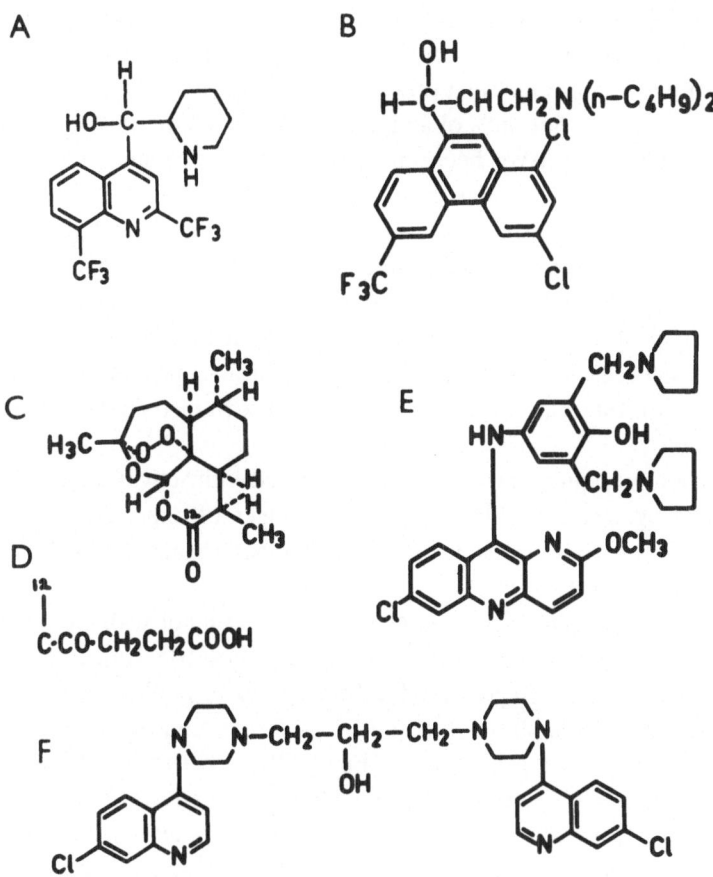

Figure 2. Chemical structures of some new antimalarials. A. mefloquine, B. halofantrine, C. artemisinine (Qinghaosu), D. artesunate, E. pyronaridine, F. hydroxypiperaquine.

mefloquine and artemisinine have been shown to produce radical cure in a high proportion of patients infected with multiple resistant *P. falciparum* [11]. Both compounds are active also against the asexual stages of *P. vivax*. Neither has any action on intrahepatic stages of either species, nor on mature gametocytes.

Because the onset of action of mefloquine may be rather slow, it has been recommended that treatment of a severe or complicated attack of falciparum malaria should be initiated with quinine [12]. Both compounds appear to share the same mode of action, interfering with membranous structures within the parasites, but whereas quinine is rapidly excreted, mefloquine remains in the body for several weeks. It has recently been shown that quinidine may replace quinine for parenteral treatment of such emergencies as cerebral malaria [13]. At present mefloquine is not recommended for prophylaxis for the reason discussed below. It has so far proved impossible to develop a formulation of mefloquine for parenteral use.

Artemisinine is administered in a lipid suspension because of its poor solubility and it too does not lend itself to intravenous administration. Unlike mefloquine, the response to an intramuscular dose of artemisinine is very rapid, but recrudescences occur in from 5 to 10% of all infections of *P. falciparum* or *P. vivax*. The reason for this has not yet been determined. In experimental rodent models strains resistant to artemisinine are readily developed [10].

A number of semi-synthetic derivatives of artemisinine have been found to be more active than the parent compound. One of these, artesunate (Figure 2D), that can be administered intravenously, has proved highly effective in the treatment of cerebral malaria and is being further studied in this indication. Experimental, toxicological and clinical studies of the artemisinine series are being guided by a joint steering committee of the Chinese Ministry of Health and WHO [10].

Several 8-aminoquinolines have been described with activity superior to that of primaquine against both blood and tissue stages of experimental malaria in rodents and monkeys [14]. None have yet been made available for clinical trial in patients with vivax malaria.

Halofantrine (Figure 1B), a 9-phenanthrenemethanol with similar mode of action to that of mefloquine, is in preliminary clinical trial [15]. It is too early to assess its possible advantages and disadvantages over mefloquine.

Two other new antimalarials have been reported in clinical trial. One of these is the Chinese compound, pyronaridine (Figure 2E), a benzonaphthyridine derivative with a Mannich base type sidechain which has been shown to retain activity against chloroquine resistant strains of *P. falciparum in vitro* and is claimed to be active also in man. A second type of compound is a bisquinoline derivative with a piperazine linkage, hydroxypiperaquine (Figure 2F) which Chinese workers claim is also active against chloroquine resistant *P. falciparum* in man [16]. It shows marked cross resistance with chloroquine in rodent models.

7. Future strategy

Three questions have to be resolved for the future: (1) How best to deploy existing antimalarial drugs?; (2) How to minimize the spread of resistance to existing compounds?; (3) How to 'protect' any new antimalarials from the problem of resistance?

7.1. Deployment of existing drugs

This topic has been considered at length in a number of basic WHO documents, particularly that by Bruce-Chwatt et al. [9]. Participants at a WHO workshop on drug-resistant malaria held in Manila [17] and at a more recent meeting in Kuala

Lumpur [18] laid stress on the necessity to consider the use of drugs as only one measure in a national control programme, emphasis being laid on the need to limit transmission by vector control measures, and to deploy primaquine as a gametocytocide especially in areas where chloroquine resistance already exists. These valuable documents should be consulted in the original.

7.2. *Minimizing the spread of resistance to existing drugs*

As suggested above, chloroquine resistant *P. falciparum*, unlike parasites resistant to dihydrofolate reductase inhibitors, appear to have biological advantages that permit them to overgrow sensitive parasite populations in the same area. Limitation of the spread of resistant parasites demands, therefore, drastic measures that must include: (1) Intensification of vector control procedures; (2) Use of alternative blood schizontocides if available; (3) Deployment of primaquine as a gametocytocide; (4) Monitoring and reporting of *in vitro* and *in vivo* responses of *P. falciparum* to chloroquine and other compounds; (5) Where indicated, monitoring and, if necessary, treatment of immigrants from areas with resistance to vulnerable areas without this problem.

Detailed recommendations on these measures are given by Bruce-Chwatt et al. [9] and WHO [18]. Wernsdorfer [19] has stressed the need for flexibility in designing appropriate measures according to the conditions prevailing in any given locality.

7.3 *'Protection' of new antimalarials*

The history of malaria chemotherapy makes it quite clear that one or more species of malaria parasites of man, and particularly *P. falciparum*, has become resistant in time to every antimalarial drug that has so far been produced [1]. The use of *appropriate* drug combinations, however, can slow down the rate at which this phenomenon develops. Stress is laid on the word *appropriate* and on the need to select combinations not empirically, but on the basis of prior experimentation in animal models. Thus the empirically selected combination of chloroquine with pyrimethamine that was extensively employed in large-scale malaria control programs in the 1950's and 1960's failed to stop *P. falciparum* becoming resistant to either compound in many areas. On the contrary, the combination of pyrimethamine with sulfadoxine 'protected' these compounds to the extent that this combination could be utilized widely for nearly 15 years before resistance to it became a problem (by contrast, resistance developed to pyrimethamine within one year of its being used on its own). Both situations could have been forecast using rodent malaria models.

Several investigators including the writer [20] have shown clearly in rodent models that a triple combination containing mefloquine, pyrimethamine and sulfadoxine significantly slows down the rate at which resistance develops to any of the components, even in a parasite that is already resistant to chloroquine. A combination of these compounds for use in man is currently being developed under WHO auspices in the hope that this will prolong the useful life of mefloquine and the other components in the field. However, because mefloquine is urgently needed for the treatment of severe falciparum malaria in areas where other drugs are failing, limited quantities of this compound will soon be released to governments for emergency use. It is important that mefloquine should not be misused, but retained for treatment only. The combination, when it becomes available, would be more suitable for prophylaxis but, even then, it should only be used for malaria control in combination with other measures, especially vector control.

The same principle should apply also to artemisinine and its derivatives, although these are currently foreseen rather as drugs for treatment than as malaria prophylactics. The same naturally should apply to other new drugs as they become available for use in endemic areas.

8. Summary

The types of antimalarial resistance found in human malaria parasites are reviewed. The most important is resistance of *P. falciparum* to chloroquine which may carry with it concomitant resistance to other compounds such as pyrimethamine, pyrimethamine-sulphonamide combinations, and quinine. Chloroquine resistance does not occur in the other species, although pyrimethamine resistance is common in *P. vivax*.

Chloroquine resistance is spreading rapidly in *P. falciparum* and resistant strains are now firmly established in East Africa. While the mechanisms involved are still uncertain, chloroquine resistant mutants appear to dominate over sensitive parasites.

Of several new drugs in development, mefloquine and artemisinine are the ones most advanced in clinical trials. Their uses and limitations are discussed briefly.

Suggestions are given for making the best use of existing antimalarials, limiting the spread of resistance, and 'protecting' new drugs by the use of appropriate drug combinations.

Acknowledgements

Studies carried out in the writer's laboratory received financial support from the CHEMAL component of the UNDP/World Bank/WHO Special Program for Research and Training in Tropical Diseases, and from the US Army Medical Research and Development Command, Department of the Army, under various contracts in collaboration with the Walter Reed Army Institute of Research, Division of Experimental Therapeutics.

References

1. Peters W: Chemotherapy and drug resistance in malaria. Academic Press, London, 1970.
2. Peters W: Antimalarial drug resistance: an increasing problem. British Medical Bulletin, 38:187–192, 1982.
3. Weniger BG, Blumberg RS, Campbell CC, Jones TC, Mount DL and Friedman SM: High-level chloroquine resistance of *Plasmodium falciparum* acquired in Kenya. New England Journal of Medicine, 30:1500–1502, 1983.
4. Kihamia CS and Gill HS: Chloroquine-resistant falciparum malaria in semi-immune native African Tanzanians. Lancet, 2:43, 1982.
5. Boudreau EF, Webster HK, Pavanand K and Thosingha L: Type II mefloquine resistance in Thailand. Lancet, 2:1335, 1982.
6. Reacher M, Campbell CC, Freeman J, Doberstyn EB and Brandling-Bennett AD: Drug therapy for *Plasmodium falciparum* malaria resistant to pyrimethamine-sulfadoxine (Fansidar). Lancet, 2:1066–1068, 1981.
7. Beale GH, Carter R and Walliker D: Genetics. In: Rodent malaria. Killick-Kendrick, R. and Peters, W. (eds.). Academic Press, London, 1978. p. 213–245.
8. WHO. Report of a section meeting of the Scientific Working Group on the Chemotherapy of Malaria. TDR/CHEMAL-SWG (MEFLO)/81.3 (WHO cyclostyled report). 1981a, WHO, Geneva.
9. Bruce-Chwatt LJ, Black RH, Canfield CJ, Clyde DF, Peters W and Wernsdorfer WH: Chemotherapy of malaria. Second edition. WHO, Geneva, 1981.
10. WHO. The development of Qinghaosu and its derivatives as antimalarial drugs. TDR/CHEMAL-SWG(QHS)/81.3 (WHO cyclostyled report). 1981b, WHO, Geneva.
11. Jiang JB, Li GO, Guo XB, Kong YC and Arnold K: Antimalarial activity of mefloquine and qinghaosu. Lancet, 2:285–288, 1982.
12. Hall AP, Doberstyn EB, Karnchanachetanee C, Samransamruajkit S, Laixuthai B, Pearlman EJ, Lampe RM, Miller CF and Phintuyothin P: Sequential treatment with quinine and mefloquine or quinine and pyrimethamine sulfadoxine for falciparum malaria. British Medical Journal, 1:1626–1628, 1977.
13. White NJ, Looareesuwan S, Warrell DA, Chongsuphajaisiddhi T, Bunnag D and Harinasuta T: Quinidine in falciparum malaria. Lancet, 2:1069–1071, 1981.
14. Davidson DE, Ager AL, Brown JL, Chapple FE, Whitmire RE and Rossan RN: New tissue schizontocidal antimalarial drugs. Bulletin of the World Health Organization, 59:463–479, 1981.
15. Cosgriff TM, Boudreau EF, Pamplin CL, Doberstyn EB, Desjardins RE and Canfield CJ: Evaluation of the antimalarial activity of the phenanthrenemethanol halofantrine (WR 171, 669). Am J Trop Med & Hyg, 31:1075–1079, 1982.
16. Howells RE: Advances in chemotherapy. British Medical Bulletin, 38:193–199, 1982.
17. WHO. Final Report. Workshop on drug-resistant malaria. 23 May to 2 June 1978, Manila ICP/MPD/006. (WHO cyclostyled report). Regional Office for the Western Pacific of WHO, Manila, 1978.
18. WHO. Drug-resistant malaria. Wernsdorfer, W. (ed.). UNDP/World Bank/WHO Special Programme for Research and Training in Tropical Diseases, Geneva, 1982.
19. Wernsdorfer WH: Drug resistance, current studies and future prospects. Scandinavian Journal of Infectious Diseases, 36 (supplement):26–30, 1982.
20. Peters W and Robinson BL: The chemotherapy of rodent malaria XXXV. Further studies on the retardation of drug resistance by the use of a triple combination of mefloquine, pyrimethamine and sulfadoxine in mice infected with *P. berghei* and '*P. berghei* NS'. Ann Trop Med Parisit (In Press), 1984.

11. Chemotherapy of babesiosis

KENNETH L. KUTTLER[1] AND
YUSUF O. ALIU[2]

[1] From the US Department of Agriculture, Agricultural Research Service, Hemo-parasitic Diseases Research Unit, Washington State University, Pullman, WA 99164.
[2] Veterinary Physiology and Pharmacology, Ahmadu Bello University, Zaria, Nigeria.

1. Introduction

Babesiosis (Texas fever, redwater, tick fever, etc.) was first described in 1893 by Smith and Kilborne as a tick-transmitted disease of cattle, characterized by anemia, fever, and hemoglobinuria [1]. Since then, however, it has been found that most domestic and many wild mammals are susceptible to a wide variety of *Babesia* species [2]. These babesias tend to be host-specific, but this is not always the case. Generally, however, the disease in a given mammalian host, referred to as babesiosis, is caused by a specific *Babesia* species. A list of different babesias and their major vertebrate hosts, as discussed in this review, is given in table 1. With the ever broadening scope of babesiosis in man and animal, increasing attention is being given to the development of appropriate treatment to moderate clinical signs in acutely infected individuals, to eliminate, and to prevent infection.

Economically, babesiosis is probably of greatest importance in cattle. With few exceptions, babesiosis is found worldwide but is of primary concern in the tropics and subtropics. In the US, treatment of cattle for babesiosis has assumed a secondary role because of a successful tick eradication program. Babesiosis virtually disappeared in the US when the one-host *Boophilus* ticks were eradicated. In most other areas of the world, however, ticks have not been eradicated, and the disease persists and is controlled by a variety of measures, including chemotherapy and chemoprophylaxis.

In recent years, a number of human cases of babesiosis have been reported, incriminating *Babesia* species that are normally found only in other mammals [2]. *Babesia microti, Babesia divergens, Babesia bovis*, and *Babesia equi* have all been suspected of causing babesiosis in man [3, 4, 5]. The pathogen most commonly involved appears to be *Babesia microti*. For years it was thought that babesiosis in man was confined to asplenic or immunosuppressed individuals, but more recently, several foci of infections have been identified in northeastern US, where the disease has become endemic, being transmitted by the hard tick, *Ixodes dammini*, from infected rodents [6, 7].

Ristic, M. et al. (eds.) *Malaria and babesiosis.*
© 1984, Martinus Nijhoff Publishers, Dordrecht/Boston/Lancaster.

Table 1. Babesia spp: Man and domestic animals

Vertebrate host	Organism (Babesia)	Average size and typical morphology
Cattle	B. bigemina	4–5 × 2.0 µm. (Large, pear-shaped, acute angle in paired form.)
	B. bovis (Syn. B. berbera and B. argentina)	2.0 × 1.5 µm. (Small, more rounded; obtuse angle in paired forms.)
	B. major	2.6 × 1.5 µm. (Similar to B. bigemina but slightly smaller.)
	B. divergens	1.5 × 1.0 µm. (Similar to B. bovis but slightly smaller.)
Sheep and goats	B. motasi	2.5–4.0 × 2.0 µm. (Large, pyriform; acute angle in paired forms.)
	B. ovis	1.5 × 1.0 µm. (Small, more rounded; obtuse angle in paired forms.)
Horses	B. caballi	3.0 × 2.0 µm. (Large, pyriform; acute angle in paired forms.)
	B. equi	1.7 × 2.0 µm. (Small and rounded; obtuse angle in paired forms; Maltese cross is characteristic.)
Swine	B. trautmanni	3.5 × 2.0 µm. (Large, narrow and long; acute angle in paired forms.)
	B. perroncitoi	0.7–2.0 µm. diameter. (Small, more rounded.)
Dogs	B. canis	5.0 × 2.5 µm. (Large, pyriform; acute angle in paired form.)
	B. gibsoni	1.2–3.2 µm diameter. (Small, more rounded, pleomorphic; similar to B. equi.)
Cats	B. felis	1.0–2.5 µm diameter. (Small, rounded.)
	B. herpailuri	2.6 × 1.3 µm. (Large, pyriform, acute angle in paired forms.)
Man	B. microti	Small, highly pleomorphic.
	B. divergens	(See above)

Babesiosis is emerging as an increasingly important disease in dogs, both in Europe and the US, where it has been introduced from endemic zones in the tropics and subtropics [8]. Babesiosis in sheep and swine has been recognized in recent years as the cause of losses in these animals [2, 9]. A problem of babesiosis in cats has been described in South Africa, which disease responds favorably to antimalarial therapy [10]. Equine babesiosis is widespread, where it occasionally produces clinical disease associated with death [2]. A major concern with this infection is the restriction it imposes on the movement of horses and the demand that carrier horses be cleared by chemotherapy before being imported into areas where the disease does not occur.

2. Treatment strategy

A large number of chemical compounds have been used in the treatment of babesiosis, with varying degrees of success. A list of some of the more commonly used compounds is presented in table 2. In addition to the use of babesiacidal compounds, supportive treatment should not be overlooked. If specific and effective treatment is given early in the course of infection, before the onset of severe anemia or nervous system disorders, recovery is the rule. If delayed, however, supportive treatment, including blood transfusions, fluids, vitamins, hematinics, and good nourishment, become essential to the patient's survival. The exertion and excitement associated with the restraint of some animals being treated may actually contribute to death. Judgment as to when and how extensively an animal is to be handled and treated must take into account the animal's temperament, location, and stage of infection. It is possible that in some instances no treatment is indicated, even though infection is advanced [11].

Treatment of babesiosis is usually concerned with moderating clinical signs, characterized by fever and anemia associated with parasitemia. Some of the babesiacidal compounds are quite effective and one injection will eliminate the causative organism. This enables a reservoir of infection to be eliminated, but in some instances may be undesirable if the animal is to be kept in an endemic zone, where reexposure will occur. Elimination of *Babesia* by treatment eventually renders the animal susceptible to reinfection [12]. If treatment eliminates infection early in the course of the disease, the level of sterile immunity is less than if treatment follows a high parasitemia. Reexposure, when sterile immunity is strong, may not result in clinical disease, and a premunizing infection is acquired [13]. But if reinfection is delayed and sterile immunity has waned, then infection may be associated with clinical signs and even death.

The establishment of drug efficacy in the treatment of babesiosis is complicated by the large number of babesias and vertebrate hosts, with differing degrees of drug susceptibility and tolerance. *Babesia rodhaini* infection in mice has been used to screen potential babesiacidal compounds [14, 15]. Caution is recommended in such trials since results can be misleading. An example is that diminazene, while highly effective against most bovine babesias, is not equally as effective against *B. rodhaini* [11]. The recent demonstration of the susceptibility of the Mongolian gerbil to *Babesia divergens* from cattle provides an additional laboratory model for babesiacidal drug screening [16]. Irvin and Young have shown that the *in vitro* uptake of tritiated purines, particularly hypoxanthine by *Babesia*, could be inhibited by babesiacidal drugs in proportion to their efficacy *in vivo* [17, 18]. This screening procedure was applicable to *B. microti* and *B. rodhaini* of mice, and *B. divergens* and *B. major* of cattle. An *in vitro* chemotherapeutic screen could probably be developed using culture techniques recently reported for the growth of *B. bovis* in bovine erythrocytes [19, 20].

The mode of action for most compounds is not entirely clear, but the acridine

154

Table 2. Products used to successfully treat babesiosis

Compound or compound group	Proprietary name	Chemical description[*]
Acridine derivatives		
Acriflavine hydrochloride (Euflavine, Trypaflavine)	Gonacrine[a]	A mixture of: 3,6-diamino-10-methylacridinium chloride, and 3,6-diamino acridine hydrochloride
Azo-Naphthalene dyes		
Trypan Blue	Congo blue, Niagara blue	3,3'-{(3,3'-dimethyl{1,1'-biphenyl}-4,4'-diyl)bis(azo)}bis{5-amino-4-hydroxy-2,7-naphthalene disulfonic acid}tetrasodium salt
Diamidine derivatives		
Aromatic:		
Diminazene diaceturate	Berenil[b]	4,4'-diamidinodiazoaminobenzene diaceturate
	Ganaseg[c]	
Pentamidine diisethionate	Lomidine[a]	4,4'-diamidinodiphenoxypentane di(beta-hydroxyethane sulfonate)
Phenamidine diisethionate	Lomadine[a]	4,4'-diamidinodiphenylether di(beta-hydroxyethane sulfonate)
Carbanilide:		
Amicarbalide diisethionate	Diampron[a]	3,3'-diamidinocarbanilide diisethionate
Imidocarb diproprionate	Imizol[d]	3,3'-bis(2-imidazolin-2yl) carbanilide dipropionate
Macrolide antibiotics		
Clindamycin phosphate	Cleosin[e]	7(S)-Chloro-7-deoxylincomycin
Phenanthridine compounds		
Isometamidium	Samorin[a]	8-{(m-Amidinophenylazo)amino}-3-amino-5-ethyl-6-phenylphenanthridinium chloride
Quinoline derivatives		
Quinuronium sulfate	Acaprin[f]	6,6;-ureylenebis(1-methylquinolinium)bis(methosulfate)
	Akiron	
	Pirevan	
	Piroplasmin	
	Babesan[g]	N,N'-di-6-quinolinylurea
8-Aminoquinolines		
Primaquine phosphate	Primaquine[g]	N⁴-(6-methoxy-8-quinolinyl)-1,4-pentanediamine

[a] May & Baker Ltd., Dagenham, England.
[b] Farbwerke-Hoechst AG, Frankfurt, West Germany.
[c] Squibb Mathieson, E.R. Squibb & Sons de Mexico, Mexico City, Mexico.
[d] Burroughs Wellcome & Co. Ltd., London, England.
[e] Upjohn, Kalamazoo, Michigan.
[f] Ludabel Farbenfabriken, Bayer, Leverkusen, West Germany.
[g] Imperial Chemical Industries Ltd., Macclesfield, Cheshire, England.
[*] Obtained when available from the Merck Index, Ninth Edition, 1976.

and diamidine derivatives are thought to combine with nucleic acids [21, 22]. There is an intercalation of the acriflavine molecule between the coils of the DNA molecule, with the amine groups of acriflavine forming bonds with adjacent thymine containing base pairs, causing partial uncoiling and denaturation of the DNA double helix. Studies of diminazene's actions on *B. herpailuri* show a dilation of membrane-bounded organelles and the perinuclear space, dissolution of the cytoplasm, and destruction of the nucleus [23].

Babesia equi in erythrocytes previously exposed to imidocarb were swollen and vacuolated, except for an area just beneath the plasma membrane, where the compressed nucleus was marginated, elongated, and clumpy. Electron microscopy revealed 4 stages of degeneration of *B. equi* in erythrocytes of ponies treated with imidocarb. The first stage showed dilation of the nuclear cisterna and clumping of chromatin. The second stage was characterized by dissolution of the nuclear envelope and passage of nuclear matrix into the cytoplasm. The third stage was associated with vacuolation of the cytoplasm and compression of the chromatin to the periphery of the cell. Degeneration continued until the organism consisted of a vacuole, and chromatin was condensed into an irregular mass of clumped material [24]. Similar ultrastructural changes were observed with *Babesia herpailuri* in the erythrocytes of cats after treatment with imidocarb, except that nuclear damage was not observed [25].

Drug-resistant babesias can be developed experimentally and probably occurs [26, 27]. This problem has not yet evolved as a major constraint in chemotherapy, but techniques of using some compounds as prophylactic agents, with sublethal, low blood levels of active drug in constant contact with the babesias could contribute to the evolution of drug-resistant organisms [27].

Generally, the small *Babesia* is more refractory to treatment. *Babesia bigemina*, *B. caballi*, and *B. canis* usually respond more readily to treatment than their small counterparts, *B. bovis*, *B. equi*, or *B. gibsoni*.

3. Bovine babesiosis

3.1. *Trypan blue*

Probably the first specific drug used to successfully treat bovine babesiosis was trypan blue. Theiler (1912) reported cures by the intravenous (IV) injection of trypan blue [28]. It was later discovered that trypan blue was not effective against the small *Babesia* such as *B. bovis*, but an IV injection of 2–3 mg/kg effectively eliminated *B. bigemina* [29]. This compound has the disadvantages of producing discolorations of the animal's flesh, body secretions, including milk, and causing severe tissue sloughing if injected extravascularly. For this reason, and because more effective drugs have been developed, it is now rarely used to treat bovine babesiosis.

3.2. *Quinoline derivatives*

For many years, the quinoline derivatives were the drugs of choice in the treatment of bovine babesiosis [30, 31]. These drugs have a low therapeutic index, and may produce transient signs of discomfort associated with the stimulation of the parasympathetic nervous system, such as excessive salivation, panting, frequent urination, and general uneasiness [32]. Such reactions usually disappear in about an hour, and may be alleviated by the administration of atropine or epinephrine [33, 34]. A fatal toxic reaction to quinuronium was observed following three daily injections of 0.5 mg/kg intramuscularly (IM) [33]. Postmortem examination revealed a volvulus at the jejunal-ilial junction. It was postulated that quinuronium was responsible for intestinal hyperperistalsis, which resulted in the volvulus.

Quinuronium is still in use, however, and one or two (24 hours apart) treatments given at the rate of 1 mg/kg subcutaneously (SC) is usually sufficient in treating both *B. bigemina* or *B. bovis* [35]. At 1 mg/kg, it was therapeutically effective in treating splenectomized calves infected with *Babesia divergens* [36]. When the drug was given one day before exposure to *B. divergens*, it had no effect on the course of the infection, but when given at the onset of fever and hemoglobinuria, the infection was arrested. Invariably, *B. divergens* recrudescence occurred two weeks after quinuronium therapy. A relatively insoluble salt, quinuronium 5,5'-methylene-bis-salicylate, given as a 1-gram implant, has been shown to prevent *B. bovis*-induced babesiosis for 21 days [37]. Similar insoluble salts injected SC at the rate of 25–50 mg/kg are reported to induce resistance to *B. divergens* challenge for up to 3–4 months [38].

3.3 *Acridine derivatives*

These compounds are reported to be effective against *B. bigemina* and *B. bovis* when given IV as a 5% solution using 4.4 ml/100 kg body weight [11, 39]. Even though they are effective, the acridine derivatives appear to have given way to the diamidine derivatives, which have become widely used in the last 15–20 years.

3.4 *Diamidine derivatives*

A wide variety of these compounds have proven effective and safe in the treatment of bovine babesiosis. Probably the most commonly used compounds are diminazene, imidocarb, amicarbalide, phenamidine, and pentamidine [11, 26, 35]. Amicarbalide administered IM has been successfully used at the rate of 5–10 mg/kg against *B. divergens* and *B. bigemina*, and phenamidine isethionate at 8–13.5 mg/kg SC against *B. bigemina* [35, 40–42]. Diminazene is usually given IM at the rate of 3–5 mg/kg, but titrations show it to be effective against *B. bigemina* at much lower levels [11, 35]. As little as 0.25 mg/kg was effective in moderating the course of *B. bigemina* infections in splenectomized calves, but a level of 0.5 mg/kg was probably the lowest safe dosage that should be used in clinical cases [11].

Pentamidine, at the level of 0.5–2.0 mg/kg administered SC to calves in the acute phase of *B. bigemina* infection, usually led to clinical recovery. As much as 5 mg/kg administered during patency did not destroy the carrier state in intact calves. Pentamidine proved ideal for use in chemoimmunization because it was effective in moderating clinical signs of infection but allowed the carrier state to persist [43].

The addition of 0.25 mg/kg of betamethasone to diminazene (3.5 mg/kg) and to quinuronium (0.9 mg/kg) failed to show any enhancing effects in the treatment of calves infected with *B. bigemina*. Treatment was administered in the acute phase of infection when animals were near death [32]. Diminazene has been successfully used with vaccine programs in South Africa and South America [12, 44]. In each instance, the diminazene is administered 7 or 10 days after vaccination with an attenuated *B. bovis*, or with a combination of *B. bigemina* and *B. bovis* [12, 44]. The drug moderates the effects of the primary infection but allows a state of premunity to develop, hence a high level of protection. When *B. bigemina* is given concurrently with the *B. bovis* vaccine, revaccination with *B. bigemina* two–three weeks later is advisable to establish solid immunity [12]. Even though diminazene has not been shown to produce extended prophylaxis, workers in South Africa have shown it to influence the onset of *B. bovis* infections for up to two weeks and up to four weeks with *B. bigemina* [12]. If, therefore, vaccination with a live agent is to follow diminazene treatment, a delay beyond the period of maximum drug action is recommended.

Babesia ovata, an immunologically distinct species, has recently been described as being pathogenic to cattle in Japan [45]. This *Babesia* morphologically resembles *B. bigemina*, and like *B. bigemina*, it is sensitive to treatment with diminazene and amicarbalide.

Imidocarb, a diamidine of the carbanilide series, is one of the more recent babesiacidal compounds found effective in the treatment and prevention of bovine babesiosis [11, 46, 47,]. Early formulations utilized the dihydrochloride salt, but the dipropionate salt is now more commonly used. This preparation appears to be less irritating to the tissues, although both are soluble and highly active therapeutically. Imidocarb is safe and effective in the recommended SC or IM levels of 1–3 mg/kg for infections due to *B. bigemina*, *B. bovis*, and *B. divergens* [11, 13, 26, 47–49]. Imidocarb is not recommended for IV use [11].

Recent work using imidocarb with *B. divergens* infections in splenectomized calves indicates that 2.4 mg/kg was effective. When given one and two weeks before infection, it had the effect of reducing the severity while not preventing infection, but when given on the day of infection, parasite multiplication was inhibited and no immunity occurred. When administered 7, 14 and 21 days after exposure, infection was eliminated, but sterile immunity was observed at a level corresponding to the length and severity of initial infection [13]. A second related study [50] showed that 3.6 mg/kg imidocarb given 14 days before exposure of splenectomized calves allowed the development of immunity while reducing the severity of infection, but 6.0 mg/kg given 14 days before infection prevented the infection and no immunity was seen. Under field conditions in France, imidocarb administered at the rate of 2 mg/kg was found effective in preventing clinical babesiosis in cattle for 6–8 weeks [51]. It also controlled an outbreak of babesiosis due to *B. divergens* in Ireland when used at 1–2 mg/kg on 682 animals [52].

Imidocarb has been used in connection with some vaccine programs. The simultaneous administration of 0.15 mg/kg imidocarb and live attenuated *B. bovis* vaccine has given satisfactory results. When the vaccine was given seven days prior to imidocarb treatment, a dose of between 0.15 and 0.6 mg/kg imidocarb was required for effective control [49]. A combined *B. bovis* and *B. bigemina* vaccine given 21 and again 61 days after a dose of 3 mg/kg allowed the development of adequate premunity to both parasites.

Treatment of intact calves with 5 mg imidocarb/kg 14 days before and 14 days after exposure to *B. bovis*-infected *Boophilus microplus* larvae not only prevented *B. bovis* infection but rendered the next generation of larvae incapable of transmitting this infection [53]. These results were not, however, duplicated using *Boophilus decoloratus* ticks infected with *B. bigemina*. Splenectomized calves treated with imidocarb at 5 mg/kg two weeks before tick infestation and with 3 mg/kg on the day of tick infestation, prevented patent infections in the calves, but did not eliminate *B. bigemina* from the *Boophilus decoloratus* ticks [54]. It should be borne in mind that *B. bovis* is not thought to persist in infective forms beyond the larval stage of *Boophilus microplus*, implying that engorging adult females must acquire the infection in each generation from an infected bovine, to complete their life cycle, and in turn infect the larvae of the next generation [55, 56]. This basic difference in the life cycle of *B. bovis* and *B. bigemina* in the tick must be considered when this drug is being used to eliminate infection in the invertebrate host.

The prophylactic effect of imidocarb has been utilized in cattle being shipped from *Babesia*-free areas to endemic zones of the tropics. In one such trial, 44 young Charolais cattle were moved from Texas to Haiti [57]. They were treated SC with 2.8 mg/kg body weight before being exposed to infected *Boophilus* ticks. After 130 days on the island, over 70% of the cattle showed serologic evidence of babesiosis, but there were no deaths due to acute babesiosis. It is probable that exposure of the cattle to *Boophilus* ticks resulted in inapparent *Babesia* infection, followed by premunition, without acute infection or death losses.

A recent unique innovation for the administration of imidocarb has been carried out in which the drug was encapsulated in bovine carrier erythrocytes with no ill effects on the carrier cells. The drug-loaded carrier cells had an *in vivo* half-life of 28–32 days, and a dose, equivalent to 0.1 mg/kg body weight imidocarb, was thought to have provided a level of protection against *Babesia* infections for at least 35 days [58].

Imidocarb is toxic under some conditions, notwithstanding a high therapeutic index for *Babesia*. Toxic reactions vary, largely due to the wide range of individual animal tolerance to the drug. Observations of imidocarb treatment on 469 adult cows at the level of 5 mg/kg IM, given two times at a two-week interval, was accompanied by 5% mortality; some, but not all, of which was shown to be drug related [59]. A study was made in calves, in which five animals in each of three groups were inoculated with 5, 10, and 20 mg/kg imidocarb 2 times at a 14-day interval[60]. All five calves receiving the 20 mg level died on days 7, 10, 11, 11, and 18 after the first inoculation. Mortality did not occur in those animals receiving the 5 and 10 mg levels. All calves showed excessive lacrimation, serous nasal discharge, and increased frequency of defecation for 30 to 40 minutes after injection. In addition to the transient reactions, persistent reactions, including sweating, diarrhea, dyspnea, and depression, occurred in one of five calves receiving the 5 mg level, two of five calves receiving the 10 mg level, and all of those inoculated with the 20 mg/kg. These reactions are attributable to an anticholinesterase activity of imidocarb. Dose-dependent injection site reactions were characterized by areas of myositis, focal areas of necrosis, edema, and granulation tissue [60]. Fatal toxicosis was associated with renal hyperemia and enlargement, pulmonary congestion, edema, hydrothorax, and hydroperitoneum. Renal lesions were mainly seen as severe cellular necrosis in the proximal convoluted tubules.

Imidocarb is very slowly metabolized and eliminated with persistent tissue residues [61, 62]. These persisting tissue residues restrict its use in food animals in some countries. Tissue assays for residues have been developed and were tested in sheep and cattle to give some indication of drug dynamics. The injection of 4.5 mg/kg IM in sheep resulted in peak plasma levels of 7.9 ug/ml within four hours, which was followed by rapid decline within the next two hours to 4.6 ug/ml and then a slow decline for several weeks [61, 62]. Average tissue levels of imidocarb 28 days after the inoculation of 1–2 mg/kg in three cattle were 2.03 ug/gm in liver, 2.13 ug/gm in kidney, 0.13 ug/gm in muscle, and 0.02 ug/gm in fat [63].

Treatment of bovine babesiosis is frequently limited to the use of specific babesiacidal drugs. In some instances, ancillary treatment is indicated. O'Neil recommends one liter of blood for each 45 kg of body weight in the treatment of acute babesiosis due to *B. divergens* [64]. Transfusions seldom exceed eight liters of blood, but this amount is recommended for a 364 kg or heavier cow. The blood is collected in sodium citrate from a mature, healthy cow, and the transfusion is made immediately. Good success has been achieved with this technique when accompanied by specific babesiacidal drug therapy.

4. Equine babesiosis

DeKock (1918) published a report in which he unsuccessfully attempted to treat nuttalliosis (*B. equi*) in horses with a large number of chemical compounds, including inorganic salts, organic arsenicals, various dyes, hyalin, formalin, quinine, hydrobromide, camphor, turpentine, etc. [65]. Included was trypan blue, which proved effective against *B. caballi* but not *B. equi*. *Babesia caballi* and *B. equi* follow a pattern of drug susceptibility similar to *B. bigemina* and *B. bovis*.

Acute equine babesiosis responds to many of the same drugs that are effective in cattle, but slightly higher dosages are usually required. The most commonly used drugs in treating equine babesiosis are amicarbalide (8 mg/kg), imidocarb (2–5 mg/kg), and diminazene (5–10 mg/kg) [11]. One injection of 2 mg/kg imidocarb is usually sufficient to bring about a clinical remission of infection due to *B. caballi*. Quinuronium sulphate was described as being ineffective in treating *B. equi* infections in splenectomized donkeys [66]. Diminazene was successfully used to treat *B. equi* infections in donkeys at the rate of 6–12 mg/kg [67]. The additon of a tetracycline at 10 mg/kg to the diminazene treatment failed to produce any potentiating effects [66]. These workers also found that imidocarb, administered at the rate of 2 mg/kg, was ineffective in treating *B. equi* infection in donkeys, but was effective when 5 mg/kg was given two times at a 48-hr interval. This latter dosage appeared effective in eliminating *B. equi* infection in these splenectomized donkeys, based on subinoculation trials [67].

Elimination of the carrier infection has assumed importance, particularly in animals being shipped from endemic zones to areas where infection is limited or does not exist. The following treatments appear effective in eliminating *B. caballi* [68, 69]:

1. diminazene, 5 mg/kg, two times 24-hr interval;
2. phenamidine isethionate, 8.8 mg/kg, two times 24-hr interval;
3. amicarbalide, 8.8 mg/kg, two times 24-hr interval;
4. imidocarb, 1–2 mg/kg, two times 24-hr interval.

Babesia equi is more refractory to treatment, particularly in the elimination of carrier infections. Amicarbalide, given at the rate of 11 mg/kg, four times at 24- and 48-hr intervals, was unsuccessful; and only four of eight horses became free of infection when they received seven daily injections of amicarbalide at 22 mg/kg, which approaches toxic levels [11]. Diminazene and imidocarb, administered at the rate of 12 mg/kg two times at a 24-hr interval, and 5 mg/kg two times at a 48-hr interval respectively, to splenectomized donkeys showing *B. equi* parasitemia, resulted in apparent remission and elimination of infection [67]. Imidocarb, given 4 mg/kg four times at 72-hr intervals, was shown to remove *B. equi* infecions in 13 of 14 horses [70]. It is recommended that this treatment (4 mg/kg) be divided into two equal doses given 30 minutes apart to minimize the undesirable acute side effects associated with imidocarb treatment.

Imidocarb, at 4 mg/kg, given four times at 72-hr intervals, caused 100% mortality in eight *B. equi*-infected donkeys [70]. The LD-50 in horses was determined to be 16 mg/kg given two times at a 24-hr interval [71]. Although horses treated with 2 mg/kg showed no adverse reactions, all horses receiving 4 mg/kg or more manifested signs compatible with excessive stimulation of the cranial and sacral portions of the parasympathetic division of the autonomic nervous system, characterized by sweating, extreme restlessness, and abdominal pain. There were increased levels of blood urea nitrogen, serum aspartate, aminotransferase, serum sorbitol dehydrogenase, serum creatine phospho-kinase, and increasing severity of renal, hepatic, and pulmonary lesions [71]. Mortalities which occurred within six days following the first injection were attributed to acute cortical tubular renal necrosis and acute periportal hepatic necrosis.

Chlortetracycline has been reported to be effective against *B. equi* if given in repeated intravenous doses early in the course of infection [72]. Six daily injections at 3-dose levels, 0.5 mg/kg, 2.5 mg/kg, and 2.6 mg/kg were described as useful in controlling multiplication of *B.equi*.

5. Canine babesiosis

Canine babesiosis is becoming increasingly widespread in Europe and North America [8, 73]. *Babesia canis* has long been recognized in the southern states (US), but recently *B. gibsoni* has been described in the New England states [8]. In reviewing treatment procedures used for canine babesiosis, Moore notes that a wide variety of ineffectual drugs such as ammonia, extract of belladonna, quinine, benzoate of soda, carbolic acid, and calomel have been tried [74]. Currently, treatment for canine babesiosis includes specific babesiacidal agents coupled with supportive treatment, including blood transfusions, fluid therapy, alkalinizing agents, liver protectants, diuretics, restricted exercise and improved nutrition [75]. Trypan blue was successfully used in 1909 for the treatment of *Babesia canis* [76]. This treatment consisted of 1 ml/kg of a 1% solution (10 mg/kg) given subcutaneously. Quinuronium is more active than trypan blue, but has a low therapeutic index and must be used with some caution. The recommended SC dose of 0.25 mg/kg of quinuronium is effective, but does not eliminate infection [74]. At 1 mg/kg, toxic signs may be observed. While trypan blue and quinuronium are effective against *B. canis*, they are not recommended for *B. gibsoni* [77].

One of the first diamidines to be recommended for the treatment of canine babesiosis was phenamidine, at a SC dose of 10 mg/kg. Although effective against both *B. canis* and *B. gibsoni*, and less toxic than quinuronium, it did not eliminate infection, and relapses were observed to occur [78]. The dose should be repeated after an interval of 24 hrs in *B. gibsoni* infection or after 6–7 days in *B. canis* infection [79, 80]. In addition to phenamidine, Klinefelter found diminazene at 7 mg/kg to be effective in treating *B. canis* [81]. Although effective against both *B. canis* and *B. gibsoni*, diminazene when used at 7.5–10.0 mg/kg as a single dose may produce some abnormal central nervous system involvement such as nystagmus, ataxia, extensor rigidity, opisthotonus, coma, and even death [73, 74, 82]. This can be avoided by using 3.0 mg/kg diminazene two times on consecutive days. As little as 2.5–3.5 mg/kg diminazene aceturate has been successful in treating *B. canis*, but 5–7 mg/kg was required for *B. gibsoni* [73, 74, 83]. Diminazene is reported to eliminate *B. canis* infections at 4–5 mg/kg in some cases and in all instances at 12 mg/kg [74]. The drug is not recommended for use over 7 mg/kg because of possible CNS changes. *Babesia gibsoni* was successfully treated with diminazene totalling 11 mg/kg, given in two doses five days apart; but chloroquine phosphate, primaquine phosphate, sodium arsenamide, and chlorguanide hydrochloride were not effective [84]. Pentamidine at the level of 16.5 mg/kg given twice on consecutive days was reported clinically effective against *B. gibsoni* and *B. canis*, but relapses commonly occurred with *B. gibsoni* [82]. Pain at the IM injection site, hypotension, tachycardia, nausea, and vomiting were observed after pentamidine treatment. The antitrypanasomal agent, isometamidium, has recently been used successfully in the treatment of *B. canis* at 2 mg/kg, IM, and compares favorably with amicarbalide and diminazene [85].

Imidocarb at 5 mg/kg has been found to be very effective against *B. canis* [86]. Following treatment, there was a rapid reduction in parasitemia and a corresponding increase in PCV. Fewer than 4% of the animals so treated relapsed with *Babesia* over a 3-month period, notwithstanding the probability of reinfection. In view of the marked prophylactic effects of imidocarb on other babesias, an effort was made to evaluate this effect on *B. canis* [87]. A single injection of 6 mg/kg imidocarb was followed by *B. canis* challenge two, three, four and five weeks later. Imidocarb did not prevent infections but may have moderated the severity of infection. The lack of definitive results suggests the need for further study. Another study reported a favorable response in *B. canis*-infected dogs following imidocarb treatment with 3 mg/kg. This treatment level was found also to prevent severe signs of infection under natural conditions for at least six weeks. When the drug is given at the time of *B. canis* exposure, carrier premunition occurred without evidence of clinical infection [88]. Field experience suggests chemoprophylaxis for at least four weeks in 75% of dogs treated with 4.8 to 6.4 mg/kg imidocarb [89].

As reported by Moore the therapeutic regime for babesiosis in dogs should vary with the severity of infection [74]. Intensive treatment is often required to counteract shock and disseminated intravascular coagulation, a common sequel in canine babesiosis. This phenomenon has also been seen in malaria. Diminazene was usually the babesiacidal drug of choice, but trypan blue was used in those patients that were categorized as severely infected, because it does not stimulate the parasympathetic nervous system and thus aggravate the medical shock which is frequently present in those critically ill patients, nor does it possess the potentially toxic effects on the central nervous system as do the diamidines. Treatment of mild cases involved using diminazene at the rate of 3.5 mg/kg in a 7% solution given SC. Each animal also received procaine penicillin, prednisolone, and vitamin B complexes. In the severe category, intravenous fluid therapy was started immediately, and the babesiacidal drug trypan blue was infused IV at the rate of 10 mg/kg in a 1% solution. The fluid infusion was followed by whole blood transfusion. Antibiotic and vitamin complexes were administered to each of the patients. In those cases that responded favorably to treatment, improvement was noted within a few hours after the initial treatment [74].

6. Feline babesiosis

There are numerous *Babesia* species in different domestic and feral cats, but among domestic cats *Babesia felis* appears to be of primary concern [10, 90]. A recent article described an unidentified *Babesia* in domestic cats in South Africa, which was tentatively identified as *Babesia herpailuri* [91]. *Babesia felis* is unique in its response to chemotherapy in that the usual drugs that are effective against other babesias fail to produce a remission of infection [10]. Primaquine phosphate administered *per os* or as an IM injection was found to be effective and was the drug of choice in the treatment of *B. felis*. The dosage used was 0.5 mg/kg body weight of primaquine base. Repeated treatment was well tolerated, but single doses in excess of 1 mg/kg are known to cause mortality in cats. Chloroquine, diminazene, phenamidine, quinuronium, euflavin, trypan blue, imidocarb, and oxytetracycline were all ineffective against *Babesia felis* [10]. *Babesia herpailuri*, on the other hand, responds to imidocarb therapy, as well as diminazene, at 5 mg/kg [23, 25, 91].

7. Human babesiosis

Babesiosis in man has reached the point when it should no longer be considered a benign medical rarity [6]. There are increasing numbers of reports in the literature of babesiosis in man. These cases do not always respond favorably to traditional therapy, which has consisted for the most part of antimalarial drugs and supportive treatment [92, 93]. Quinine sulphate and chloroquine are generally ineffective in reducing *Babesia* parasitemias. The principal cause of babesiosis in man is *Babesia microti* [4]; however, reports of *B. divergens* from Europe are not uncommon [93]. In one instance, the cause of a human case of babesiosis was assumed to be *B. equi*. In this instance, the infection appeared to respond to pyrimethamine [3]. When a 65-year-old man, infected with *B. microti*, failed to respond to supportive and antimalarial treatment, he was successfully treated with diminazene [92]. Treatment consisted of a 3-day course of 2 mg/kg a day, given IM. This was preceded by one experimental dose of 50 mg to determine tolerance to treatment. Following the third dose, the patient became and remained afebrile, and the *Babesia* parasitemia disappeared. Some time after his recovery from babesiosis, the patient developed acute idiopathic polyneuritis (Landry-Guillian-Barre Syndrome). A splenectomized man infected with *B. divergens* died after treatment with chloroquine and pyrimethamine, plus supportive treatment [93]. In two cases of *B. microti* infection, pentamidine at 4 mg/kg given IM for 14 days was successful in eliminating parasitemia with eventual recovery [94]. In the third case, recovery occurred after only seven inoculations. *Babesia microti* was recovered five weeks after the last treatment in one case, but in the other, no *Babesia* was isolated in hamsters or mice 6 months after treatment. There was considerable persisting discomfort at the site of the pentamidine injection.

Recently, Rowin has described the use of clindamycin for the treatment of *B. microti* infections in hamsters [95]. Clindamycin, at the rate of 150 mg/kg IM, was reasonably successful in eliminating parasitemias and bringing about a remission of *B. microti* infections. It has also been used successfully in a near-fatal case of babesiosis in man, which occurred following blood transfusion from a *Babesia* carrier [96]. Because of enterocolitis which may accompany treatment with clindamycin alone, it has been necessary to use it in combination with vancomycin given at the rate of 100 mg/kg body weight. The addition of oral quinine (250 mg/kg/day for seven days) to the clindamycin/vancomycin therapy enhances the efficacy of this treatment. Many cases of human babesiosis can be effectively handled with symptomatic and supportive care, but these treatment regimes generally fail to produce results comparable to those seen in animals when specific babesiacidal compounds are used [97].

8. Ovine and porcine babesiosis

Babesia motasi and *Babesia ovis* in sheep, and *Babesia trautmanni* and *Babesia perroncitoi* in swine are susceptible to treatment using the same general compounds previously mentioned and following the same general rules of susceptibility as described for other domestic animals [11]. *Babesia ovis* was shown to be relatively resistant to a single injection of the usual levels of quinuronium and imidocarb, but treatment with 2 mg/kg imidocarb SC three times at 24-hr intervals was successful [98, 99]. The large, *Babesia motasi* has been reported from northern Europe and north Wales [100, 101]. Babesiosis occurring as a result of this infection can be successfully treated with amicarbalide at the rate of 5 mg/kg and also diminazene at 5.5 mg/kg [101].

An outbreak of porcine babesiosis in Senegal caused by *B. perroncitoi* resulted in 318 deaths [9]. Over 4000 swine were treated IM with diminazene at 5 mg/kg body weight. This was followed by decreased death rate and clinical cures, although parasitemia was still detectable in some animals.

9. Conclusions

With the exception of *B. felis*, most babesias are susceptible to one or more of the recognized babesiacidal drugs. Instances of drug resistance have been reported, but this has not to date evolved as a major problem. It is probable that greater emphasis is needed in areas of chemoprophylaxis and the study of the so-called 'sterile immunity' which may occur and persist for differing periods following radical cures.

Chemotherapy is playing an increasingly frequent role with the use of live vaccines to moderate the vaccinal reaction. Chemoprophylaxis alone might be feasible when used to prevent fatal tick-acquired infections by susceptible cattle introduced into endemic zones where exposure occurs on a continuing basis. Theoretically, a point will be reached when drug levels are sufficiently low to allow infection to occur, but still high enough to prevent a fulminating infection, clinical signs, and death. Such animals may then develop carrier or premune status without undergoing severe or fatal reactions.

Often, the availability of highly specific and effective chemotherapeutic agents has contributed to the practice of excessive reliance on these drugs in the treatment of infection to the extent that little attention has been paid to the need for supportive and symptomatic treatment. With the increasing number of babesiosis cases occurring in man and companion animals, greater emphasis is being given to supportive and symptomatic treatment. The extrapolation of these techniques to large food-producing animals is probably indicated in selected cases.

Additional pharmacokinetic studies are indicated on the more commonly used drugs to determine safe and effective doses and establish the effect of treatment intervals in cases where multiple doses are indicated.

Recent studies involving *B. equi* have revealed a number of unique characteristics which have placed some doubt as to the validity of its classification as a *Babesia* [102]. The presence of lymphocytic schizonts [103], and the absence of transovarial tick transmission both resemble a *Theileria*. The marked difference of *B. equi* in response to treatment plus the apparent unique response to tetracycline therapy further contribute to the idea of differences. The failure of *B. felis* to respond to traditional babesiacidal compounds suggests the need to further study the taxonomic classification of this hemoparasite. A careful evaluation of drug response by the large and small babesias may well contribute to our future understanding of these organisms.

Table 3. Suggested treatment regimen in babesiosis

Disease and Drug used[a]	Dose (mg/kg) and route[b]	Number of treatments	Dosing interval
Bovine babesiosis:			
Curative			
Amicarbalide	5–10 IM	1	–
Diminazene	3–5 IM	1	–
Imidocarb	1–3 IM or SC	1	–
Quinuronium	1 SC	1–2	24 h
Prophylaxis			
Imidocarb	2.8 SC	1	–
Chemo-immunization			
Imidocarb	3 IM	1	9 days after parasite inoculation or parasite inoculated 21 and and 61 days after imidocarb treatment
Diminazene	1.5 IM	1	10 days after parasite inoculation
Equine babesiosis:			
Curative			
B. caballi			
Amicarbalide	8.8 IM	2	24 h
Diminazene	5 IM	2	24 h
Imidocarb	2 IM	2	24 h
Phenamidine	8.8 SC	2	24 h
B. equi			
Diminazene	12 IM	2	24 h
Imidocarb (donkeys)	5 IM	2	48 h
Imidocarb (horses)	4 IM	4	72 h
Canine babesiosis:			
Curative			
Diminazene	3–5 IM or SC	2	24 h
Imidocarb	5 IM	1–2	24 h
Phenamidine	10 SC	1–2	24 h in *B. gibsoni*, and 6–7 days in *B. canis* infection
Trypan blue	10 IV	1	–
Feline babesiosis:			
Curative			
B. felis			
Primaquine	0.5 IM or PO	2	24 h
B. herpailuri			
Diminazene	5 IM	1	–
Imidocarb	5 IM	1	–
Ovine babesiosis:			
Curative			
B. motasi			
Amicarbalide	5 IM	1	–
Diminazene	5.5 IM	1	–

B. ovis					
Imidocarb	2	SC	3	24 h	
Porcine babesiosis:					
Curative					
Diminazene	5	IM	1	–	
Human babesiosis:					
Curative					
Clindamycin	20	IM	7	24 h	
Diminazene	2	IM	3	24 h	
Pentamidine	4	IM	7–14	24 h	

[a] Aqueous solutions of:
Amicarbalide diisethionate
Clindamycin phospate, 15%
Diminazene diaceturate, 3.5 ® –7%
Imidocarb dipropionate, 12%
Pentamidine diisethionate, 10%
Phenamidine diisethionate, 40% in horses and cattle; 5% in dogs
Primaquine phosphate
Quinuronium sulfate, 5%
Trypan blue, 1%

[b] IM = intramuscular; IV = intravenous; PO = *per os*; SC = subcutaneous

Table 4. Relative efficacy of the more commonly used babesiacidal compounds

	Dimi-nazene	Imido-carb	Amicar-balide	Phena-midine	Quinu-ronium	Trypan blue	Penta-midine	Clinda-mycin	Prima-quine
Cattle:									
Babesia bigemina	++++	++++	++++	++	+++	++	++		
B. bovis	+++	+++	++	++	++	– –			
B. divergens	++	+++	++		+	– –			
Horses:									
B. caballi	+++	++++	+++	+++	++	++			
B. equi	++	+++	+	++	– –	– –			
Dogs:									
B. canis	+++	+++	++	+++	++	+	++		
B. gibsoni	++			++	– –	– –	++		
Cats:									
B. herpailuri	+++	+++							
B. felis		– –		– –	– –	– –			+++
Sheep:									
B. motasi	+++		+++		+	+			
B. ovis	+	++			±	– –			
Swine:									
B. trautmanni				++	++	++			
B. perroncitoi	+++				++	– –			
Man:									
B. microti	+						++	++	

168

Mention of a trademark or proprietary product does not constitute a guarantee or warranty of the product by the US Department of Agriculture and does not imply its approval to the exclusion of other products that also may be suitable.

References

1. Smith T, Kilbourne FL: Investigations into the nature, causation and prevention of Texas or Southern cattle fever. US Dept Agriculture, Bureau of Animal Industry, Bull. No. 1, 1–301, 1893.
2. Purnell RE: Babesiosis in various hosts. In Babesiosis, pp. 25–63. Ristic M, Kreier JP, eds. New York: Academic Press, 1981.
3. Bredt AB, Weinstein WM, Cohen S: Treatment of babesiosis in asplenic patients. J Am of Med Assoc 245:1938–1939, 1981.
4. Brocklesby DW: Human babesiosis. J S Afr Vet Assoc 50:302–307, 1979.
5. Skrabalo Z, Deonovic Z: Piroplasmosis in man. Report on a case. Doc Med Georgr et Trop 9:11–16, 1957.
6. Zaino EC, Amelkin S: Babesiosis: A potentially grave disease for the immunosuppressed. N Y State J Med 81:384, 1981.
7. Filstein MR, Benach JL, White DJ, Brody BA, Goldman WD, Bakal CW, Schwartz RS: Serosurvey for human babesiosis in New York. J Infect Dis 141:518–521, 1980.
8. Anderson JF, Magnarelli LA: Canine *Babesia*, new to North America. Science 204:1431–1432, 1979.
9. Vercruysse J, Parent R: Report of an account of porcine babesiosis due to *Babesia perroncitoi* in Senegal. Afrique Medicale 20 (192):435–437, 1981.
10. Potgieter FT: Chemotherapy of *Babesia felis* infection: Efficacy of certain drugs. J S Afr Vet Assoc 52:289–293, 1981
11. Kuttler KL: Chemotherapy of babesiosis: A review. In Babesiosis, pp. 65–85. Ristic M, Kreier JP, eds. New York: Academic Press, 1981.
12. DeVos AJ: Epidemiology and control of bovine babesiosis in South Africa. J S Afr Vet Assoc 50:357–362, 1979.
13. Lewis D, Purnell RE, Francis MA, Young ER: The effect of treatment with imidocarb diproprionate on the course of *Babesia divergens* infections in splenectomized calves and on their subsequent immunity to homologous challenge. J Comp Path 91:285–292, 1981.
14. Beveridge E: *Babesia rodhaini*: A useful organism for the testing of drugs designed for the treatment of piroplasmosis. Ann Trop Med Parasit 47:134, 1953.
15. Lucas JMS: The chemotherapy of experimental babesiasis in mice and splenectomized calves. Res Vet Sci 1:218–225, 1960.
16. Lewis D, Williams H: Infection of the Mongolian gerbil with the cattle piroplasm, *Babesia divergens*. Nature 278:170, 1979.
17. Irvin AD, Young ER: Possible *in vitro* test for screening drugs for activity against *Babesia* and other blood protozoa. Nature 169:407–409, 1977.
18. Irvin AD, Young ER: Further studies on the uptake of tritiated nucleic acid precursors by *Babesia spp.* of cattle and mice. Int J Parasitol 9:109–114, 1979.
19. Erp EE, Gravely SM, Smith RD, Ristic M, Osorno BM, Carson CA: Growth of *Babesia bovis* in bovine erythrocyte cultures. Am J Trop Med Hyg 27:1061–1064, 1978.
20. Levy MG, Ristic M: Continuous cultivation in a microaerophilous stationary phase culture. Science 207:1218–1220, 1980.
21. Newton BA: Interaction of berenil with deoxyribonucleic acid and some characteristics of the berenil-deoxyribonucleic acid complex. Biochem J 105:50–51, 1967.

22. Neville DM: The interaction of acridine dyes with DNA. An x-ray diffraction and optical investigation. J Molec Biol 17:57–74, 1966.

23. Hebel R, Dennig HK: Licht und Elektronenmikroskopische Untersuchungen an *Babesia herpailuri* nach Behandlung mit 4,4′Diamidinodiazoamino-benzol (Berenil). Z Parasitenkd 33:1–20, 1969.

24. Simpson CF, Neal FC: Ultrastructure of *Babesia equi* in ponies treated with imidocarb. Am J Vet Res 41:267–271, 1980.

25. Göbel E, Dennig HK: Die Ultrastruktur der Trophozoiten und Merozoiten von *Babesia herpailuri* in Erythrozyten der Hauskatze nach Behandlung mit Imidocarb (3,3′-bis-2-imidazolin-2-yl)-carbanilid. Z Parasitenkd 49:97–112, 1976.

26. Joyner LP: The chemotherapy of protozoal infections of veterinary importance. J Protozool 28:17–19, 1981.

27. Dalgliesh RJ, Stewart NP: Tolerance to imidocarb induced experimentally in tick-transmitted *Babesia argentina*. Austr Vet J 53:176–180, 1977.

28. Theiler A: The treatment of Redwater in cattle with trypan blue. Vet J 68:64–73, 1912.

29. Rees CW: Characteristics of the piroplasms *Babesia argentina* and *Babesia bigemina* in the United States. J Agric Res 48(5):427–438, 1934.

30. Legg J: The treatment of piroplasmosis (*P. bigeminum*) with akiron. Aust Vet J 12:227–230, 1936.

31. Legg J: The treatment of babesiellosis (*B. argentina*) with acaprin. Aust Vet J 15:121–123, 1939.

32. Löhr FK, Otieno PS, Gacanga W: Therapy trial using betamethasone in addition to specific treatment with a diamidine and quinuronium derivate in cattle experimentally infected with *Babesia bigemina*. Bull Anim Hlth Prod XXIV, 199–205, 1976.

33. Vanzini VR, Gomez MR, Hadani A, Bermudez AC, Luciani CA, Guglielmone AA, Angold AJ: A case of intestinal torsion in a cow, apparently caused by administration of acaprin as a babesiacide. Rev Med Vet Argentina 6:503–506, 1981.

34. Eyre P: Some pharmacodynamic effects of the babesicidal agents quinuronium and amicarbalide. J Pharm Pharmacol 19:509–519, 1967.

35. Barnett SF: The chemotherapy of *Babesia bigemina* infection in cattle. Res Vet Sci 6:397–415, 1965.

36. Purnell RE, Lewis D, Young ER: Quinuronium sulphate for the treatment of *Babesia divergens* infections of splenectomized calves. Vet Rec 108:538–539, 1981.

37. Newton LG, O'Sullivan PJ: Chemoprophylaxis in *Babesia argentina* infection in cattle. Aust Vet J 45:404–407, 1969.

38. Ryley JF: A chemoprophylactic approach to babesiasis. Res Vet Sci 5:411–418, 1964.

39. Riek RF: Babesiosis. In Infectious Blood Diseases of Man and Animals, pp. 219–268. Weinman D, Ristic M, eds. New York: Academic Press, 1968.

40. Adam KMG, Blewett DA, Collins TJ, Edgar JT: Outbreaks of babesiasis on two farms in Scotland. Br Vet J 134:428–433, 1978.

41. Pipano E, Weisman Y, Raz A, Klinger I: Immunity to *Babesia bigemina* in calves after successful babesicidal treatment of a previous infection. Refuah Vet 29:1–8, 1972.

42. Collins JD, Nuallain TO, Ferguson AR: Observations on bovine babesiosis in Ireland. Irish Vet J 24:42–51, 1970.

43. Pipano E, Jeruhan I, Frank M: Pentamidine in chemoimmunisation of cattle against *Babesia bigemina* infections. Trop Anim Hlth Prod 11:13–16, 1979.

44. Thompson KC, Todorovic RA, Mateus C, Adams LG: Methods to improve the health of cattle in the tropics: immunisation and chemoprophylaxis against haemoparasitic infections. Trop Anim Hlth Prod 10:75–81, 1978.

45. Minami T, Ishihara T: *Babesia ovata* sp.n. isolated from cattle in Japan. Nat I Anim Hlth Q (Jpn) 20:101–113, 1980.

46. Todorovic RA, Vizcaino OG, Gonzalez EF, Adams LG: Chemoprophylaxis (Imidocarb)

against *Babesia bigemina* and *Babesia argentina* infections. Am J Vet Res 34:1153–1161, 1973.

47. Callow LL, McGregor W: The effect of imidocarb against *Babesia argentina* and *Babesia bigemina* infections of cattle. Aust Vet J 46:195–200, 1970.

48. Purnell RE, Rae MC, Deuk SM: Efficacy of imidocarb dipropionate and primaquine phosphate in the prevention of tickborne disease in imported Hereford heifers from South Korea. Trop Anim Hlth Prod 13:123–127, 1981.

49. Taylor RJ, McHardy N: Preliminary observations on the combined use of imidocarb and *Babesia* blood vaccine in cattle. J S Afr Vet Assoc 50:326–329, 1979.

50. Purnell RE, Lewis D, Young ER: Investigations on the prophylactic effect of treatment with imidocarb diproprionate on *Babesia divergens* infections in splenectomized calves. Brit Vet J 136:452–456, 1980.

51. Euzeby J, Rancien P, Simon PH: Outbreak of *Babesia* infection in the Charolles region of France. 3. Chemoprophylaxis by imidocarb. B Soc Sci Vet Med Comp de Lyon 76(6):423–426, 1974.

52. Haigh AJB, Hagan DH: Evaluation of imidocarb dihydrochloride against redwater disease in cattle in Eire. Vet Rec 94:56–69, 1974.

53. Kuttler KL, Graham OH, Trevino JL: The effect of imidocarb treatment on *Babesia* in the bovine and the tick (*Boophilus microplus*). Res Vet Sci 18:198–200, 1975.

54. Gray JS, Potgieter FT: The retention of *Babesia bigemina* infection by *Boophilus decoloratus* exposed to imidocarb dipropionate during engorgement. Onderst J Vet Res 48:225–227, 1981.

55. Mahoney DF, Mirre GB: A note on the transmission of *Babesia bovis* (syn. *B. argentina*) by the one host tick, *Boophilus microplus*. Res Vet Sci 26:253–254, 1979.

56. Potgieter FT: The life cycle of *Babesia bovis* and *Babesia bigemina* in ticks and in cattle in South Africa. Ph.D. Thesis, Rand Afrikaans University, Johannesburg, S. Africa, 1977.

57. Day WC, Kuttler KL: Animal health considerations involved in the movement of US cattle to Haiti. SW Vet 28:229–232, 1975.

58. DeLoach JR, Wagner GG, Craig TM: Imidocarb dipropionate encapsulation and binding to reseal carrier bovine erythrocytes for potential babesiosis chemotherapy. J Appl Biochem 3:254–262, 1981.

59. Kuttler KL: Use of imidocarb to control anaplasmosis. SW Vet 28:47–52, 1975.

60. Adams LG, Corrier DE, Williams JD: A study of the toxicity of imidocarb dipropionate in cattle. Res Vet Sci 28:172–177, 1980.

61. Aliu YO: Absorption, distribution, and excretion of imidocarb dipropionate (3,3'-bis-(2-imidazolin-2-yl)carbanilide) in sheep. Ph.D. dissertation. Texas A&M University, College of Veterinary Medicine, College Station, Texas, 1974.

62. Aliu YO, Davis RH, Camp BJ, Kuttler KL: Absorption, distribution and excretion of imidocarb dipropionate in sheep. Am J Vet Res 38:2001–2006, 1977.

63. Wood JC: The activity of imidocarb against *Babesia* infections of cattle. Irish Vet J 25:254–257, 1971.

64. O'Neill AR: Blood transfusions in cattle with particular reference to 'Redwater' (Babesiosis). Irish Vet J 33:1–7, 1979.

65. DeKock GDW: Drug treatment in *Nuttalliosis*. Union of S.A., Dept of Agric 7th and 8th Reports, Dir Vet Res 639–675, April 1918.

66. Malhotra DV, Gautam OP, Banerjee DP: A note on chemotherapeutic trials against *Babesia equi* infection in donkeys. I J Anim Sc 49:75–77, 1979.

67. Singh B, Banerjee DP, Gautam OP: Comparative efficacy of diminazine diaceturate and imidocarb dipropionate against *B. equi* infections in donkeys. Vet Parasit 7:173–179, 1980.

68. Frerichs WM, Holbrook AA: Treatment of equine piroplasmosis (*B. caballi*) with imidocarb dipropionate. Vet Rec 95:188–189, 1974.

69. Kirkham WW: The treatment of equine babesiosis. J Am Vet Med Assoc 155:457–460, 1969.

70. Frerichs WM, Allen PC, Holbrook AA: Equine piroplasmosis (*Babesia equi*): Therapeutic

trials of imidocarb dihydrochloride in horses and donkeys. Vet Rec 93:73–75, 1973.

71. Adams LG: Clinicopathological aspects of imidocarb dipropionate toxicity in horses. Res Vet Sci 31:54–61, 1981.

72. Jansen BC: The parasiticidal effect of Aureomycin (Lederle) on *Babesia equi* (La Veran 1899) in splenectomized donkeys. Onderst J Vet Res 26:175–182, 1953.

73. Dennig Von HK, Centurier C, Göbel E, Weiland G: Ein Beitrag zur Babesiose des Hundes und ihrer Bedeutung in der Bundesrepublik Deutschland und Berlin-West. Berl Münch Tierärztl Wschr 93:373–379, 1980.

74. Moore DJ: Therapeutic implications of *Babesia canis* infection in dogs. J S Afr Vet Assoc 50:346–352, 1979.

75. Button C: Metabolic and electrolyte disturbances in acute canine babesiosis. J Am Vet Med Assoc 175:475–479, 1979.

76. Nuttall GHF, Hadwen S: The successful drug treatment of canine piroplasmosis, together with observations upon the effect of drugs on *Piroplasma* canis. Parasitol 2:156–191, 1909.

77. Groves MG, Dennis GL: *Babesia gibsoni*: Field and laboratory studies of canine infections. Exp Parasit 31:153–159, 1972.

78. Groves MG, Vanniasingham JA: Treatment of *Babesia gibsoni* infections with phenamidine isethionate. Vet Rec 86:8–10, 1970.

79. Ruff MD, Fowler JL, Fernau RC, Matsuda K: Action of certain antiprotozoal compounds against *Babesia gibsoni* in dogs. Am J Vet Res 34:641–645, 1973.

80. Joyner LP, Davies SFM, Kendall SB: Chemotherapy of babesiosis. In *Experimental Chemotherapy*, Vol. I, pp. 603–624. Schnitzer RJ, Hawking F, eds. New York, Academic Press, 1963.

81. Klinefelter MR: Cause, diagnosis, and treatment of canine piroplasmosis. Vet Med/SAC 77:1505–1508, 1982.

82. Farwell GE, LeGrand EK, Cobb CC: Clinical observations on *Babesia gibsoni* and *Babesia canis* infections in dogs. J Am Vet Med Assoc 180:507–511, 1982.

83. Breitschwerdt EB, Malone JB, MacWilliams P, Levy MG, Qualls CW, Prudish MJ: Babesiosis in the greyhound. J Am Vet Med Assoc 182:978–982, 1983.

84. Fowler JL, Ruff MD, Fernau RC, Furusho Y: *Babesia gibsoni*: Chemotherapy in dogs. Am J Vet Res 33:1109–1114, 1972.

85. Stewart CG: A comparison of the efficacy of isometamidium, amicarbalide, and diminazene against *Babesia canis* in dogs and the effect on subsequent immunity. J S Afr Vet Assoc 54:47–51, 1983.

86. Ogunkoya AB, Adeyanju JB, Aliu YO: Experiences with the use of imizol in treating canine blood parasites in Nigeria. J Sm Anim P 22:775–777, 1981.

87. Uilenberg G, Verdiesen PA, Zwart D: Imidocarb: A chemoprophylactic experiment with *Babesia canis*. Tijdschr. Diergeneesk 106:118–123, 1981.

88. Euzeby J, Moreau Y, Chauve C, Gevrey J, Gauthey M: Experimentation des proprietes antipiroplasmiques de l'Imidocarb sur *Babesia canis*, agent de la piroplasmose canine en Europe. B Aca Vet de France 53:475–480, 1980.

89. Coll JL, Descamps H, Fayette JP, Feraud JP, Villemin P: Essai de chimo-prevention de la Babesiose canine avec l'imidocarbe. Rec Med Vet 158:791–798, 1982.

90. Futter GJ, Belonje PC: Studies on feline babesiosis. I. Historical Review. J S Afr Vet Assoc 50:105–106, 1980.

91. Stewart CG, Hackett KJW, Collett MG: An unidentified *Babesia* of the domestic cat (*Felis domesticus*). J S Afr Vet Assoc 51:219–221, 1980.

92. Ruebush TK II, Rubin RH, Wolpow ER, Cassaday PB, Schultz MG: Neurologic complications following the treatment of human *Babesia microti* infection with diminazene aceturate. Am J Trop Med Hyg 28:184–189, 1979.

93. Entrican JH, Williams H, Cook IA, Lancaster WM, Clark JC, Joyner LP, Lewis D: Babesiosis in man: Report of a case from Scotland with observations on the infecting strain. J Infection 1:227–234, 1979.

94. Francioli PB, Keithly JS, Jones TC, Brandstetter RD, Wolf DJ: Response of babesiosis to pentamidine therapy. Ann Int Med 94:326–330, 1981.
95. Rowin KS, Tanowitz HB, Wittner M: Therapy of experimental babesiosis. Ann Int Med 97:556–558, 1982.
96. Wittner M, Rowin KS, Tanowitz HB, Hobbs JF, Saltzman S, Wenz B, Hirsch R, Chisholm E, Healy GR: Successful chemotherapy of transfusion babesiosis. Ann Int Med 96:601–604, 1982.
97. Gombert ME, Goldstein EJC, Benach JL, Tenebaum MJ, Grunwaldt E, Kaplan MH, Eveland LK: Human babesiosis, clinical and therapeutic considerations. JAMA 248:3005–3007, 1982.
98. Michael SA, Refaii AH: The effect of imidocarb dipropionate on *Babesia ovis* infection in sheep. Trop Anim Hlth Prod 14:1–2, 1982.
99. Hashemi-Fesharki R: Studies on imidocarb dihydrochloride in experimental *Babesia ovis* infection in splenectomized lambs. Br Vet J 133:609–614, 1977.
100. Lewis D, Herbert I: A large *Babesia* of sheep from north Wales. Vet Rec 107:352–353, 1980.
101. Uilenberg G, Rombach MC, Perie NM, Zwart D: Blood parasites of sheep in the Netherlands. II. *Babesia motasi (Sporozoa babesiidae)*. Vet Q 2: 3–14, 1980.
102. Friedhoff KT: The piroplasms of equidae-significance for international commerce. Berl Münch Tierärztl Wschr 95:368–374, 1982.
103. Schein E, Rehbein G, Voigt WP, Zweygarth E: *Babesia equi* (Laveran 1901) 1. Development in horses and in lymphocyte culture. Tropenmed P 32:223–227, 1981.

12. Malaria epidemiology

WALTHER H. WERNSDORFER*

Research and Technical Intelligence, Malaria Action Programme, World Health Organization, Geneva, Switzerland.

1. Introduction

In this chapter it is not intended to give an account of the many factors governing malaria transmission since such a review has been provided in the chapter on 'The Importance of Malaria in the World' in Vol. 1 of *Malaria* (ed. J. Kreier, Academic Press, 1980). However, an attempt is made here to cover the current malaria situation in the world, and recent results of applied research which have relevance to the epidemiology of malaria. A section is also devoted to the distribution of drug resistant *Plasmodium falciparum* as this problem is becoming one of the most serious obstacles to curbing mortality and suffering from malaria.

2. Malaria in the world

Reliable data on the incidence of malaria are hard to provide as the efficiency of diagnosis and notification has shown a serious deterioration since the beginning of the 1970s. Coverage in space and time has undergone a substantial reduction as a consequence of diminishing national efforts to combat malaria. These developments may be ascribed, in part, to political decisions but the main contributory factors were of a financial, social and economic nature such as static government budgets, inflationary cost increases of manpower and commodities, and personal inconvenience associated with field work in rural areas.

Of a total world population of 4 574 million in 1982, some 1 292 million (28%) were living in areas which were naturally free from malaria or where the disease had disappeared spontaneously; approximately 807 million people (18%) lived in areas which were freed from malaria as a result of specific antimalaria measures; some 2 111 million people (46%) lived in areas which were under malaria risk and where some form of malaria control was being applied; the remainder (8%) resided without specific protection in malarious areas which include a large part of tropical Africa.

Ristic, M. et al. (eds.) *Malaria and babesiosis.*
© 1984, Martinus Nijhoff Publishers, Dordrecht/Boston/Lancaster.

In 1981 some 7.7 million malaria cases were reported to the World Health Organization [1] as against 8.0 million in 1980 and 7.0 million in 1979 [2]. The provisional figure for 1982 is 6.3 million [1]. These data do not include information from Africa south of the Sahara. In view of the above mentioned considerations it is unlikely that the figure for 1982 represents a true reduction of malaria incidence in the world. The global distribution of malaria is illustrated in Figure 1. There has been no major change in this distribution over the last decade.

There are, of course, important regional differences in the intensity of malaria transmission. These are expressed in the wide variations observed in the malaria incidence or prevalence (Table 1), with a very low incidence being found in North-West Africa and the highest prevalence in tropical Africa which has remained the world's hard core area of malaria. In the past, malaria incidence used to be lower in Central and South America as compared to Asia, but recently the trend appears to be reversed.

The European Continent (with the exception of Turkey), Australia and the United States of America have succeeded in maintaining a malaria free status in spite of a massive importation of malaria cases which could have given rise to the reestablishment of autochthonous transmission. Similarly, most of the other countries which achieved malaria eradication have maintained this status, with the exception of Mauritius, where malaria reestablished itself after a series of natural disasters.

Plasmodium falciparum is by far the leading parasite species. It is deeply entrenched in tropical Africa (Table 1), and globally, it accounts for approximately 80% of all infections, followed by *P. vivax* which is the leading species in many American and Asian countries. *P. malariae* has a worldwide incidence of < 1%, but it reaches substantially higher levels in tropical Africa. *P. ovale* has its main distribution in West Africa, but the species is also encountered in other tropical African countries, and sporadically in eastern Asia although it remains unclear whether closely related simian plasmodia are responsible for the 'ectopical' infections in Asia.

The following regional reviews of the malaria situation are largely based on data provided by the World Health Organization [1, 2, 3].

Incidence data are related to the population in the malarious areas only.

2.1. *Africa*

In Africa north of the Sahara, some 73 million people out of a total population of 96 million live in originally malarious areas. Malaria incidence is generally very low and transmission is focalized. In 1982 the reported malaria incidence showed a slight increase over 1981 (475 cases as compared to 464). Tunisia has become virtually free of malaria, while in Algeria, Morocco and Libya malaria incidence has become very low, with transmission being restricted to few foci. The only

175

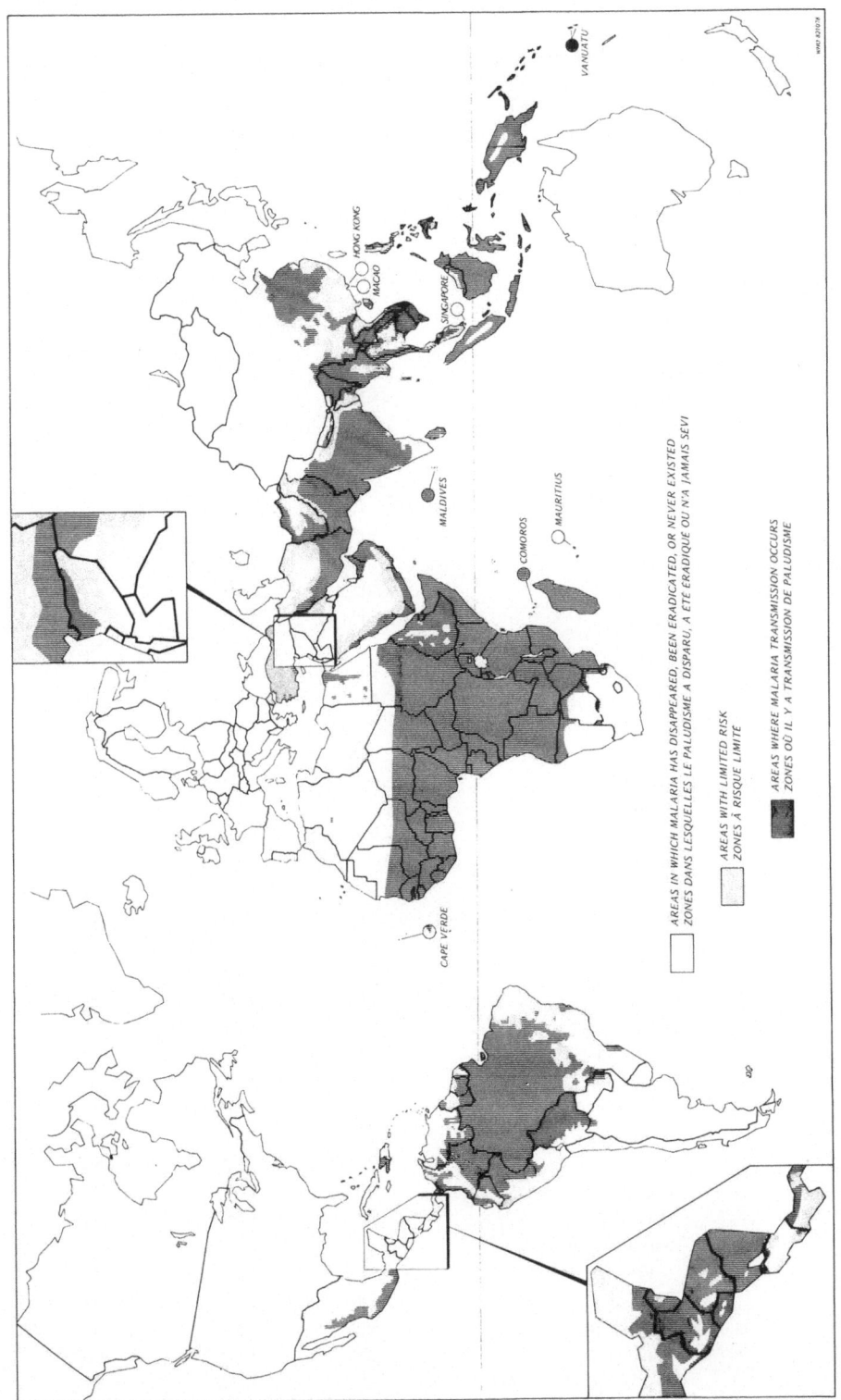

Fig. 1. Epidemiological assessment of status of malaria, 1981.

ÉVALUATION ÉPIDÉMIOLOGIQUE DU PALUDISME, 1981

AREAS IN WHICH MALARIA HAS DISAPPEARED, BEEN ERADICATED, OR NEVER EXISTED
ZONES DANS LESQUELLES LE PALUDISME A DISPARU, A ÉTÉ ÉRADIQUÉ OU N'A JAMAIS SÉVI

AREAS WITH LIMITED RISK
ZONES À RISQUE LIMITÉ

AREAS WHERE MALARIA TRANSMISSION OCCURS
ZONES OÙ IL Y A TRANSMISSION DE PALUDISME

Table 1. Malaria Incidence or Prevalence and Proportion of *Plasmodium falciparum* by geographical area and country

Area	Country	Annual* malaria incidence per 1000 pop.	Malaria prevalence**	Frequency sequence of plasmodia	*P. falciparum* as % of all positives
North Africa	Algeria	<0.01		VM	0
	Egypt		<1%	VFM	4%
	Libya	<0.1		VMF	<1%
	Morocco	<0.01		VMF	<1%
	Tunisia	0	–	–	–
Africa south of the Sahara	Angola		>50%	FMOV	>90%***
	Benin		>50%	FMO	90%***
	Botswana		<50%	FMV	95%***
	Burundi		<50%	FMOV	80%
	Cape Verde	? (low)		?	?
	Central Afr. Republic		>50%	FMO	85%***
	Chad		>50%	FMO (V)	85%***
	Comoros		>50%	FMOV	90%***
	Congo		>50%	FMO	90%***
	Djibouti	<10		FMV	80%***
	Equatorial Guinea		>50%	FMO	85%***
	Ethiopia		>50%	FMV	80%***
	Gabon		>50%	FMO (V)	95%***
	Gambia		>50%	FMO (V)	85%***
	Ghana		>50%	FMO	85%***
	Guinea		>50%	FMO	90%***
	Guinea-Bissau		>50%	FMO (V)	90%***
	Ivory Coast		>50%	FMO	90%***
	Kenya		>50%	FMOV	85%***
	Liberia		>50%	FMO (V)	90%***
	Madagascar		<50%	FMV	85%***
	Malawi		>50%	FMV (O)	90%***
	Mali		>50%	FMO	85%***
	Mauritania		>50%	(O)	10%
	Mauritius	<1	–	V	0%
	Mozambique		>50%	FMV	95%***
	Namibia		<10%	FMV	90%***
	Niger		>50%	FMO	80%***
	Nigeria		>50%	FMO	85%***
	Rwanda		>50%	FMO	90%***
	Sao Tome and Principe		>50%	FMV (O)	?
	Senegal		>50%	FMO (V)	85%***
	Sierra Leone		>50%	FMO	80%***
	Somalia		<25%	FMV	95%***
	South Africa	1-2		FMV	99%***

Table 1. Continued

Area	Country	Annual* malaria incidence per 1000 pop.	Malaria prevalence**	Frequency sequence of plasmodia	*P. falciparum* as % of all positives
	Sudan		>50%	FMVO	90%***
	Swaziland	1		FM	99%
	Togo		>50%	FMO	85%***
	Uganda		>50%	FMO	85%***
	United Rep. of Cameroon		>50%	FMO	85%***
	United Rep. of Tanzania		>50%	FMVO	80%***
	Upper Volta		>50%	FMO	85%***
	Zaire		>50%	FMO	90%***
	Zambia		>50%	FMV	90%***
	Zimbabwe		>50%	FMV	90%***
Central America	Belize	2.5		V	0%
	Costa Rica	< 0.1		VF	5%
	Dominican Republic	0.8		F (V)	>99%
	El Salvador	20		VF	12%
	Guatemala	27		VF	10%
	Haiti	15		F	100%
	Honduras	16		VF	7%
	Mexico	1.3		VFM	1%
	Nicaragua	5.3		VF	8%
	Panama	< 0.2		FV	55%
South America	Argentina	< 0.2		V	0%
	Bolivia	2.9		VF	13%
	Brazil	4.1		VF (M)	43%
	Colombia	4.5		VFM	41%
	Equador	2.7		VF	21%
	French Guiana	19		FV	87%
	Guyana	1.8		VF	25%
	Paraguay	< 0.05		VF	29%
	Peru	2.4		V (M)	0%
	Suriname	8.5		FV	90%
	Venezuela	0.4		VFM	15%
Europe incl. USSR and Turkey	Turkey	1.2		VMF	< 0.1%
	USSR (only area with transmission. 460 000 pop.)	0.66		V	0%

178

Table 1. Continued

Area	Country	Annual* malaria incidence per 1000 pop.	Malaria prevalence**	Frequency sequence of plasmodia	*P. falciparum* as % of all positives
Asia west of Burma	Afghanistan	11.5		VFM	< 1%
	Bangladesh	0.4		VFM	43%
	Bhutan	?		?	?
	Dem. Yemen	3.6		FV	Approx. 50%
	India	3.1		VFM	20%
	Iran	1.3		VFM	20%
	Iraq	0.2		VFM	< 1%
	Maldives	0.7		VF	1%
	Nepal	1.8		VF	14%
	Pakistan	0.7		VFM	23%
	Saudi Arabia	4.5		FV	Approx. 50%
	Sri Lanka	3.5		VFM	4%
	Syria	0.3		VFM	< 1%
	United Arab Emirates	7.9		FV	55%
	Yemen	7.7		FV	Approx. 50%
Eastern Asia and Oceania	Burma	1.2		FVM (O)	80%
	China	2.2		VFM	<10%
	Dem. Kampuchea	?		FV	>70%
	East Timor	?		?	?
	Indonesia	0.5 (Java)	? (Other Isl.)	VF	40%
	Lao People's Dem. Rep.		Aprox 10%	FV	70%
	Malaysia Peninsular	0.9		FVM (O)	77%
	Sabah	55		FVM	72%
	Sarawak	0.5		VFM	31%
	Papua New Guinea	41	?	FVM	73%
	Philippines	6.2		FVM	69%
	Solomon Islands	244		VF	30%
	Thailand	9.7		VFM (O)	49%
	Vanuatu	53		VF	10%
	Viet Nam	11		FVM	Approx. 50%

* Refers to areas under risk only, autochthonous cases (most recent data, usually 1982 or 1981)

** In unprotected areas with a high endemicity of malaria; these data refer to young children during peak seasons

*** Approximate data, subject to seasonal variation, *P. falciparum* reaching lowest levels during the dry season.

Key: F = *Plasmodium falciparum;* M = *P. malariae;* O = *P. ovale;* V = *P. vivax.*

country showing increased incidence is Egypt where the number of cases rose from 298 in 1981 to 365 in 1982. In these areas *P. vivax* is the main *Plasmodium* species.

In Africa south of the Sahara some 47 million of the total population of 397 million live in areas which are naturally free of malaria or where malaria has been eliminated. These areas include Cape Verde, Lesotho, Réunion, St. Helena, the Seychelles, large parts of South Africa, and high altitude areas (generally above 2500 m) in various countries. In Mauritius malaria reestablished itself in the late 1970s following natural disasters. The 669 cases reported in 1982 (all *P. vivax*) were distributed in 155 foci throughout the island, but energetic measures have apparently succeeded in halting the epidemic.

Most of tropical Africa is affected by stable, holo- or hyperendemic malaria, with *P. falciparum* as the leading species. *Anopheles gambiae* s.l. and *A. funestus* are the principal vectors in these areas. In the semiarid fringe areas malaria tends to be meso- or hypoendemic and of medium or low stability. This accounts for an epidemic occurrence of the disease which is not seen in areas with highly stable malaria. Recently, droughts in the Sahel belt have destabilized malaria in parts of West Africa, thus changing its pattern to an epidemic pattern which is also characteristic of the high altitude fringes.

Depending on environmental factors, the malaria situation may widely vary within the same country, and from season to season. Such differences are particularly marked in the presence of specific malariogenic factors, e.g. irrigation schemes such as the one in the Ruzizi plain of Burundi [4].

In Malumfashi, Nigeria, a wet season parasite rate of 93% was recorded in children 5–9 years of age [5]. The dry season parasite rate was 76%. *P. falciparum* fluctuated between 74 and 96% of all infections, *P. malariae* between 4 and 25%; *P. ovale* accounted for 0.3%.

In the same area a point prevalence survey yielded parasite rates of 32% in infants (0–1 year), 87% in children 5–9 years of age, and 40% in persons 15–20 years of age [6]. Spleen rates were highest in the 2–4 year age group (72%), declining to 24% in the 15–20 year olds.

Stronger seasonal variations of the parasite rate were seen in the northern savanna area of Upper Volta (recently renamed BurKina Faso), with a dry season rate of 40% and nearly 100% at the end of the wet season in young children [7].

In the past, many of the urban areas in tropical Africa used to be little affected by malaria, but rapid and chaotic urbanization on the outskirts of cities has brought malaria increasingly to this environment.

A positivity rate of 29% among 500 febrile children was observed in Libreville, Gabon (13% in infants 0–6 months old, 42% in children 2–4 years old), with *P. falciparum* accounting for 97% of the infections [8].

East Africa is often considered to be less malarious than Central or West Africa. This may be true with regard to the intensity of transmission, but there is obviously little difference in prevalence and clinical manifestations. In Rwanda malaria is estimated to account for 20% of attendances at dispensaries. In Malawi, a dry season survey in schools (8–18 year age group) showed a parasite rate of 70.5% with 94.4% of the slides being positive for *P. falciparum*, 6.2% for *P. malariae*, and 3.6% for *P. ovale* – an unusually high prevalence of *P. ovale* for an East African country [9], but a significant, though lesser prevalence of this species was also recorded in Zambia where the malaria prevalence was generally lower [10].

2.2. *The Americas*

Some 245 million of the Americas' total population of 637 million live in originally malarious areas; 120 million reside in areas which have been freed from the disease, 59 million in areas with a very limited malaria risk, and 66 million in areas with a significant degree of malaria transmission. The USA and the Caribbean (with the exception of the Dominican Republic and Haiti) have maintained a malaria free status. Malaria incidence in the Americas has shown a continuous upward trend from 280 000 cases in 1973 to 709 000 cases in 1982, and the slide positivity rate has risen from 3.0% in 1973 to 8.1% in 1982.

Central American countries, namely Guatemala, El Salvador, and Honduras had in 1982 an average malaria incidence of 16–27 per thousand, the highest recorded in the Americas; in these countries technical problems such as insecticide multi-resistance of the local vector mosquitos are combined with political destabilization and population migration, rendering adequate malaria control virtually impossible. Countries unaffected by these factors, e.g. Costa Rica and Panama, were able to maintain effective malaria control and recorded in 1982 a malaria incidence of <0.2 per thousand. *P. vivax* is the leading parasite species in Central America, with the exception of Haiti where only *P. falciparum* occurs (the population is of predominantly West African origin). The parasite incidence in Haiti was 15 per thousand in 1982. The neighbouring Dominican Republic is a major recipient of imported falciparum malaria from Haiti.

In the South American countries, the annual malaria incidence (1982) was generally well under 5 per thousand (1982) with the exception of French Guiana (19/1000) and Suriname (8.5/1000), the only South American countries where *P. falciparum* is the leading parasite species. Paraguay maintained highly efficient control reflected in an annual parasite incidence of 0.05/1000 in 1982. The number of cases increased slightly in Brazil, Ecuador and Venezuela, but malaria shows a tendency to focalization in these countries. Colombia and Peru are facing major problems in malaria control, but Bolivia has recently achieved a significant reduction of malaria incidence from approximately 8/1000 in 1980 to 3/1000 in 1982.

When considering incidence data from Amazonian countries one should be aware of the existing gaps of coverage in space and time. Thus, a parasite rate of 79.2%, a high prevalence of *P. malariae* (89% of all positives), and an absence of

P. falciparum were observed in a remote area of the Peruvian Amazon jungle [11].

2.3 *Asia, Australia, Oceania*

Out of a total population of 2 640 million, some 2 234 live in originally malarious areas (1982). Malaria has been eradicated from areas with a population of 321 million; 1 913 million people are still exposed to various degrees of malaria risk – generally lowest in western Asia and highest in the Solomon Islands and probably Kampuchea.

In Asia west of India, a malaria free status was maintained in Cyprus, Jordan, Lebanon, Kuwait and Qatar; Israel recorded four cases and Bahrain two of autochthonous malaria in 1982, but the foci were quickly brought under control. In most countries the malaria incidence rose in 1982, with the exception of the United Arab Emirates. In Saudi Arabia improved case detection may account for an apparently increased malaria incidence. Several countries in western Asia are exposed to a heavy influx of malaria from abroad; for example Syria receives cases from Turkey, and the Gulf States from southern and eastern Asia. In the latter case this constitutes also a major risk of having drug resistant *P. falciparum* introduced into vulnerable and receptive areas. Among the malarious countries of western Asia, Iraq has the lowest parasite incidence (0.2/1000 in 1982), while Afghanistan has the highest (11.5/1000). *P. vivax* is the leading malaria parasite species in most countries, but *P. falciparum* is the most prevalent species in Saudi Arabia, the United Arab Emirates and the two Yemens.

None of the countries of middle south Asia has become malaria free as yet, but practically all of the population residing in that part of the world is covered by malaria control. Malaria incidence is lowest in Bangladesh and the Maldives (0.4/ 1000 and 0.7/1000 respectively in 1982), and highest in Bhutan (between 22 and 40 per thousand during 1978–1982), followed by Sri Lanka and India (3.5/1000 and 3.1/1000 respectively in 1982). In Bangladesh malaria is concentrated in the southeastern region, in India urban areas account for a large part of the malaria incidence which dropped from 6.5 million cases in 1976 to approximately 2.2 million in 1982, following the strengthening of control operations. However, a rise of the proportion of *P. falciparum* from 15% in 1978 to 25% in 1982 raises some doubts as to the accuracy of case detection data. Similarly, a decreased incidence was reported from Sri Lanka, but here also the proportion of *P. falciparum* rose from 2.6% in 1981 to 4.2% in 1982, a tendency which was further accentuated in 1983. In Pakistan the malaria incidence showed a more than fourfold increase between 1979 and 1982 (from 12 300 to 56 700 cases). A major urban focus exists in Karachi. *P. vivax* is now the leading malaria parasite species in all countries of middle southern Asia. Originally, *P. falciparum* was the most prevalent species in some areas, e.g. in parts of West Bengal, but in the course of intensive malaria control the proportion of *P. falciparum* dropped [12] and *P. malariae* virtually disappeared, a sequence of events also experienced in Karnataka and Tamil Nache States of India [13]. A limited outbreak of human *P. cynomolgi* infections has occurred in the Greater Nicobar Islands, India [14]. This has been ascribed to the environment which is shared between man and the local *Macaca*, with *A. sundaicus* frequenting them both. Nevertheless, other studies seem to suggest that the risk of zoonotic malaria in other parts of India is very limited since simian malaria is ecologically well separated from man [15].

In eastern Asia and Oceania, Brunei, the Democratic People's Republic of Korea, Hongkong, Japan, Macao, the Republic of Korea, Singapore, and large parts of China have maintained a malaria free status. Oceania east of 170° E is naturally free of malaria. The lowest malaria incidence has been recorded in Sarawak, Malaysia (0.5/1000 in 1981), the highest in the Solomon Islands (244/1000 in 1981), but there are countries and areas where malaria endemicity is high and where incidence data have little significance. Such areas comprise Papua New Guinea, East Timor, several Indonesian islands, Democratic Kampuchea and the Lao People's Democratic Republic. In China, the number of cases dropped from 3.06 million in 1981 to 2.04 million in 1982. Similarly, a substantial decrease of malaria incidence was recorded in Java, Indonesia, and Thailand, while little change was observed in Burma, and a further deterioration had taken place in Sabah, Malaysia, and Vanuatu (malaria incidence 55/1000 and 53/1000 respectively in 1981). *P. falciparum* is the leading malaria parasite species in Burma, Democratic Kampuchea, Lao People's Democratic Republic, Peninsular Malaysia, Sabah (Malaysia), the Philippines and Viet Nam. In Thailand it accounts for almost half the cases. *P. vivax* represents the large majority of infections (90% or more) in China and Vanuatu. *P. ovale* is sporadically found in eastern Asia. Earlier reports have mentioned Southern China and the Indochinese Peninsula, the Philippines and the island of New Guinea. The species occurs apparently also in Burma [16]. In western Timor, Indonesia [17], it was observed during a cross sectional survey which revealed a general parasite rate of 34%, with *P. falciparum* as the leading species. Yet higher parasite rates, 52% in children 2–9 years of age, and a high proportion of *P. falciparum* were observed in Irian Jaya, Indonesia [18].

Continental Australia has maintained a malaria free status although it is subject to a heavy influx of malaria cases from abroad, especially from Papua New Guinea and malarious areas of Oceania.

2.4 *Europe (including Asian parts of Turkey and USSR)*

Apart from two cases of local transmission near Brussels Airport (likely to have originated from imported, infected mosquitos) and one introduced case in Greece, autochthonous malaria was restricted to Turkey and a small area in the

Asian part of the USSR. In Turkey malaria had almost disappeared by 1968, but an epidemic developed subsequently in the Çukurova plain (Asia Minor), reaching in 1977 a peak with 115 000 cases. Control measures brought the malaria incidence down to 29 000 cases in 1979, but since then it has risen again, reaching 62 000 cases in 1982 and now affects also other parts of Turkey. The malaria focus in the Asian part of the USSR remained practically static, producing 304 cases in 1981. The overall number of imported malaria cases in Europe showed no appreciable change over the last three years, levelling close to 4000 *per annum.*

3. Drug resistance in Plasmodium falciparum

The term drug resistance has been defined as the 'Ability of a parasite strain to multiply or to survive in the presence of concentrations of a drug that normally destroy parasites of the same species or prevent their multiplication. Such resistance may be relative (yielding to increased doses of the drug tolerated by the host) or complete (withstanding maximum doses tolerated by the host) [19]. Observations on the response of *P. falciparum* to quinine in Brazil early in the 20th century suggest that complete resistance to this drug had occurred at least in this part of the world [20, 21]. Fortunately, quinine resistance has not shown a pronounced tendency to spread, and its biological selection may have been relatively limited on account of the drug's short half life. There was, at any rate, no major operational problem with quinine resistance while this drug was the only one available for the treatment and suppression of malaria. Mepacrine, the first synthetic blood schizontocidal drug, introduced in the 1930s, was probably in use not long enough to produce large-scale resistance since it was superseded in the late 1940s by a new generation of suppressive and therapeutic drugs. These were the dihydrofolate reductase (DHFR) inhibitors proguanil and pyrimethamine, and a very potent group of drugs, the 4-aminoquinolines such as chloroquine and amodiaquine.

Resistance to DHFR inhibitors was observed within two years of their widespread use, but this event gave rise to little concern at the time since response to the 4-aminoquinolines remained satisfactory. However, in 1960, resistance to chloroquine was reported almost simultaneously from Colombia and Thailand. This marked the onset of a problem the full dimensions of which it has not yet been possible to determine precisely, especially as the selection for and the spread of chloroquine resistance are still in progress. The consequences of chloroquine resistance, particularly in tropical Africa, have to be seen in the light of the cost of alternative drugs which is outside the financial possibilities of many a government.

3.1. *Field assessment of drug response*

Before the advent of *in vitro* tests, drug response of *P. falciparum* could only be assessed *in vivo*, using standard dose regimens of drugs. The appropriate procedures have been described in WHO publications [22, 23]. The *in vivo* response can be classified as follows:

S (sensitive	clearance of asexual parasitaemia within 7 days of initiation of treatment, without subsequent recrudescence
RI (Resistant I)	clearance of asexual parasitaemia as in sensitivity, followed by recrudescence
RII (Resistant II)	marked reduction of asexual parasitaemia (<25% of pre-treatment level), but no clearance
RIII (Resistant III)	no marked reduction of asexual parasitaemia

The post-treatment observation period required for the differentiation of S and RI responses has been estimated at 28 days for the 4-aminoquinolines. It is higher for drugs with a long half life, e.g. mefloquine where the observation needs to be extended to eight weeks.

In vivo tests, though essential, are cumbersome to conduct; their results may not be conclusive if they are conducted while there is active malaria transmission. The results may also be influenced by the individual's immune response and thus not be indicative of the parasite's true drug sensitivity. This is evident from *in vivo* studies in areas with highly endemic malaria, where the drug response in young children is markedly different from that in adults.

The introduction of an *in vitro* test [24] was therefore a milestone in the assessment of drug response. The technique is based on the measurement of schizont maturation and its suppression by ascending concentrations of chloroquine using defibrinated blood in vials fortified with glucose. The method and the essential material were subsequently standardized and extended to assess also the response to mefloquine. A disadvantage of this 'macrotechnique' was the need for relatively advanced ring forms in the patient's blood, and for drawing blood through venepuncture. Based on the elements for the continuous cultivation of *P. falciparum* [25] a microtechnique was described [26] which was subsequently adapted to field use, standardized and validated [27, 28, 29, 30]. The microtechnique requires only a small quantity of blood which can be drawn by finger prick; its success rate is higher than that of the macrotechnique, and it does not require advanced ring stages. The microtechnique has been adapted to test parasite sensitivity to chloroquine, amodiaquine, mefloquine and quinine, and has by now largely replaced the macrotechnique. Current studies aim at the development of a field test for the assessment of the sensitivity of *P. falciparum* to sulfadoxine and pyrimethamine.

Probit analysis of logdose/response is probably the most convenient method of processing the results of the *in vitro* tests. An appropriate programme for the calculation of the regression parameters and the estimation of the effective concentration levels has been described [31].

3.2. *Distribution of drug resistant* P. falciparum

The distribution of chloroquine resistant *P. falcipaum* in the world is given in Figure 2 and Table 2. In Asia and Oceania chloroquine resistance is observed now in a solid band of countries from Vanuatu – the easternmost malarious country – to central India. In South America, chloroquine resistant *P. falciparum* is found in all malarious countries with the exception of Argentina ad Paraguay. In Africa the first reports on chloroquine resistance date from 1978, when nonimmune travellers had contracted infections with resistant *P. falciparum*. Since then, chloroquine resistance has occurred in eight more African countries, and it is suspected to exist also in Somalia and Gabon.

There are marked differences in frequency and degree of chloroquine resistance, both being highest in the 'hard-core' areas on the Indochina Peninsula. In the border area of Thailand and Kampuchea more than 90% of all *P. falciparum* isolates are resistant to chloroquine, and RII and RIII *in vivo* responses are now more common than RI. In the marginal areas of its distribution, chloroquine resistance is usually low both in frequency and degree, e.g. in western India. The northernmost limit of the distribution of chloroquine resistant *P. falciparum* has remained stationary at the Panama Canal since 1969, but recent observations [32] point to an incipient loss of sensitivity in Haiti.

Generally, the degree of chloroquine resistance is higher in Asia and Oceania than in South America. The situation is still unclear in East Africa since the situation is continuously evolving. However, recent studies in Tanzania indicate a very rapid loss of sensitivity of *P. falciparum* to chloroquine resulting in an increased proportion of resistant isolates [33]. Decreasing response of the individual isolates was obviously accelerated by the use of extensive mass drug administration.

In large parts of Asia, Oceania and South America chloroquine has lost its usefulness and reliability in the treatment of falciparum malaria. This has not yet occurred in East Africa, where chloroquine usually still eliminates *P. falciparum* in semi-immunes. However, the efficacy of this drug in groups with little immunity, such as infants and young children, is becoming increasingly compromised, and alternative drugs will be required for therapeutic use in these vulnerable groups.

Alternative drugs, of which the first is the combination of sulfadoxine and

186

Fig. 2. Distribution of chloroquine resistant *Plasmodium falciparum* in the world. Status of mid-1983.

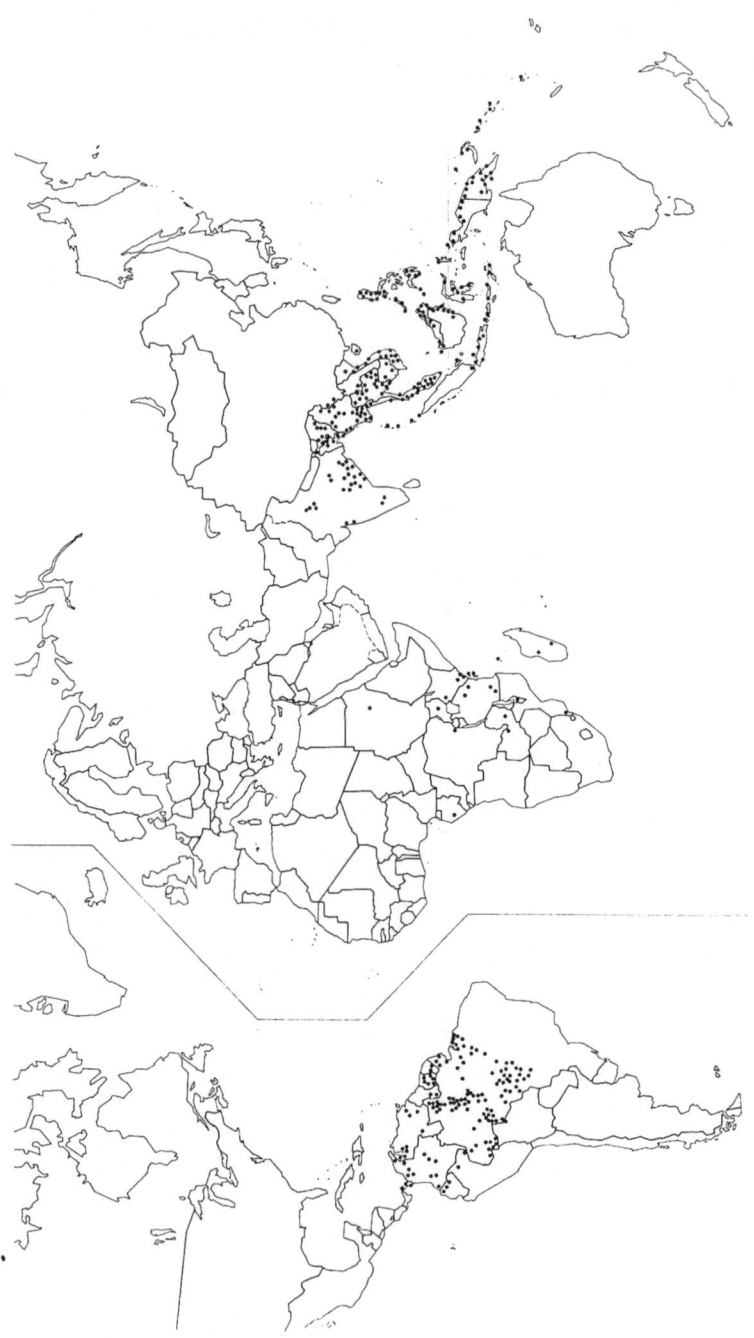

Table 2. Countries with autochthonous chloroquine resistant falciparum malaria

Area	Country	First notification of resistance	Degree of resistance
Africa	Burundi	1983	R (unspec.)
	Comoro Islands	1978	RI
	Kenya	1979	RI, RII
	Madagascar	1980	RI, RII
	Malawi	1983	RI, RII
	Sudan	1983	RI, RII
	Tanzania (United Republic of)	1980	RI, RII
	Uganda	1981	R (unspec.)
	Zaire	1983	RI, RII, RIII
	Zambia	1980	RI, RII, RIII
The Americas	Bolivia	1980	R (unspec.)
	Brazil	1961	RI, RII, RIII
	Colombia	1961	RI, RII, RIII
	Ecuador	1976	RI, RII
	French Guiana	1975	R (unspec.)
	Guyana	1969	R (unspec.)
	Panama (south)	1969	RI, RII
	Peru	1980	R (unspec.)
	Suriname	1972	RI, RII
	Venezuela	1960	RI, RII, RIII
Asia & Oceania	Bangladesh	1970	RI, RII, RIII
	Burma	1978	RI, RII, RIII
	China (Hainan)	1979	RI, RII, RIII
	Democratic Kampuchea	1962	RI, RII, RIII
	India	1973	RI, RII, RIII
	Indonesia	1973	RI, RII, RIII
	Lao People's Democratic Republic	1980	RI, RII, RIII
	Malaysia	1963	RI, RII, RIII
	Papua New Guinea	1976	RI, RII, RIII
	Philippines	1974	RI, RII, RIII
	Solomon Islands	1980	R (unspec.)
	Thailand	1961	RI, RII, RIII
	Timor (East)	1982	RI, RII
	Vanuatu	1980	RI, RII, RIII
	Viet Nam	1962	RI, RII, RIII

pyrimethamine, are increasingly being used to treat chloroquine resistant falciparum malaria. This combination gives good results as long as the parasite has not acquired a high degree of pyrimethamine resistance since sulfadoxine potentiates the effect of pyrimethamine. It fails, however, if pyrimethamine resistance has reached a high level, e.g. in some areas of the Indochina Peninsula, Brazil and Colombia, and East Africa. This may appear to indicate primary pyrimethamine resistance in parts of Africa where the use of alternative antimalarials was very limited; it is likely that non-target selection pressure of DHFR inhibitors and dihydropteroate synthase inhibitors (used as antibacterial drugs) in the presence of intensive transmission is responsible for this phenomenon.

Quinine and tetracycline are being used for the treatment of infections with multiresistant *P. falciparum*. Even in the hardcore areas of multiresistance, response to these drugs has generally remained satisfactory, but the use of quinine and tetracycline is cumbersome and poses problems of patient compliance. These constraints could be overcome through the introduction of a drug requiring only single dose administration. Mefloquine (formulated in combination with sulfadoxine and pyrimethamine) will probably meet this requirement. This compound has undergone extensive trials which demonstrated its high efficacy and safety. Nevertheless, there are two reports of primary drug resistance [34, 35] which point to the need for taking measures to protect the efficacy of the new drug.

P. vivax, P. ovale and *P. malariae* are still responding fully to chloroquine which remains the drug of choice for the clinical treatment of infections with these parasites. Pyrimethamine resistant *P. vivax* occurs in Asia and South America.

4. Applied research relevant to epidemiology

It is not intended to give a detailed review of recent applied research, but only to highlight a few points in areas which are of major epidemiological importance. This summary review will include entomological, parasitological, physio-pathological and epidemiological aspects.

4.1. *Entomological research*

Cytological studies of anopheline chromosomes have permitted the identification of individual species of the *A. gambiae* complex, differentiating so far a total of 6 species. The development of methods for the starch gel electrophoresis of mosquito enzymes [36, 37, 38] has also facilitated species differentiation since there are distinct species-specific enzyme and isoenzyme patterns. The biochemical methods are however less cumbersome and time consuming than cytological procedures.

Species complex status has been confirmed for *A. culicifacies* [39, 40, 41, 42, 43, 44, 45] in which four distinct species have been identified. The Leucosphyrus group was subject to extensive studies in eastern Asia [46, 47, 48, 49, 50, 51, 52] confirming full species status for *A. dirus* (formerly *A. balabacensis balabacensis*) and *A. takasogoensis* as well as the Fraser's Hill and Perlis forms of *A. balabacensis*. Studies on *A. albimanus* [53], *A. funestus/A. aruni* [54], *A. maculatus* [55], *A.*

punctulatus [56]; *A. stephensi* [57] and *A. subpictus* [58] strongly indicate the presence of species complexes.

Mosquito susceptibility to plasmodial infection is becoming recognized as an important epidemiological factor. All genetic variants of *A. albimanus* tested were found to be less susceptible to *P. falciparum* than to *P. vivax*, and less susceptible to both species than *A. freeborni* [59]. *A. freeborni* proved to be the most susceptible species to infection with the El Salvador/Santa Lucia isolate of *P. falciparum* [60], followed by *A. maculatus*, *A. dirus* and *A. albimanus* (infection rates of 86.9%, 46.7%, 40.5% and 25.1%). *A. nuñeztovari* in Venezuela was more susceptible to *P. falciparum* (37.7% infection rate) than to *P. vivax* (4.4% infection rate) [61]. This observation merits follow-up. *A. pseudopunctipennis* from El Salvador proved to be refractory to infection with *P. falciparum* and *P. vivax* [62]. An isolate of *P. falciparum* from China proved to be most infective to *A. dirus* from Thailand, followed by *A. stephensi*, *A. maculatus* and *A. culicifacies*. Two *A. gambiae* s.l. strains from East and West Africa were least susceptible to this Chinese isolate [63]. *A. sinensis*, a member of the Hyrcanus group, was found to be highly susceptible to infection with *P. vivax* from China, with infections developing in more than 60% of the mosquitos tested [64]. *A. atroparvus* in the USSR was almost equally susceptible to *P. vivax* from Africa, America and Asia, with an average infection rate of 36%. *A. messeae* and *A. sacharovi* were also susceptible to *P. vivax*, but none of the three anophelines developed infections with *P. falciparum* from Africa [65]. *A. atroparvus* was also refractory to infections with *P. malariae* and *P. ovale* from West Africa [66]. Of major epidemiological importance is the observed correlation between chloroquine resistance and infectivity of *P. falciparum* to mosquitos. A positive correlation was found in *A. dirus* and *A. stephensi*, suggesting a biological advantage of chloroquine resistant *P. falciparum* [67].

Laboratory studies on the longevity of *P. cynomolgi*-infected *A. dirus* [68] suggest that the early mortality rates in infected and noninfected mosquitos are similar, but there is a significantly higher mortality of infected *A. dirus* as from day ten after infection, reducing the mean longevity by eight days.

Studies on the breeding of *A. nuñeztovari* showed a wide adaptability of this species to changes of water temperature, pH, oxygen tension and CO_2 content [69]. In Bangladesh *A. dirus* eggs and larvae were found to be remarkably resistant to drying [70].

Major species-specific differences in resting heights of local anopheline species, were demonstrated in Central Java, Indonesia [71]. *A. stephensi*, mainly an urban vector, was found to rest indoors at heights over 2.5 m, and in wells deeper than 8 m [72]. Flight level studies of *A. melas* in the Gambia [73, 74] showed maximum movement at ground level and decreasing numbers with increasing height, but a significant yield was still obtained at 8 m. The flight speed of *A. ziemanni* was found to be 1.8 m/s, that of *A. gambiae* s.l., *A. pharoensis* and *A. squamosus* 1.4 m/s [75], and that of *A. melas* of the *A. gambiae* group 1.1 m/s [73].

Flight ranges are largely species specific. A relatively high range of 4.5 km was observed in *A. stephensi mysorensis* [76]. Flight may be triggered by irritation. *A. arabiensis* and *A. gambiae* s.s. were found to adopt a 'bite and run technique' in the presence of DDT, with *A. gambiae* flying for twice as long a time as *A. arabiensis* after such irritation [77].

The duration of the gonotrophic cycle is largely species specific and temperature dependent. *A. darlingi* in Amazonian Brazil shows a 48-hour cycle [78], a pattern prevailng also in *A. gambiae* in the Congo [79], whereas *A. nili* in the Congo has a 3-day cycle [80]. In *A. culicifacies*, the gonotrophic cycle was observed to vary from 2 days at 28° C to 5½ days at 18° C [81]. These variations are of great epidemiological significance since they determine the frequency at which infections can be contracted or imparted.

Biting habits of anophelines are another epidemiologically important factor. Using haptoglobins as markers, the frequency of multiple feeds was found to be 10% in *A. gambiae* s.l. in Nigeria [82]. Marked differences in the human blood ratio of *A. gambiae* s.s. from the Gambia were observed [83] in specimens collected from bednets (0.88), inside houses (0.67) and outside houses (0.15). In the Congo, *A. gambiae* biting rates were observed to be dependent on the host's age; adults being bitten three times more frequently than infants. There was no sex difference in host frequentation [84]. In Maharashtra villages, India, the local anophelines were found to prefer biting on legs (95%) as compared to hands (3%) and other parts of the body [85]. Contrary to earlier presumptions, *A. nili* proved to be highly anthropophilic in the Congo [86], with a human blood ratio of 0.96 which suggests that this species is an important malaria vector in this part of Africa.

Hitherto most bloodmeal identifications have been made with the precipitin technique. However, preliminary studies with a gel diffusion method [87] and an enzyme linked immunosorbent assay (ELISA) [88] suggest that these procedures offer good prospects for the development of rapid and inexpensive tests for bloodmeal identification.

4.2 *Research related to the parasite and the human host*

Studies in the Liutum area, Liaoning Province, China [89], indicate the presence of *P. vivax* with a long incubation period (average 9.5 months), while in eastern Henan, China, 49% of all *P. vivax* infections developed relapses after an interval of 186–342 days even when effective blood schizontocidal treatment had been given [90]. This long interval is characteristic of some *P. vivax* strains of the temperate regions. However, relatively long latency, between eight and 52 weeks with a mean of 25 weeks, was also found in El Salvador [91], where one would have expected a short interval pattern common in tropical *P. vivax*. In Northern Nigeria, the prevalence of *P. malariae* increased towards the end of the dry season when *P. falciparum* transmission was at its lowest [92]. *P. falciparum* suppressed *P. malariae*, but no such interaction was found with *P. ovale*.

The characterization of *P. falciparum* isolates has been greatly facilitated by the introduction of continuous cultivation *in vitro*. Enzyme typing of the isolates [93, 94] was the first method utilized for this purpose, but antigenic differentiation and DNA typing seem to offer better prospects.

In an area with a high endemicity of malaria in Nigeria immunity was shown to increase the natural rate of recovery from infection by a factor which could be as high as 10, reducing also the periods of patent parasitaemia [95]. Malaria control in such an environment led to a rapid decrease of IgM levels, whereas the IgG levels showed little change [96]. Observations in Gambian children [97] indicate a possible relationship between a positive direct antiglobulin test (DAT) and protective immunity. A significant association of ahaptoglobinaemia and parasitaemia was observed in village populations of the Gambia [98]. However, a group working in Upper Volta came to the conclusion that haptoglobin levels cannot be used as a reliable indicator for past or present infections in this part of Africa, where a large proportion of the population has low haptoglobin levels [99]. Serum and lymphocytes from Gambian children were shown to induce gametocytogenesis *in vitro* to a more marked degree than those from European subjects [100]. A possible relationship has been suggested between complement C3b and gametocytaemia in Nigerian children [101].

The passive transfer and waning in offspring of the maternal antibodies directed against asexual blood forms is a well-known phenomenon in hyperendemic areas. Studies in the Gambia [102] show that antisporozoite antibodies are also maternally transmitted. Of 20 mothers examined, 18 had antisporozoite antibodies; 17 infants had antisporozoite antibodies at birth, but the antibody levels decreased and became undetectable generally before six months. In contrast, the mothers maintained their antisporozoite antibody levels.

Anaemia is commonly associated with malaria and is in part the result of the destruction of red blood cells by the parasite. In chronic malarial infections, however, immunopathological factors are believed to be responsible for the accelerated erythrocyte destruction and for reduced erythropoiesis [103]. An association was found between anaemia and high IgG 1 levels in the absence of IgG 4 [104]. Anaemia is often concomitant with malaria during pregnancy, especially in primipara in hyperendemic areas [105].

The relative protective role against *P. falciparum* of the sickle cell trait in heterozygotes seems to have been established earlier. This factor is apparently responsible for the selection of a gene which is clearly deleterious in the homozygous state. *In vitro* studies indicate a significantly lesser invasion rate and growth of *P. falciparum* in AS and SS cells as compared to normal erythrocytes [106]. However, a number of field studies have yielded inconclusive results on the protective effect of the sickle cell trait [107, 108]. On the other hand, persons with HbAS attained only significantly lower IgM levels as compared to normal individuals [109] and a consistently lower parasitaemia was found in Nigerian children with HbAS as compared to those with HbAA [110]. A higher survival rate of young individuals with HbAS and HbAC, as compared to those with HbAA, was also reported from Ghana [111], whereas no difference in parasite density and serological reaction was found between individuals with HbAC and HbAA in Nigeria [112]. HbAS individuals had a higher survival rate as compared to persons with HbAA also in the Cameroons [113]. Ovalocytes were found to be less susceptible to invasion by *P. falciparum* merozoites [114, 115]. Apart from New Guinea this trait is also found in Sulawesi, Indonesia [116] where its epidemiological significance needs to be investigated.

In a study in Gambian children no association was found between the A B O blood groups and malaria infection [117]. Similar results were also obtained in Nigeria with regard to the M, MN, N, S, Sa, U-, U, Fy^a, Fy^b, Fy^a-Fy^b and FyFy blood groups [118], but the studies were conducted essentially in the absence of *P. vivax*. Observations in India [119] showed a significantly higher incidence of vivax malaria in persons of blood group A, and a lower one in those of group O. This would merit further investigation. Earlier observations of the refractoriness to *P. vivax* of Duffy negative individuals have been further strengthened by parasitological and serological field investigations in Honduras [120] and Ethiopia [121].

In contrast, the potentially protective effect of phenotypic G-6-PD deficiency against *P. falciparum* has not been conclusively proven. Retrospective studies in Bulgaria [122] seem to indicate that malaria was a selection factor, while investigations in Sardinia, Italy [123, 124] give little support to this hypothesis and correspond with observations made in Cameroon [113]. However, other studies indicated significantly lower parasitaemias in heterozygous girls with the genotype B for G-6-PD deficiency [110]. This may explain a malaria-induced rise of gene frequency which would otherwise be difficult to reconcile with the apparent absence of survival advantage in G-6-PD deficient individuals.

Placental infection with malaria parasites is frequent in hyperendemic areas. No association was found between placental malaria and still birth in the Gambia, but the birth weight of the infants was 170 g below average with primigravidae [125]. Further studies in the same country [126] showed that all babies with a birth weight below 2500 g were born from mothers who showed evidence of placental infection. Congenital infection of newborns in hyperendemic countries is not as rare as previously thought. In Senegal 35 out of 450 newborns were infected with *P. falciparum*, but all infections disappeared spontaneously within 30 days following treatment and most of them within only nine days [127]. In studies conducted in Nigeria 43% of infant cord blood slides were positive for *P. falciparum* [128]. The rarity of overt manifestations of malaria in the newborn and the fast spontaneous disappearance of parasites underline the importance of passively transferred maternal immunity.

4.3. *Epidemiological studies*

Little progress has been made with regard to direct parasitological diagnosis of malaria in blood. Concentration techniques with density gradient centrifugation of blood [129] have only a limited application in the field laboratory. Fluorescent staining of parasites and examination by fluorescence microscopy are more rapid and reliable than the screening of Romanovsky stained blood slides, but the appropriate equipment is expensive and difficult to maintain, and parasite species diagnosis from fluorescence slides is not easy [130]. A recently developed radiometric assay [131] is expected to improve considerably the assessment of sporozoite infections in anopheline mosquitos. In addition to its species specificity it permits quantitation of the sporozoites which is a prerequisit for studies on parasite inoculation.

There have been few recent developments in the area of serological tests for the detection of malaria antibodies. The indirect fluorescent antibody (IFA) test is recognized as the most sensitive of the commonly applicable tests; no major improvements have been made with regard to indirect haemagglutination (IHA) and enzyme linked immunosorbent assay (ELISA) so that their field application has remained quite restricted. In a comparative study of IFA, IHA and ELISA, using *P. falciparum* antigens from four Thai and one Gambian isolate, no differences in reactivity were observed in the IFA, but in tests using soluble antigens (IHA and ELISA) the Gambian antigen produced the highest titres. A correlation existed between IFA and IHA readings, but none between the ELISA and the others [132]. In an outbreak of quartan malaria in Grenada, producing a total of 59 cases, 16% of all parasitologically negative blood samples yielded IFA titres of $1/>16$ with *P. brasilianum* [133].

Immunodiagnostic tests for malaria antigen in patient blood could become a useful tool in the future. A radioimmunoassay for the detection of *P. falciparum* has been developed and adapted to an ELISA system which proved to be quite sensitive and specific [134, 135]. The system will require further improvement and validation in the field, but it offers substantial advantages for the rapid processing of large numbers of blood specimens, without imposing major technical sophistication.

The quantitation of malaria transmission poses problems to which no simple solution has as yet been found. Estimation of the inoculation rate in suitable populations is one way of arriving at estimates, the other is to assess the vectorial capacity. The latter is a composite function of mosquito density, frequentation of man, longevity and also the gametocyte reservoir which are all subject to seasonal variation. This may explain the substantial rise in the infection rate of *A. albimanus* during a vivax malaria epidemic in El Salvador [136]. Low human blood indices are not *per se* an indication of low vectorial capacity if mosquito densities and longevity are high as seen in the example of *A. annularis* in Nepal which was responsible for a serious epidemic in spite of a human blood index of only 0.035.

Mosquito longevity is a major determinant of vectorial capacity. In the Gambia *A. melas* attained a sporozoite rate of only 0.35% as compared to 3.5% in *A. gambiae* s.s., a fact explained by the shorter life expectancy and lesser anthropophilic index of *A. melas* [137]. The intensity of transmission may be high in spite of a low gametocyte rate. Transmission was found to be fully maintained in the Congo when the gametocyte rates were as low as 1.34% – but there was a biting rate of 80–100 per night (*A. gambiae*) [138]. Differences in the frequentation of man were found to be mainly responsible for differences in the sporozoite rates between *A. arabiensis* (0.33%) and *A. gambiae* s.s. (5.3%) in the Kisumu area, Kenya [139]. Environmental changes may, of course, influence vector propagation and bionomics, requiring a follow-up of the entomological situation. Thus, a survey of the anopheline fauna undertaken in coastal villages of Pondicherry and Tamil Nadu because of continued transmission revealed the presence of *A. annularis*, *A. hyrcanus*, *A. pallidus*, *A. subpictus* and *A. vagus* which were hitherto not recognized as malaria vectors in the area. Conclusive proof was found on the role of *A. subpictus* as a vector of malaria [140]. Environmental changes such as deforestation may render the habitat unsuitable for local vectors such as *A. dirus* in Hainan, China [141].

The elucidation of low-grade malaria transmission often requires extraordinary efforts and may result in unexpected findings such as the detection of *A. aruni*, a member of the *A. funestus* complex in Transvaal [142] or the discovery of spring transmission of *P. vivax* by *A. stephensi* in Rajasthan, Northern India [143].

Seasonal changes of malaria transmission are also quite marked in the tropical African environment, being most marked of course in areas with major seasonal meteorological fluctuations. Thus malaria transmission in Cape Verde, Senegal, was found to be restricted to September–February, with a mean annual vectorial capacity of 2.8, and a seasonal peak of 35.9 in October [144]; *A. arabiensis* was apparently the only vector present, with an unusually high human blood index of 0.99. In Upper Volta the density of *A. gambiae* s.l. in rice cultivation areas was 4–5 times higher than in the savanna, but the sporozoite rates were significantly lower (0.4% as compared to 2.4%) [145]. This can be explained by an absence of dry-season transmission in the rice growing area, whereas dry-season transmission in the savanna is maintained by *A. funestus*. The savanna fauna is, moreover, reinforced by *A. nili*.

While entomological indices such as those derived from the estimation of vector anopheline populations [146] and life table characteristics of vectors [147] may be very useful in developing an early warning system for malaria epidemics, it seems that the continuous monitoring of parasitological data, as proposed on a district basis in Thailand [148], is more practical. It is also less demanding since it can be integrated within the normal malaria surveillance activities, with an adequate coverage in space and time which would be difficult to achieve with entomological investigations. In particular environmental circumstances, other indices may be used as warning signals, e.g. discharge rates of streams or rivers in areas where the formation of remaining river pools favours mosquito breeding. Data on the cyclical occurrence of epidemics may also be useful for forecasting and preventing epidemics [149].

Several new mathematical models for the estimation of malaria transmission have been described, but most of them have only been in a very limited range of situations so that validation is still pending. A more widely tested and very interesting mathematical-statistical model for the analysis of cross-sectional serological data has been developed [150]. This provides a new dimension to the epidemiological evaluation of serological data.

Environmental changes of a rather abrupt nature usually accompany the construction of dams or irrigation schemes. In tropical and subtropical areas they often result in renewed or increased malaria transmission and prevalence such as in the area of the Sathanaur Reservoir in Tamil Nadu, India [151], in Thailand [152] and in southern Cameroon [153]. The situation may be different in areas where malaria is already holoendemic as on River Benue in northern Cameroon [154], but there are other water-associated diseases which may be more important in this context. Less perceptible environmental changes related to land use, industrial effluents and other factors are also apt to change the anopheline fauna. Thus, *A. sacharovi* has disappeared from Romania, *A. atroparvus* is much reduced as compared to earlier years, and only *A. messeae* has about maintained its usual densities [155]. Similarly, *A. labranchiae* has disappeared from Spain, thereby reducing receptivity for malaria [156]. Still, the reintroduction of the habitual vectors or the introduction of new ones may be a danger associated with the development of communications, such as the risk of importing *A. arabiensis* into North Africa along the Trans-Sahara Highway [157].

Urban malaria plays an important role in many townships of India, where *A. stephensi* is the exclusive or main vector [158, 159], but *A. culicifacies* has started to penetrate the inner core of Delhi, a city with a substantial malaria incidence [160].

Part of the problem of urban malaria, especially in the large cities of tropical Africa, may stem from migration which brings new malaria reservoirs to the urban centres and perimeters. But also in rural areas which were freed from malaria immigration of malarious persons may lead to the reestablishment of the disease as in Tamil Nadu, India [161]. Also tropical aggregations of labour are constituting a major risk factor, e.g. in the sugar cane plantations of western Thailand [162]. Population movement was also responsible for a fundamental change of the malaria situation in Papua New Guinea. The disease was imported by infected visitors from the malarious lowlands to the hitherto malaria free and very isolated highland populations where it firmly established itself, leading within a short time to considerable degrees of endemicity [163].

In spite of a reawakened interest in malaria as a disease, relatively little has been done recently to evaluate its impact on the human population apart from some demographic yet rather imcomplete studies. Very interesting observations in New Guinea [164] brought evidence of a correlation between malaria prevalence and growth stunting. In Zambia, an association was found between malaria and malnutrition which was significant in weight for age, serum albumin, haemoglobin, urinary riboflavin and urea indices [165]. In this area *P. falciparum* is the prevalent species, followed by *P. malariae*. A highly evident indicator of the impact of malaria came from an insecticide trial project in Kenya, where the infant mortality was 157/1000 live births prior to spraying. Within two years from the start of 3-monthly applications of fenitrothion the rate in the protected area had dropped to 93/1000 [166]. This and similar observations should be of value in selecting the appropriate armamentarium for malaria control on a rational basis independent of considerations of relevance to areas with little or no anthropod borne diseases.

Acknowledgement

The author thanks Dr P.I. Trigg and Mrs N. Valabrègue for reviewing the manuscript, Mrs J. Brass for secretarial assistance, and Mr J. Hempel for providing Figure 2. Thanks are also expressed to the World Health Organization for permitting reproduction of Figure 1.

References

1. World Health Organization: World Malaria Situation 1982. World Health Statistics Quarterly, 37:130–161, 1984.
2. World Health Organization: World Malaria Situation 1981. WHO Weekly Epidemiological Record 58:189–192, 198–199, 206–209, 214–216, 222–224, 232–233, 1983.
3. World Health Organization: Status of Malaria Programs in the Americas. XXXI. Report. WHO Document No. DC 29/INF/2 (AMRO/PAHO), 1983.
4. Coosemans M, Storme B, Wery M: Recherche épidémiologique d'un paludisme plus stable en Afrique centrale: prospection géographique dans la plaine de la Ruzizi; perspectives de control. In: Abstracts of Papers: 2nd International Conference on Malaria and Babesiosis, 19–22 September 1983, Annecy, France, p 193.
5. Williamson WA, Gilles HM: Malumfashi endemic diseases research project. II. Malariometry in Malumfashi, Northern Nigeria. Annals of Tropical Medicine and Parasitology 72:323–328, 1978.
6. Osuhor PC, Ereme DVE: Malariometric indices of infants, children and young adults (under 20 years) in Malumfashi, northern Nigeria. Journal of Communicable Diseases 9:143–149, 1977.
7. Gazin P, Ovazza L, Brandicourt O, Ouari B, Legros F: Etudes transversales sur le paludisme dans plusieurs villages de la région de Bobo-Dioulasso. XXIIIème Conférence technique de l'OCCGE, 11 au 15 avril 1983 Ouagadougou No. 8224/83/Doc.Techn.OCCGE, 1983.
8. Richard-Lenoble D, Kornbila M, Chandenier J: Paludisme au Gabon: Résultats d'enquêtes récentes menées en milieu urbain et rural. XIVe Conférence Technique, Yaoundé, 20–23 avril 1982. OCEAC, Yaoundé, pp 67–69.
9. Chabasse D, Dumon H, Tounkara A, Maiga A, Ranque P: Indices paludométriques chez 938 enfants et adolescents en savane humide au sud du Mali. Bulletin de la Société de Pathologie exotique 73:254–258, 1980.

10. Wenlock RW: The incidence of *Plasmodium* parasites in rural Zambia. East African Medical Journal 55:268–276, 1978.

11. Sulzer AJ, Cantella R, Colichon A, Gleason NN, Walls KW: A focus of hyperendemic *Plasmodium malariae – P. vivax* with no *P. falciparum* in a primitive population in the Peruvian Amazon jungle. Bulletin of the World Health Organization 52:273–278, 1975.

12. Hati AK, Mukhopadhyay NC: Distribution of *Plasmodium falciparum* in West Bengal. Transactions of the Royal Society of Tropical Medicine and Hygiene 74:420–421, 1980.

13. Roy RG, Shanmugham CAK, Chakrapani KP, Madesayya NM, Ghosh RB: Distribution of human plasmodia in Karnataka and Tamil Nadu States in the reappearing phase of malaria in 1970 and 1975. Indian Journal of Medical Research 69: 53–59, 1979.

14. Kalra NL: Emergence of malaria zoonosis of simian orgin as natural phenomenon in Greater-Nicobars, Andaman and Nicobar Islands – a preliminary note. Journal of Communicable Diseases 12:49–54, 1980.

15. Choudhury DS: Investigation on simian malaria in India and its potential as a source of zoonosis. Indian Journal of Malariology 18:28–34, 1981.

16. Somboon P, Sivasomboon C: A case of *Plasmodium ovale* malaria acquired in Burma. Transactions of the Royal Society of Tropical Medicine and Hygiene 77:567, 1983.

17. Gundelfinger BF, Wheeling CH, Lien JC, Atmosoedjono S, Simanjuntak CH: Observations on malaria in Indonesian Timor. American Journal of Tropical Medicine and Hygiene 24:393–396. 1975.

18. Lee VH, Atmosedjono S, Aep S, Swaine CD: Vector studies and epidemiology of malaria in Irian Jaya, Indonesia. Southeast Asian Journal of Tropical Medicine and Public Health 11:341–347, 1980.

19. World Health Organization: Terminology of Malaria and Malaria Eradication. WHO, Geneva, 1963.

20. Neiva A: Über die Bildung einer chininresistenten Rasse des Malaria parasiten. Memorias do Instituto Oswaldo Cruz 2: 131–140, 1910.

21. Nocht B, Werner H: Beobachtungen über relative Chininresistenz bei Malaria aus Brasilien. Deutsche Medizinische Wochenschrift 36:1557–1560, 1910.

22. World Health Organization: Chemotherapy of Malaria and Resistance to Antimalarials. WHO Technical Report Series No. 529, 1973.

23. Bruce-Chwatt LJ, Black RH, Canfield CJ, Clyde DF, Peters W, Wernsdorfer WH: Chemotherapy of Malaria. WHO, Geneva, 1981.

24. Rieckmann KH, McNamara JV, Frischer H, Stockert TA, Carson PE, Powell RD: Effects of chloroquine, quinine and cycloguanil upon the maturation of asexual erythrocytic forms of two strains of *Plasmodium falciparum in vitro*. American Journal of Tropical Medicine and Hygiene 17:661–671, 1968.

25. Trager W, Jensen JB: Human malaria parasites in continuous culture. Science 193:673–675, 1976.

26. Rieckmann KH, Campbell GH, Sax CJ, Mrema JE: Drug sensitivity of *Plasmodium falciparum*. An *in vitro* microtechnique. Lancet 1:22–23, 1978.

27. Lopez Antuñano FJ, Wernsdorfer WH: *In vitro* response of chloroquine resistant *Plasmodium falciparum* to mefloquine. Bulletin of the World Health Organization 57:663–665, 1979.

28. Wernsdorfer WH: Field evaluation of drug resistance in malaria. *In vitro* micro test. Acta Tropica 37:222–227, 1980.

29. Kouznetsov RL, Rooney W, Wernsdorfer WH, El Gaddal AA, Payne D, Badalla RE: Use of the *in vitro* microtechnique for the assessment of drug sensitivity of *Plasmodium falciparum* in Sennar, Sudan. Bulletin of the World Health Organization 58:785–789, 1980.

30. Myint-Lwin, Min-Zaw, Rooney W: Comparative study of the micro *in vitro* and the *in vivo* tests of the response of *Plasmodium falciparum* to chloroquine in Burma. Unpublished document WHO/MAL/82.982, 1982.

31. Grab B, Wernsdorfer WH: Evaluation of *in vitro* tests for drug sensitivity in *Plasmodium*

198

falciparum: probit analysis of logdose/response test from 3–8 points assay. Unpublished document WHO/MAL/83.990, 1983.

32. Magloire R, Nguyen-Dinh P: Chloroquine susceptibility of *Plasmodium falciparum* in Haiti. Bulletin of the World Health Organization 61:1017–1020, 1983.

33. Draper CC, Brubaker G, Geser A, Kilimali VAEB, Wernsdorfer WH: Serial studies on the evolution of chloroquine resistance in an area of East Africa receiving intermittent chemosuppression, 1984 (In press).

34. Boudreau EF, Webster HK, Pavanand K, Thosingha L: Type II mefloquine resistance in Thailand. Lancet 2:1335, 1982.

35. Bygbjerg IC, Schapira A, Flachs H, Gomme G, Jepsen S: Mefloquine resistance of falciparum malaria from Tanzania enhanced by treatment. Lancet 1:774–775, 1983.

36. Mahor RJ, Green CA, Hunt RH: Diagnostic allozymes for routine identification of adults of the *Anopheles gambiae* complex (Diptera: Culicidae). Bulletin of Entomological Research 66:25–31, 1976.

37. Miles SJ: Enzyme variation in the *Anopheles gambiae* Giles group of species (Diptera: Culicidae). Bulletin of Entomological Research 68:85–96, 1978.

38. Miles SJ: A biochemical key to adult members of the *A. gambiae* group of species (Diptera: Culicidae). Journal of Medical Entomology 15: 297–299, 1979.

39. Baker RH: *Anopheles culicifacies*: mating behaviour and competitiveness in nature of males carrying a complex chromosomal aberration. Annals of the Entomological Society of America 73:581–588, 1980.

40. Green CA, Miles SJ: Chromosomal evidence for sibling species of the malaria vector *Anopheles (Cellia) culicifacies* Giles. Journal of Tropical Medicine and Hygiene 83:75–78, 1980.

41. Jayaprakash, Chowdaiah BN: Chromosome studies of oriental *Anopheles*. V. Polytene chromosomes of *Anopheles culicifacies*. Parasitologia 22:165–171, 1980.

42. Miles SJ: Unidirectional hybrid male sterility from crosses between species A and species B of the taxon *Anopheles (Cellia) culicifacies* Giles. Journal of Tropical Medicine and Hygiene 84:13–16, 1981.

43. Subbarao SK: Distribution of sibling of the taxon *Anopheles culicifacies*. Journal of Communicable Diseases 14:219, 1982.

44. Subbarao SK, Adak T, Sharma VP: *Anopheles culicifacies*: Sibling species distribution and vector incrimination studies. Journal of Communicable Diseases 12:102–104, 1980.

45. Suguna SG, Tewari SC, Mani TR, Hiriyan J, Reuben R: *Anopheles culicifacies* species complex in Thenpennaiyar reverine tract, Tamil Nadu. Indian Journal of Medical Research 77:455–459, 1983.

46. Baimai V, Harrison BA, Nakavachara V: The salivary gland chromosomes of *Anopheles (Cellia) dirus* (Diptera: Culicidae) of the southeast Asian *Leucosphyrus* group. Proceedings of the Entomological Society of Washington 82:319–328, 1980.

47. Baimai V, Harrison A, Somchit L: Varyotype differentiation of three anopheline taxa in the balabacensis complex of Southeast Asia (Diptera: Culicidae). Genetica 57:81–86, 1981.

48. Baimai V, Wibowo S, Andre RC: Heterochromatin and sex chromosome differentiation of four taxa in the *Anopheles balabacensis* complex. In: Abstracts of Papers, Conference on Malaria Research, Pattaya, 25–27 April 1983, Bangkok, Ministry of Public Health p 66, 1983.

49. Kanda T, Chiang GL, Ito K, Tumurasvin W, Loong PK: Cytogenetic observations on *Anopheles dirus* of the leucosphyrus complex. Mosquito News 40:585–592, 1980.

50. Kanda T, Cheong WH, Oguma Y, Takai K, Chiang GL, Sucharit S: Systematics and cytogenetics of the *hyrcanus* group, *leucosphyrus* group and *pyrethophorus* group in East Asia. In: Recent developments in the genetics of insect disease vectors. Champaign, I.L. Stipes, p 506–522, 1982.

51. Kanda T, Takai K, Chiang GL, Loong PK, Sucharit S, Cheong WH: Phylogenetic interpretation and chromosomal polymorphism among nine strains of human malaria vectors of the *Anopheles leucosphyrus* group. Japanese Journal of Genetics 58:193–208, 1983.

52. Sucharit S, Choochote W, Pratchyanusorn N, Limsuwan W, Apiwathnasorn C, Kanda T: Esterase patterns of *Anopheles dirus* (Bangkok strain) and *Anopheles balabacensis* (Perlis form) in the laboratory. Southeast Asian Journal of Tropical Medicine and Public Health 14:127–132, 1983.

53. Warren M, Richardson BH, Collins WH: Pupal pleomorphism in a strain of *Anopheles albimanus* from El Salvador. Mosquito News 35:549–551, 1975.

54. De Meillon B, Van Eeden GJ, Coetzee L, Coetzee M, Meiswinkel R, Du Toit CLN, Hansford CF: Observations on a species of the *Anopheles funestus* subgroup, a suspected exophilic vector of malaria parasites in northeastern Transvaal, South Africa. Mosquito News 37:657–661, 1977.

55. Green CA, Baimai V, Harrison BA, Andre RG: Chromosomal evidence for a complex of genetic species within *Anopheles maculatus*. In: Abstracts of Papers, Conference on Malaria Research, Pattaya, 25–27 April 1983, Bangkok, Ministry of Health, p 65, 1983.

56. Kanda T: Report on a visit to Papua New Guinea, 19 January to 8 February 1979. Unpublished WPR document ICP/MPD/002.E:PNG/MPD/001.E of 20 April 1979.

57. Suguna SG: Inversion (2)R, in *Anopheles stephensi*, its distribution and relation to egg size. Indian Journal of Medical Research 73(Suppl.):124–128, 1981.

58. Suguna SG: Cytological and morphological evidence for sibling species in *Anopheles subpictus* Grassi. Journal of Communicable Diseases 14:1–8, 1982.

59. Warren M, Collins WE, Richardson RB, Skinner JC: Morphologic variants of *Anopheles albimanus* and susceptibility to *Plasmodium vivax* and *P. falciparum*. American Journal of Tropical Medicine and Hygiene 26:607–611, 1977.

60. Collins WE, Warren M, Skinner JC, Richardson BB, Kearse TS: Infectivity of the Santa Lucia (El Salvador) strain of *Plasmodium falciparum* to different anophelines. Journal of Parasitology 63:57–61, 1977.

61. Scorza JV, Tallaferro E, Rubiano H: Comportamiento y susceptibilidad de *Anopheles nuneztovari* Gabaldon, 1940 a la infeccion con *Plasmodium falciparum* y *Plasmodium vivax*. Boletin de la direccion de malariologia y saneamiento ambiental 16:129–136, 1976.

62. Warren M, Collins WE, Jeffery GM, Richardson BB: *Anopheles pseudopunctipennis*: laboratory maintenance and malaria susceptibility of a strain from El Salvador. American Journal of Tropical Medicine and Hygiene 29:503–506, 1980.

63. Collins W, Nguyen-Dinh P, Skinner JC, Sutton BB: Infectivity of a strain of *Plasmodium falciparum* from Hainan, People's Republic of China, to different anophelines. American Journal of Tropical Medicine and Hygiene 30:538–540, 1981.

64. Shi DY: Experimental infection of *Anopheles sinensis* of Zhengzhou and Xinyang districts with *Plasmodium vivax*. Chinese Journal of Preventive Medicine 16(2):85 (In Chinese, with English abstract), 1982.

65. Daskova NG: New data on the susceptibility of *Anopheles* mosquitos of the USSR fauna to imported strains of the causative agents of human malaria. Meditsinskaya parazitologiya i parazitarnye bolezni 46:652–657 (In Russian), 1977.

66. Daskova NG, Rasnicyn SP: Review of data on susceptibility of mosquitos in the USSR to imported strains of malaria parasites. Bulletin of the World Health Organization 60:893–897, 1982.

67. Sucharit S, Surathin K, Tumrasvin W, Sucharit P: Chloroquine resistant *Plasmodium falciparum* in Thailand: susceptibility of *Anopheles*. Journal of the Medical Association of Thailand 60:648–654, 1977.

68. Klein TA, Harrison BA, Andre RG, Whitmire RE, Inlao I: Detrimental effect of *Plasmodium cynomolgi* infections on the longevity of *Anopheles dirus*. Mosquito News 42:265–271, 1982.

69. Segini SE, Scorza JV, Anez N: Variaciones diurnas de algunos factores fisico-quimicos en un criadero de larvas de *Anopheles nuneztovari*, Gabaldon, 1940. Boletin de la direccion de malariologia y saneamiento ambiental 19:1–1, 1979.

70. Rosenberg R: Forest malaria in Bangladesh. III. Breeding habits of *Anopheles dirus*. American Journal of Tropical Medicine and Hygiene 31:192–201, 1982.

71. Damar T, Fleming GA, Gandahusada S, Bang YH: Nocturnal indoor resting heights of the malaria vector *Anopheles aconitus* and other anophelines (Diptera: Culicidae) in Central Java, Indonesia. Journal of Medical Entomology 18:362–365, 1981.

72. Batra CP, Reuben R, Das PK: Studies of day-time resting places of *Anopheles stephensi* Liston in Salem (Tamil Nadu). Indian Journal of Medical Research 69:583–588, 1979.

73. Snow WF: Field estimates of the flight speed of some West African mosquitos. Annals of Tropical Medicine and Parasitology 74:239–242, 1980.

74. Snow WF: Further observations on the vertical distribution of flying mosquitos (Diptera: Culicidae) in West African savanna. Bulletin of Entomological Research 72:695–708, 1982.

75. Gilles MT, Wilkes TJ: Field experiments with a wind tunnel on the flight speed of some West African mosquitoes (Diptera: Culicidae). Bulletin of Entomological Research 71:65–70, 1981.

76. Manouchehri AV, Javadian E, Eshghy N, Motabar M: Ecology of *Anopheles stephensi* Liston in southern Iran. Tropical and Geographical Medicine 28:228–232, 1976.

77. Gerold JL: Evaluation of some parameters of house-leaving behaviour of *Anopheles gambiae* s.l. Acta Leidensia 45:79–90, 1977.

78. Roberts DR, Alecrim WD, Tavares AM, McNeill KM: Field observations on the gonotrophic cycle of *Anopheles darlingi* (Diptera: Culicidae). Journal of Medical Entomology 20:189–192, 1983.

79. Carnevale P, Bosseno MF, Molinier M, Lancien J, Le Pont F, Zoulani A: Etude du cycle gonotrophique d'*Anopheles gambiae* (Diptera: Culicidae) (Giles, 1902) en zone de forêt dégradée d'Afrique centrale. Cahiers ORSTOM. série entomologie médicale et parasitologie 17:55–75, 1979.

80. Carnevale P, Bosseno MF, Zoulani A: Etude du cycle gonotrophique d'*Anopheles nili* (theo.) 1904. Cahiers ORSTOM. série entomologie médicale et parasitologie 16:43–52, 1977.

81. Mahmood F, Reisen WK: Duration of the gonotrophic cycles of *Anopheles culicifacies* Giles and *Anopheles stephensi* Liston, with observations on reproductive activity and survivorship during winter in Punjab Province, Pakistan. Mosquito News 41:41–50, 1980.

82. Boreham PFL, Lenahan JK, Boulzaguet R, Storey J, Ashkar TS, Nambiar R, Matsushima T: Studies on multiple feeding by *Anopheles gambiae* s.l. in a Sudan savanna area of north Nigeria. Transactions of the Royal Society of Tropical Medicine and Hygiene 73:418–423, 1979.

83. Boreham PFL, Port GR: The distribution and movement of engorged females of *Anopheles gambiae* Giles (Diptera: Culicidae) in a Gambian village. Bulletin of Entomological Research 72:489–495, 1982.

84. Carnevale P, Frezil JL, Bosseno MF, Le Pont F, Lancien J: Etude de l'agressivité d'*Anopheles gambiae* A en fonction de l'âge et du sexe des sujets humains. Bulletin of the World Health Organization 56:147–154, 1978.

85. Vittal M, Deo RR: A note on the feeding behaviour of mosquitos in Maharashtra villages. Indian Journal of Malariology 19:63–64, 1982.

86. Carnevale P, Boreham PFL: Etudes des préférences trophiques d'*Anopheles nili* (Theo.) 1904. Cahiers d'ORSTOM série entomologie médicale et parasitologie 16:17–22, 1978.

87. Collins RT, Dash BK, Agarwala RS, Dhal KB: An adaptation of the gel diffusion technique for identifying the source of mosquito bloodmeals. Unpublished document WHO/MAL/83.992; WHO/VBC/83.873, 1983.

88. Edrissian GH, Hafizi A: Application of enzyme-linked immunosorbent assay (ELISA) to identification of *Anopheles* mosquito bloodmeals. Transactions of the Royal Society of Tropical Medicine and Hygiene 76:54–55, 1982.

89. Dai GJ: Preliminary observation on vivax malaria of long incubation in Liutum area, Donggou Xian, Liaoning Province. Zhonghua neike zazbi 18:411 (In Chinese), 1979.

90. Yang BL: Studies on the relapse patterns of tertian malaria in eastern Henan. Chinese Journal of Epidemiology 3(2):65 (In Chinese), 1982.

91. Mason J: Patterns of *Plasmodium vivax* recurrence in a high incidence coastal area of El Salvador C.A. American Journal of Tropical Medicine and Hygiene 24:581–585, 1975.

92. Molineaux L, Storey J, Cohen JE, Thomas A: A longitudinal study of human malaria in the West African savanna in the absence of control measures: relationship between different *Plasmodium* species, in particular *P. falciparum* and *P. malariae*. American Journal of Tropical Medicine and Hygiene 29:725–737, 1980.

93. Sanderson A, Walliker D, Molez JF. Enzyme typing of *Plasmodium falciparum* from African and some other Old World countries. Transactions of the Royal Society of Tropical Medicine and Hygiene 75:263–267, 1981.

94. Thaithong S, Sueblinwong T, Beale GH: Enzyme typing of some isolates of *Plasmodium falciparum* from Thailand. Transactions of the Royal Society of Tropical Medicine and Hygiene 75:268–270, 1981.

95. Bekessy A, Molineaux L, Storey J: Estimation of incidences and recovery rates of *Plasmodium falciparum* from longitudinal data. Bulletin of the World Health Organization 54:685–693, 1976.

96. Cornille-Brøgger R, Mathews HM, Storey J, Ashkar TS, Brøgger S, Molineaux L: Changing patterns in the humoral immune response to malaria before, during, and after the application of control measures: a longitudinal study in the West African savanna. Bulletin of the World Health Organization 56:579–600, 1978.

97. Abdalla S, Weatherall DJ: The direct antiglobulin test in *P. falciparum* malaria. British Journal of Haematology 51:415–425, 1982.

98. Boreham PFL, Lenahan JK, Port GR, McGregor IA: Haptoglobin polymorphism and its relationship to malaria infections in the Gambia. Transactions of the Royal Society of Tropical Medicine and Hygiene 75:193–200, 1981.

99. Monjour L, Trape JF, Druilhe P, Bourdillon F, Fribourg-Blanc A, Palminteri R, Gentilini M, Kyelem JM: Malaria and haptoglobin content of serum in a rural population in Upper Volta. Annals of Tropical Medicine and Parasitology 76:105–107, 1982.

100. Smalley ME, Brown J: *Plasmodium falciparum* gametocytogenesis stimulated by lymphocytes and serum in infected Gambian children. Transactions of the Royal Society of Tropical Medicine and Hygiene 75:316–317, 1981.

101. Ade-Serrano MA, Ejezie GC, Kassim OO: Correlation of *Plasmodium falciparum* gametocytaemia with complement titres in rural Nigerian school children. Journal of Clinical Microbiology 13:195–198, 1981.

102. Nardin EH, Nussenzweig RS, Bryan JH, McGregor IA: Congenital transfer of antibodies against malarial sporozoites detected in Gambian infants. American Journal of Tropical Medicine and Hygiene 30:1159–1163, 1981.

103. Abdalla S, Weatherall DJ, Wickramasinghe SN, Hughes M: The anaemia of *P. falciparum* malaria. British Journal of Haematology 46:171–183, 1980.

104. Facer CA: Direct antiglobulin reactions in Gambian children with *P. falciparum* malaria. III. Expression of IgG subclass determinants and genetic markers and association with anaemia. Clinical and Experimental Immunology 41: 81–90, 1980.

105. Reinhardt MC: Maternal anaemia in Abidjan – its influence on placenta and newborn. Helvetica paediatrica Acta 33(Suppl.)41:43–63, 1978.

106. Pasvol G: The interaction between sickle haemoglobin and the malaria parasites *Plasmodium falciparum*. Transactions of the Royal Society of Tropical Medicine and Hygiene 74:701–705, 1980.

107. Michel R, Carnevale P, Bosseno MF, Molez JF, Brandicourt O, Zoulani A, Michel Y: Le paludisme à *Plasmodium falciparum* et le gène de la drépanocytose en République populaire du Congo. I. Prévalence du paludisme et du trait drépanocytaire en milieu scolaire dans la région Brazzavilloise. Médecine tropicale 41:403–411, 1981.

108. Vaisse D, Michel R, Carnevale P, Bosseno MF, Molez JF, Peelman P, Loembe MT, Nzingoula S, Zoulani A: Le paludisme à *Plasmodium falciparum* et le gène de la drépanocytose en République Populaire du Congo. II. Manifestations cliniques du paludisme selon la parasitémie et le génotype hémoglobinique. Médecine tropicale 41:413–423, 1981.

109. Cornille-Brøgger R, Fleming AF, Kagan I, Matsushima T, Molineaux L: Abnormal

haemoglobins in the Sudan savanna of Nigeria. II. Immunological response to malaria in normals and subjects with sickle cell trait. Annals of Tropical Medicine and Parasitology 73:173–183, 1979.

110. Guggenmoos-Holzmann I, Bienzle U, Luzzatto L: *Plasmodium falciparum* malaria and human red cells. II. Red cell genetic traits and resistance against malaria. International Journal of Epidemiology 10:16–22, 1981.

111. Ringelhann B, Hathorn MKS, Jilly P, Grant F, Parniczky G: A new look at the protection of hemoglobin AS and AC genotypes against *Plasmodium falciparum* infection: a census tract approach. American Journal of Human Genetics 28:270–279, 1976.

112. Storey J: Abnormal haemoglobins in the Sudan Savanna of Nigeria. IV. Malaria immunoglobulins and malaria antibodies in haemoglobin AC individuals. Annals of Tropical Medicine and Parasitology 73:311–315.

113. Bernstein SC, Bowman JE, Noche LK: Population studies in Cameroon. Haemoglobin S, glucose-6-phosphate dehydrogenase deficiency and falciparum malaria. Human Heredity 30:251–258, 1980.

114. Kidson C, Lamont G, Saul A, Nurse GT: Ovalocytic erythrocytes from Melanesians are resistant to invasion by malaria parasites in culture. Proceedings of the National Academy of Sciences of the United States of America 78:5829–5832, 1981.

115. Castelino D, Saul A, Myler P, Kidson C, Thomas H, Cooke R: Ovalocytosis in Papua New Guinea – dominantly inherited resistance to malaria. Southeast Asian Journal of Tropical Medicine and Public Health 12:549–555, 1981

116. Stafford EE, Dennis DT, Masri S, Sudomo M: Intestinal and blood parasites in the Torro Valley, Central Sulawesi, Indonesia. Southeast Asian Journal of Tropical Medicine and Public Health 11:468–472, 1980.

117. Facer CA: ABO blood groups and falciparum malaria. Transactions of the Royal Society of Tropical Medicine and Hygiene 73:599–600, 1979.

118. Martin SK, Miller LH, Hicks CU, David-West A, Ugbode C, Deane M: Frequency of blood group antigens in Nigerian children with falciparum malaria. Transactions of the Royal Society of Tropical Medicine and Hygiene 73:216–218, 1979.

119. Gupta M, Chowdhuri ANR: Relationship between ABO blood groups and malaria. Bulletin of the World Health Organization 58:913–915, 1980.

120. Spencer HC, Miller LH, Collins WE, Knud-Hansen C, McGinnis MH, Shiroishi K, Lobos RA, Feldman RA: The Duffy blood group and resistance to *Plasmodium vivax* in Honduras. American Journal of Tropical Medicine and Hygiene 27:664–670, 1978.

121. Mathews HM, Armstrong JC: Duffy blood groups and vivax malaria in Ethiopia. American Journal of Tropical Medicine and Hygiene 30:299–303, 1981.

122. Tzoneva M, Bulanov AG, Mavrudieva M, Lalchev S, Toncheva D, Tanev D: Frequency of glucose-6-phosphate dehydrogenase deficiency in relation to altitude: a malaria hypothesis. Bulletin of the World Health Organization 58:659–662, 1980.

123. Gloria-Bottini F, Falsi AM, Mortera J, Bottini E: The relations between G-6-PD deficiency, thalassemia and malaria. Further analysis of data from Sardinia and the Po Valley. Experientia 36:541–543, 1980.

124. Brown PD: New considerations on the distribution of malaria, thalassaemia, and glucose-6-phosphate dehydrogenase deficiency in Sardinia. Human Biology 53:357–382, 1981.

125. McGregor IA, Wilson ME, Bullewicz WZ: Malaria infection of the placenta in the Gambia, West Africa: its incidence and relationship to stillbirth, birthweight and placental weight. Transactions of the Royal Society of Tropical Medicine and Hygiene 77:232–244, 1983.

126. Watkinson M, Rushton DI: Plasmodial pigmentation of placenta and outcome of pregnancy in West African mothers. British Medical Journal 287:251–254, 1983.

127. Diallo S, Victorius A, Ndir O, Diouf F, Bah IB, Bah MD: Prévalence et évolution du paludisme congénital en zone urbaine: cas de la ville de Thiès (Sénégal). Unpublished document WHO/MAL/81.947, 1981.

128. Emajuaiwe SO: Some evidence for the occurrence of congenital malaria infections in ports of Nigeria. Nigerian Journal of Medical Science 2:81–90, 1979.

129. Le Bras J, Ricour A, Savel J, Payet M: Diagnostic parasitologique du paludisme par concentration des hématies parasitées: technique et résultats préliminaires. Bulletin de la Société de Pathologie exotique 70:605–614, 1977.

130. Midha N, Ichhpujani RL, Singh P, Arora DR, Arora B, Chugh TD: Evaluation of fluorescent microscopy for the identification of malaria parasites. Journal of Communicable Diseases 13:241–243, 1981.

131. Zavala F, Gwadz RW, Collins FH, Nussenzweig RS, Nussenzweig V: Monoclonal antibodies to circumsporozoite proteins identify the species of malaria parasites in infected mosquitoes. Nature 299:737–738, 1982.

132. Tharavanij S, Tantivanich S, Chongsa-Nguan M, Prasertsiriroj V: Comparison of various serological test results using antigens from different strains of *Plasmodium falciparum*. Southeast Asian Journal of Tropical Medicine and Public Health 13:174–180, 1982.

133. Tikasingh E, Edwards C, Hamilton PJS, Commissiong LM, Draper CC: A malaria outbreak due to *Plasmodium malariae* on the island of Grenada. American Journal of Tropical Medicine and Hygiene 29:715–719, 1980.

134. Mackey L, McGregor IA, Lambert PH: Diagnosis of *Plasmodium falciparum* infection using a solid-phase radioimmunoassay for the detection of malaria antigens. Bulletin of the World Health Organization 58:439–444, 1980.

135. Mackey LJ, McGregor IA, Paounova N, Lambert PH: Diagnosis of *Plasmodium falciparum* infection in man: detection of parasite antigens by ELISA. Bulletin of the World Health Organization 60:69–75, 1982.

136. Warren M, Mason J, Hobbs J: Natural infections of *Anopheles albimanus* with *Plasmodium* in a small malaria focus. American Journal of Tropical Medicine and Hygiene 24:545–546, 1975.

137. Boyan JH: *Anopheles gambiae* and *A. melas* at Brefet, the Gambia and their role in malaria transmission. Annals of Tropical Medicine and Parasitology 77:1–12, 1983.

138. Carnevale P, Bosseno MF: Le paludisme humain à *Plasmodium falciparum* dans le Sud-Ouest de la République populaire du Congo en fonction du biotype et du vecteur. Médecine d'Afrique noire 26:29–40, 1979.

139. Highton RB, Bryan J, Boreham PFL, Chandler JA: Studies on the sibling species *Anopheles gambiae* Giles and *Anopheles arabiensis* Patton (Diptera: Culicidae) in the Kisumu area, Kenya. Bulletin of Entomological Research 69:43–53, 1979.

140. Panioker KN, Bai MG, Rao USB, Viswam K, Murthy US: *Anopheles subpictus*, vector of malaria in coastal villages of south-east India. Current Science 50:694–695, 1981.

141. Anon: Studies on the ecological characteristics of the chief malaria vector *Anopheles balabacensis balabacensis* in Hainan Island and the effects of control experiments. Chinese Journal of Preventive Medicine 14(3):129 (In Chinese), 1980.

142. Smith A, Hansford CF, Thompson JF, Malaria along the southernmost fringe of its distribution in Africa: epidemiology and control. Bulletin of the World Health Organization 55:95–103, 1977.

143. Sharma SK, Wattal BL, Singh K, Bhargava YS: Spring transmission of malaria in Alwar Region (Rajasthan). Journal of Communicable Diseases 14:125–129, 1981.

144. Vercruysse J, Jancloes M: Etude entomologique sur la transmission du paludisme humain dans la zone urbaine de Pikine (Sénégal). Cahiers ORSTOM, série entomologie médicale et parasitologie 19:165–178, 1981.

145. Carnevale P, Robert V, Hervy JP, Legros F, Ovazza L, Hurpin C: La transmission du paludisme en zone rizicole et en zone de savane. XXIIIème Conférence technique de l'OCCGE, 11 au 15 avril 1983, Ouagadougou, No. 8224/83/Doc.Tech.OCCGE, 1983.

146. Reisen WK, Mahmood F: Relative abundance, removal sampling and mark-release-recapture estimates of population size of *Anopheles culicifacies* and *A. stephensi* in diurnal resting sites in rural Punjab Province, Pakistan. Mosquito News 41:22–30, 1981.

204

147. Reisen WK, Mahmood F: Horizontal life table characteristics of the malaria vectors *Anopheles culicifacies* and *Anopheles stephensi* (Diptera: Culicidae). Journal of Medical Entomology 17:211–217, 1980.

148. Cullen JR, Chitprarop U, Doberstyn EB, Sombatwattanangkul K: An epidemiological early warning system for malaria control in northern Thailand. Unpublished document WHO/MAL/ 83.994, 1983.

149. De Zulueta J, Miytaba SM, Shah IH: Malaria control and long-term periodicity of the disease in Pakistan. Transactions of the Royal Society of Tropical Medicine and Hygiene 74:624–632, 1980.

150. Van Druten JAM: A mathematical-statistical model for the analysis of cross-sectional serological data, with special reference to the epidemiology of malaria. M.D. thesis, Catholic University of Nijmegen, The Netherlands, 1981.

151. Hyma B, Ramesh A: The reappearance of malaria in Sathanaur Reservoir and environs: Tamil Nadu, India. Social Science and Medicine 14:337–344, 1980.

152. Bunnag T, Sornmani S, Pinithpongse S, Harinasuta C: Surveillance of water-borne parasite infections and studies of the impact of ecological changes on vector mosquitoes of malaria after dam construction. Southeast Asian Journal of Tropical Medicine and Public Health 10:656–660, 1979.

153. Atangana S, Foumbi J, Charlois M, Ambroise-Thomas P, Ripert C: Etude épidémiologique de l'onchocercose et du paludisme dans la région du lac de retenue de Bamendjin – Cameroun. Médecine tropicale 39:537–543, 1979.

154. Ripert C, Same-Ekobo A, Enyong P, Palmer D: Evaluation des répercussions sur les endémies parasitaires (malaria, bilharziose, onchocercose, dracunculose) de la construction de 57 barrages dans les monts Mandara (Nord-Cameroun). Bulletin de la Société de Pathologie exotique 72:324–339, 1979.

155. Bîlbîe I, Enescu A, Tâcu V, Giurcă I, Nicolescu G, Velehorschi N, Petrescu S: Date actuale de biologie si comportament fată de insecticide a faunei anopheline din fostele zone endemice de malarie situate in sudul tărîi. Revista a Societatea de Bacteriologie, Virusologie, Parazitologie, Epidemiologie 27:23–27, 1982.

156. Blazquez J, De Zulueta J: This disappearance of *Anopheles labranchiae* from Spain. Parassitologia 22:161–163, 1980.

157. Stafford Smith DM: Mosquito records from the Republic of Niger, with reference to the construction of the new Trans-Sahara Highway. Journal of Tropical Medicine and Hygiene 84:95–100, 1981.

158. Menon PKB, Rajagopalan PK: Seasonal changes in the density and natural mortality of miniature stages of the urban malaria vector, *Anopheles stephensi* (Liston) in wells in Pondicherry. Indian Journal of Medical Research 70(Suppl.):123–127, 1979.

159. Das PK, Reuben R, Batra CP: Urban malaria and its vectors in Salem (Tamil Nadu): Natural and induced infection with human plasmodia in mosquitos. Indian Journal of Medical Research 69:403–411, 1979.

160. Pattanayak S, Rahman SJ, Samnotra KG, Kalra NL: Changing patterns of malaria transmission in urban Delhi. Journal of Communicable Diseases 9:150–158, 1977.

161. Dutta HM, Duth AK, Vishnukumari G: The resurgence of malaria in Tamil Nadu. Social Science and Medicine 13D:191–194, 1979.

162. Kanjanpan W: Health effects of labour mobility. A study of malaria in Kanchanaburi Province, Thailand. Southeast Asian Journal of Tropical Medicine and Public Health 14:54–57, 1983.

163. Radford AJ, Van Leeuwen H, Christian SH: Social aspects in the changing epidemiology of malaria in the highlands of New Guinea. Annals of Tropical Medicine and Parasitology 70:11–23, 1976.

164. Sharp PT, Harvey P: Malaria and growth stunting in young children of the highlands of Papua New Guinea. Papua New Guinea Medical Journal 23:132–140, 1980.

165. Wenlock RW: The epidemiology of tropical parasitic diseases in rural Zambia and consequences for public health. Journal of Tropical Medicine and Hygiene 82:90–98, 1979.
166. Payne D, Grab B, Fontaine RE, Hempel JHG: Impact of control measures on malaria transmission and general mortality. Bulletin of the World Health Organization 54:369–377, 1976.

13. Epidemiology of babesiosis

RONALD D. SMITH

College of Veterinary Medicine, University of Illinois, 2001 South Lincoln, Urbana, IL 61801.

1. Introduction: species, geographic distribution and economic importance of the babesioses

1.1. Babesial species

Levine [1] identified 71 species within the genus *Babesia*. Our knowledge of the epidemiology of these organisms and the diseases that they may cause varies from scanty (only described in the vertebrate host) to extensive, including qualitative and quantitative data on transmission, reservoir mechanisms and factors predisposing to disease outbreaks. The paucity of epidemiologic studies on most species reduces, by default, the number of species which this chapter will focus upon.

Many of our concepts of babesial transmission have changed in the 25 odd years since Neitz [2, 3] published his classic reviews of the piroplasms and other tick-borne parasites. The validity of some of the earlier work has been questioned [4]. This is due in part to periodic redefinition or consolidation of babesial species. For example, the number of commonly recognized species of bovine babesiae has been reduced to four: *B. bovis* (syn. *B. argentina, B. berbera, B. colchica*), *B. bigemina, B. divergens* (syn. *B. caucasica, B. occidentalis, B. karelica*) and *B. major* [5]. This number may again increase. Purnell [6] has argued for the inclusion of a fifth genus, *B. jakimovi* [7], while Japanese [8] and South African [9] workers would include two more, *B. ovata* and *B. ocultans*, respectively.

Among the relatively small number of species of veterinary and/or zoonotic importance, *B. bovis* and its boophilid tick vectors have been the focus of epidemiologic study throughout the world. Other species, including *B. divergens, B. bigemina* and *B. major* have received some attention whereas less information is available on babesiae of horses (*B. caballi* and *B. equi*) and dogs (*B. gibsoni* and *B. canis*).

Epidemiologic studies of the rodent babesia, *B. microti*, are relatively recent and reflect the zoonotic importance of this species. At least 57 species of rodents

Ristic, M. et al. (eds.) *Malaria and babesiosis.*
© 1984, Martinus Nijhoff Publishers, Dordrecht/Boston/Lancaster.

have been reported to be naturally infected with *Babesia,* making it the second most common hemoprotozoan genus parasitizing rodents after the genus *Hepatozoon* [10].

1.2. *Geographic distribution*

The Animal Health Yearbook provides yearly updates on the worldwide distribution of several diseases of veterinary importance. In 1981 bovine babesiosis was reported to occur in 120 (70%) of the 171 reporting countries [11]. For comparison, babesiae of other animal species were reported by approximately 11% (equine babesiosis) to less than 1% of countries. These figures underestimate the actual occurrence of babesiae, but probably reflect the importance which each country places on the disease. In the United States, for example, only bovine babesiosis is reported despite frequent reports of canine and equine babesiosis outbreaks in the literature [12, 13]. Although babesiosis is frequently considered a 'tropical' disease, outbreaks occur in many temperate regions. Infections among cattle and/or sheep have recently been reported in Britain [14, 15], the Netherlands [16] and Switzerland [17].

1.3. *Economic importance*

It is difficult to separate economic losses due to tick-borne diseases from those caused by the ticks themselves. A breakdown of economic losses caused by the cattle tick by Gee [18] provides an idea of the nature of losses (Table 1).

Only 7% of losses summarized in Table 1 are due to mortality. A significant portion of losses are incurred by periodic roundup and acaricide treatments to reduce tick burdens.

The economic impact of these losses has been estimated for cattle in the Americas [19]. Approximatley 250 million cattle reside in Central and South

Table 1. Breakdown of losses incurred from ticks and tick-borne diseases of cattle in Queensland, Australia [18]

	% of total loss
Increased labor costs	36
Loss of beef	20
Loss in dairy production	16
Cost of acaricides	11
Loss by death	7
Hide damage	5
Increased drought loss	5

America and approximately 175 million (70%) are in tick-infested regions. Based upon estimates from Argentina, Mexico and Australia, a minimum of five U.S. dollars per head annual loss due to ticks and tick-borne diseases can be expected. This represents a total loss of 875 million US dollars per year for the cattle industry throughout Latin America.

Further costs are incurred in administering official tick control programs (Argentina, Mexico, United States) and from restricted movement of animals to and from tick-infested regions, thereby limiting potential markets.

As a result of successful application of integrated pest management (IPM) for the control of many agricultural pests, veterinary scientists, extensionists and livestock producers are receptive to appication of similar integrated strategies for control of tick-borne diseases and their vectors. Mathematical models of tick and babesial populations and their interaction have recently been developed to design and test optimal disease control strategies [20, 21, 22].

In keeping with this trend, this chapter will focus on life history and epidemiologic data which can be used for predictive purposes. The *B. bovis/Boophilus microplus* system will be used for illustrative purposes. Aside from its economic importance, the natural history of disease caused by this species is sufficiently clear for epidemiologic modeling. Those seeking additional information are referred to recent reviews [4, 5, 23, 24]. It is hoped that this review will encourage similar studies of the dynamic relationship among vector, parasite and host in other babesial systems.

2. Qualitative aspects of transmission

2.1. *Routes of transmission and infection*

With one exception, all of the known vectors of babesiae are ticks of the family Ixodidae, or hard ticks. The exception is *B. meri* which is transmitted by the argasid tick *Ornithodoros erraticus*. Unlike other arthropod vectors such as mosquitoes or flies, ixodid ticks feed only once between each instar. Thus, infections are acquired by one instar and, after a period of development in the tick, are transmitted to the vertebrate host by one or more subsequent instars.

The terminology used to describe the transmission of babesiae to and from the vertebrate host and between tick stages has not always been consistent. Unless otherwise stated, 'infection' will refer to the infection of a given tick stage, whether from the vertebrate host or a previous ticks stage. 'Transmission' will refer to tranmission to the vertebrate host. Tick stages may acquire infections during feeding (= alimentary infection), from a previous stage (= transstadial infection), or from the engorged female to the offspring via the egg (= transovarial infection).

Transovarial infection produces two distinct infection rates [25]: the 'tran-

210

sovarial infection rate' is the percentage of female ticks that pass microorganisms to their progeny whereas the 'filial infection rate' is the percentage of infected progeny derived from an infected female. These rates vary considerably with babesial vector-parasite-host systems, the level of infection in the blood meal, the stage of ovipositioning (egg-laying) and environmental factors [4]. In some cases infection persists in all tick stages by continuous transstadial and transovarial infection without apparent alimentary infection. This may occur over many generations and is referred to as 'vertical infection' [4].

Table 2 summarizes data available on routes of infection and transmission of selected babesiae by one-, two- and three-host ticks following the format used by Neitz [2, 3]. To date *Bo decoloratus* is the only one-host tick species shown capable of both alimentary and vertical infection with babesiae [26]. Other one-host tick species become infected transovarialy from alimentary infections acquired in the previous generation. The actual tick stage which transmits infection to the vertebrate host depends upon the particular vector-parasite system.

Table 2. Transmission patterns of some babesial species by 1-, 2- and 3-host ticks

Babesial species	Tick vectors	Number of hosts	Tick stage					Reference
			Adult	Egg	Larva	Nymph	Adult	
Bigemina	Bo. microplus	1	0————————————>>——>					4***, 26
Bigemina	Bo. decoloratus	1	0————————————>>——>>					26, 32
Bovis	Bo. microplus	1	0————————>					4, 33
Caballi	A. nitens	1	0————————>>——>>——>?					30
Ovis	R. bursa	2	0————————————>>*——>>					4
Bigemina	R evertsi	2	0————————————>					26
Divergens	I. ricinus	3	0————————>>——>>——>>					4
Divergens+	I. ricinus	3	0————————>?					34
Canis	R. sanguineus	3	0————————>>——>>——>>					4
Major	H. punctata	3	0————————>>——>>——>?					4
Merionis	Rhipicephalus spp	3			0——>			4
	Hyalomma spp.							
Microti	I. scapularis**	3			0——>			35
Microti	I. pacificus	3			0——>			35
Microti	I. dammini	3			0——>			36, 37
Microti	I. ricinus	3			0——>			38
Microti	D. andersoni	3				0——>		39

0 = Acquisition of infection by tick
> = Transmission of infection to vertebrate host
>> = Continuing vertical transmission in absence of alimentary infection
* = Depends on tick strain
** = May have been I. dammini
*** = Review
+ = Human strain

An additional means of transmission results from interrupted feeding of male ticks. *Babesia bigemina* [27, 28], *B. equi* [29] and *B. caballi* [30] may be transmitted to more than one host by transfer of male ticks between bovine (*Bo microplus, Bo decoloratus*) or equine (*Anocentor nitens*) hosts. It appears that male *Bo microplus* ticks must acquire the infection transovarialy, as alimentary infection of nymphal or adult male *Bo microplus* with *B. bigemina* could not be demonstrated [27]. Whether this is also true of *B. equi* and *B. caballi* is not known. Under field conditions larvae of the one-host tick *Bo microplus* may be more likely to transfer between hosts than adult males [31]. This could conceivably lead to multiple infections caused by individual larvae.

2.2. *The reservoir mechanism*

2.2.1. *Vertebrate host*

The duration of the babesial carrier state measured in domestic animal species has been reported to last from 12 months or less for the rodent babesiae *B. rodhaini, B. hylomysci* and *B. microti* to several years or lifelong in some large animal species [40]. The transmissibility of babesiae between domestic animal species and other mammals, which may represent 'wildlife reservoirs', has been reviewed [5, 41]. Since many of these transmissions have only been demonstrated by needle passage, their epidemiologic significance is unclear.

Fauna may be more important as reservoirs of vector tick populations than babesiae. Marshall et al. [42] provide a vivid account of the controversy surrounding the role of white-tailed deer (*Odocoileus virginianus*) as alternate hosts for the tropical cattle tick, *Bo microplus*, during the US eradication program in Florida. The question has never been properly resolved because intensive (2-week interval) dipping of cattle, horses and mules was being carried out at the same time as deer depopulation. Other states were able to eradicate the tick by cattle dipping alone, without deer depopulation. It would appear that although *Bo microplus* and *Bo annulatus* can complete their life cycles on deer [43] these infestations result from a 'spill-over' of the tick population from cattle and that deer alone would not support a *Boophilus* population. However, white-tailed deer are probably more numerous now in the southeast than at any time in recent history. Should *Bo microplus* be introduced into these areas there is a very real danger that deer would facilitate its spread geographically.

A much different relationship exists between white-tailed deer and *Ixodes dammini* the vector of *B. microti* to humans. Some authors feel that prior to the growth of the white-tailed deer population on Nantucket and Martha's Vinyard Islands off the Massachusetts coast, *B. microti* infections were restricted to certain rodent and lagomorph hosts, including *Peromyscus leucopus* and *Microtus pennsylvanicus* [44, 45, 46]. Infections were probably transmitted to these species by *Ixodes scapularis*. Growth of deer populations on these islands after

1940 permitted introduction and survival of *I. dammini* the adults of which feed primarily on deer, but will also parasitize man and dogs [47]. Consequently, white-tailed deer populations support populations of a vector species capable of transmitting rodent babesiae to man. As in the case of the *Boophilus/Babesia* controversy described above, white-tailed deer are not considered reservoirs of babesiae, but rather the ticks that transmit infection.

2.2.2. *Invertebrate host*

The efficiency of ticks as reservoirs of babesiae depends upon their ability to survive in the absence of suitable hosts and the persistence of babesial infection in their tissues. Ticks may be important reservoirs when the lifespan of the vertebrate host is short. For example, survival of *B. microti* in Massachusetts appears to depend primarily upon overwintering of larvae infected in the fall with subsequent transmission the following spring. The short lifespan of *P. leucopus* which is generally less than one year, assures a high proportion of nonimmunes in the mouse population during the spring [46]. A similar relationship has been reported for *B. microti* and *I. triaguliceps* which serves as a reservoir of babesiae from season to season for small mammals in Britain [48].

In contrast, non-parasitic stages of larvae of the cattle tick *Bo microplus* seldom survive more than a few weeks on pasture [49] and infections could conceivably disappear were it not for the continual reinfection of ticks from carrier cattle [22].

The vector and reservoir potential of non-parasitic ticks also depends upon their 'environmental experiences'. Thus, it has been shown that the infection rate and *in vivo* infectivity of *B. bovis* -infected *Bo microplus* larvae was enhanced by exposure to a temperature of 14 C prior to feeding [50]. Higher temperatures initially stimulated babesial development but prolongued exposure (37 C for 5 days or 31 C for 14 days) actually depleted the number of infective forms and reduced larval infectivity. Infectivity could conceivably be lost before larvae lose their ability to attach and feed [51].

Tick reservoirs of vertically-transmitted babesiae are a special case. It is conceivable that an infected tick population, which is capable of surviving by feeding on alternate hosts considered refractory to babesial infection, could remain infective in the absence of the definitive host for a number of generations [4]. Another exception may be male ticks which, unlike immature stages and females, do not engorge and may remain on the host for months.

3. Quantitative aspects of transmission

The preceeding section has dealt with babesiosis epidemiology primarily in conceptual terms. Numerous investigators have also attempted to describe the vector-parasite-host cycle in quantitative terms and a number of rates or indices have been developed. Many of the details of the maintenance of babesiae in their vertebrate and invertebrate hosts were reviewed by Friedhoff and Smith [4]. Additional aspects are discussed below using the *B. bovis*/*Bo microplus* system as a model.

3.1. *Tick infection rate*

The influence of the route of infection, phase of ovipositioning, parasitemia in the vertebrate host and phase of parasitemia upon infection of feeding ticks and transmission to the next stage were discussed in detail by Friedhoff and Smith [4]. The optimum infective dose for ticks is well below the high levels observed in the blood of splenectomized animals and is probably $=< 0.1\%$ parasitized erythrocytes [4]. Ingestion of large numbers of babesiae may have a negative effect upon female tick survival and reproduction [52] and lead to reduced filial infection rates in larvae [53].

Some authors report that the phase of parasitemia has a greater influence on infectivity of babesiae for engorging ticks than the degree of parasitemia [4]. In other systems, however, alimentary infection rates appear to be directly related to degree of parasitemia [54]. Hemolymph infections are generally higher in tick species infected by both vertical and alimentary routes [4].

Babesia bovis parasitemia appears to bear little if any relationship to filial infection rates in *Bo microplus* larval progeny [53, 55]. Babesial infection of daily egg batches is not uniform as ovipositioning usually commences before significant numbers of babesiae gain access to developing ova via the hemolymph. Infection rates of daily egg batches usually increase as ovipositioning proceeds [55]. Under field conditions environmental factors probably exert a much greater influence on tick infectivity than host parasitemia. Temperatures below 20 C are reported to completely inhibit alimentary and transovarial infection of *Bo microplus* with *B. bigemina* and *B. bovis* (= *argentina*), although female ticks are capable of egg production at this temperature [56, 57]. However, infections in eggs and larvae are not adversely affected when held at even lower temperatures and babesial development may actually be enhanced [50]. The development of babesiae in ticks is temperature dependent [50, 51, 58, 59]. Incubation of larvae or even eggs at temperatures simulating that found on vertebrate skin surfaces 'activates' babesiae by accelerating development to the infective form [58, 59].

The epidemiologic significance of the above findings for estimates of *B. bovis* and *B. bigemina* tick infection rates in field collected *Bo microplus* ticks [50, 51] and *B. microti* in *I. dammini* [37] has been discussed.

3.2. *Tick burden*

The risk of babesial infection is directly related to the tick burden, or average

214

number of ticks completing engorgement per day on each animal. Interest in obtaining accurate estimates of tick burdens has come primarily from tick control or eradication programs where detection of low tick burdens is fundamental for monitoring program success. The difficulty of obtaining accurate estimates of tick burden at low infestation levels has been discussed [60].

Due to the relatively long feeding period of ixodid ticks, the actual number of ticks completing engorgement may not accurately reflect the number which initially attached. Tick mortality occurs at variable rates throughout the feeding period [61]. The principal determinant of feeding success is the degree of host resistance. Other factors, such as competition for predilection sites, may also reduce feeding success. Accurate assessment of the effect of feeding success and tick burdens upon babesial transmission depends upon knowledge of the life cycle of the babesial parasite, specifically the tick stage actually responsible for transmission.

3.3. Inoculation rate

The inoculation rate is the daily probability of transmission of babesiae from ticks to any member of the susceptible population. The numerical value of the inoculation rate affects the size and age structure of the uninfected segment of the vertebrate population. It also provides a means for comparing the risk of contracting infections among different populations or regions and for predicting when and where outbreaks may occur [4, 22].

The inoculation rate can be estimated directly from the size of the infected tick population. This technique requires accurate detection of babesiae in a statistically significant sample of the tick population and accurate estimates for the daily tick burden. Since many ticks die or are removed before they have had a chance to transmit infection, estimation of inoculation rates from tick exposure must be approached with caution.

The inoculation rate 'h' can also be estimated by fitting the equation

$$P = 1-e\cdot(-ht)$$

to serologic prevalence data in different age groups where 'P' = serologic prevalence in a group of animals with average age 't', the latter corrected for the time required following infection for a detectable antibody response to develop.

3.4. Recovery rate

The recovery rate is defined as the proportion of infected animals which, having received one infective inoculum only, will recover from infection in one day.

Recovery may be defined as an absence of detectable parasitemia (and therefore non-infectivity of the vertebrate host for ticks) or as freedom from infection. Microscopically detectable infections with *B. bovis* have been shown to persist for up to 4 years following a single infection whereas *B. bigemina* becomes undetectable after 6 months to 1 year [62, 63, 64]. If we assume that after the above time periods 99% of carrier cattle are free of infection, and that the infection rate (I) in the herd at any time 't' following a single tick-borne infection of all members of the herd is given by the equation

$$I = e \cdot (-rt)$$

then by rearranging and substitution

$r = (-\ln.01)/t$
$r = (-\ln.01)/1460 \text{ days} = .0032 \text{ for } B. \text{ bovis and}$
$r = (-\ln.01)/180 \text{ days} = .0256 \text{ for } B. \text{ bigemina}$

The herd parasite rate (see 3.6. below) has also been used to estimate *B. bovis* and *B. bigemina* recovery rates [62]. If exposure to and recovery from babesial infections occur at a constant rate then an equilibrium parasite rate should eventually be achieved at which the numbers of new infections and recoveries are equal. The proportion of the herd infected at equilibrium is dependent upon values for the inoculation and recovery rates. Since the time at which equilibrium occurs depends only on the recovery rate [62], it can be used to estimate the numerical value of this parameter. Corresponding values for 'r' calculated by this method were .0085 for *B. bovis* and .02 for *B. bigemina*. These estimates were then used to estimate the respective inoculation rates in the herd, whose values could be compared with values derived from serologic prevalence or tick infection rate data.

Since both of the above methods relie upon the assumption that 99% of animals in the herd have either recovered or reached equilibrium, there is a significant margin for error. An additional factor which cannot yet be accurately estimated is the degree to which superinfections increase the recovery rate [65]. Notwithstanding, the respective values for *B. bovis* and *B. bigemina* recovery rates estimated by the two techniques are reasonably close and provide a means for quantitative comparison of the two parasites.

3.5. Herd infection rate

As discussed in the previous section, this rate is the proportion of cattle actually infected with the parasite. It is determined by the rate at which infections are acquired by herd members exposed to tick infestations and the rate of recovery from infection through immune removal of the parasite. In an earlier paper by the author [4] 'infection rate' was defined as the serological prevalence of infection. A distinction must be made, however, since infection rate is intended to represent that portion of the herd serving as a reservoir of infection for ticks.

Theoretically, infection rates seldom if ever reach 100%. In addition to natural recovery from infection, addition of noninfected animals and superinfection of animals already infected favor stabilization of infection rates below 100%, even at high inoculation rates.

3.6. *Herd parasite rate*

The parasite rate is the proportion of animals within defined groups with detectable parasitemia. *Babesia* – infected cattle experience periodic parasite recrudescences throughout the infection [62] which determine the probability of detecting parasites in the blood of infected cattle at any given point in time. Repeated sampling of the same group over a period of time would yield a more accurate estimate of the proportion of the herd actually infected. As a result, a distinction must be made between the parasite rate, defined as the percentage of animals with detectable parasitemia at a point in time, and the age-group prevalence of parasitemia measured over a period of time in a defined age group [22, 23, 62, 66, 67]. The latter index is most frequently used in epidemiologic studies since it reflects the actual proportion of the herd which serves as a source of infection for ticks.

The method used to detect parasitemia will influence estimates of the parasite rate and therefore must be consistent throughout a survey. Thick blood films are preferable to thin films. The probability of detecting parasites in an animal also depends upon the frequency of superinfections with heterologous strains. Superinfections with other strains tend to increase parasite rates until the antigenic pool of the parasite population has been exhausted [66]. The influence of immunologic mechanisms upon *B. bovis* herd parasite rates has been explored with a computer simulation model [65].

As discussed in section 3.4. bove, parasite rates have been used to derive estimates of parasite inoculation and recovery rates. Owing to the large number of variables influencing the parasite rate, estimation of inoculation rates from serologic prevalence data may be more precise.

4. Dynamics of transmission; mathematical or simulation models

The dynamics of babesiosis transmission is dependent upon a number of variables affecting the three major components of the life cycle: tick vector, babesial parasite and bovine host. Disease transmission can be interrupted at several points. Some of the variables and the stage at which they influence the life cycle are:

Tick vector
    a. climatic variations
    b. chemical control methods
    c. resistance of cattle to tick feeding
    d. density-dependent factors affecting host-finding
    e. abundance of alternate hosts
    f. pasture rotation interval

Babesial parasite
    a. use of chemotherapeutic agents
    b. level of herd immunity
    c. climatic variations affecting the life cycle in the vector
    d. species of parasite
    e. breed susceptibility of cattle
    f. infection rate in tick vector population
    g. infection rate in bovine host population

Bovine host
    a. rate of entries into and removals from the herd
    b. age structure of the herd

Several types of mathematical models have been developed which describe individual components of the vector-parasite-host relationship in bovine babesiosis [23]. Mahoney and co-workers laid the foundation for these efforts in a series of articles culminating with a model which related inoculation rates to tick numbers [62, 66, 67, 68]. Although numerical estimates for major variables were used, the model was limited by the fact that tick infection rates were fixed and not allowed to respond to changing parasite rates and tick burdens in the herd. Nor were recovery rates incorporated into the interactive model. Consequently, the model tended to overestimate the inoculation rate, especially at low tick burdens [69, 70, 71].

Ross and Mahoney [65] simulated fluctuations in *B. bovis* parasite rates in cattle based on spontaneous appearance and subsequent immunologic clearance of parasite populations from a 'pool' of antigenic types. Tick population dynamics and infection rates were not included in the model. Blewett and co-workers [72] described a model which used herd serologic prevalence data, adjusted for antibody decay, to estimate transmission rates.

Sutherst, Utech and co-workers have developed weather-driven models of *Bo microplus* tick populations both on and off the animal [20, 21, 49]. Breed resistance and seasonal survivability of free-living stages on pasture are used to derive optimal management strategies for tick control. Rates of babesial transmission by ticks are not included in this model.

In the following sections the dynamic interaction among variables discussed in section 3 above will be used to develop a mathematical model of bovine babesiosis [22]. The model will be developed in stages as outlined by MacDonald [73].

4.1. *A biological picture of transmission: life cycle of* **B. bovis** *in* **Bo microplus**

Within 24 hours of inoculation of infective *B. bovis* sporozoites by *Bo microplus* larvae, babesiae appear in the blood and invade circulating erythrocytes where they multiply. Cell rupture releases parasites which reinvade other erythrocytes.

Susceptibility of *Bo microplus* to infection is restricted to the initial and recrudescent parasitemias in the bovine host, and then only during the last 24 hours of tick feeding, corresponding to the period of rapid engorgement. Parasites multiply in the gut epithelium, followed by invasion of the ovary and developing ova. The babesial parasites continue to multiply in gut epithelial cells of the larval progeny, after which they invade and multiply in salivary gland cells. Here the infective sporozoite is formed within 3–4 days of larval tick attachment and inoculated with salivary fluids to initiate the cycle anew.

Babesia bovis parasites do not persist in an infective form in ticks beyond the larval stage. Unless the female tick is reinfected during the period of rapid engorgement, the progeny will be free of infection. The life cycle of *B. bovis* in *Bo microplus* is depicted in Figure 1.

4.2. *Identification of factors directly or indirectly involved in transmission*

The components of the babesial life cycle which influence transmission and for which numerical estimates are needed must now be identified. *Independent variables* are defined as those parameters which are either biologic properties of the vector-parasite-host system and whose values are determined by climatic

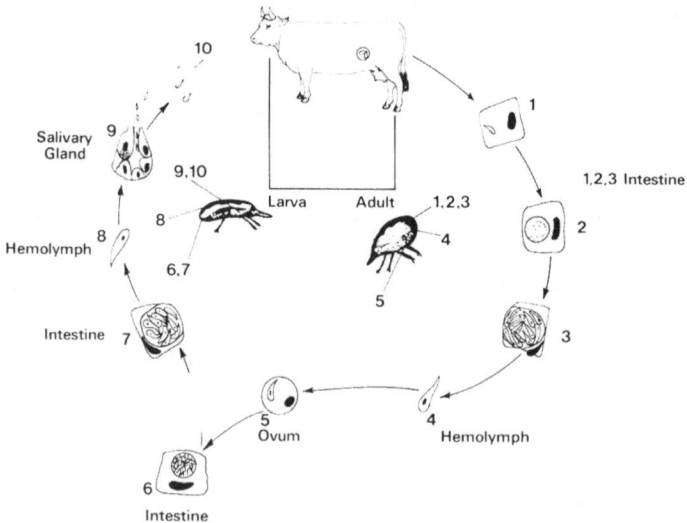

Figure 1. Developmental cycle of *Babesia bovis* in *Boophilus microplus*.

conditions, genetic characteristics of host cattle, tick vector, or babesial parasite, or reflect management practices such as tick control, chemotherapy, or immunoprophylaxis. Their values may change, but not in response to the progress of the vector-parasite-host cycle. *Dependent variables,* in contrast, do not have any predifined numerical value but rather are generated during each tick generation by predictive equations from both independent and previous dependent variables.

The factors affecting the *B. bovis* transmission cycle and which are reflected in the values chosen for independent and dependent variables are depicted in Figure 2. The cyclic nature of transmission between vertebrate and invertebrate host is apparent as is the interdependence of tick and bovine infection rates with *B. bovis.*

4.3. *Conversion of the biological picture into quantitative terms*

Some of the key independent variables used in the model and the points at which they influence the transmission cycle are depicted in Figure 3. Their derivation is explained elsewhere [22] together with relevant predictive equations and resulting dependent variables.

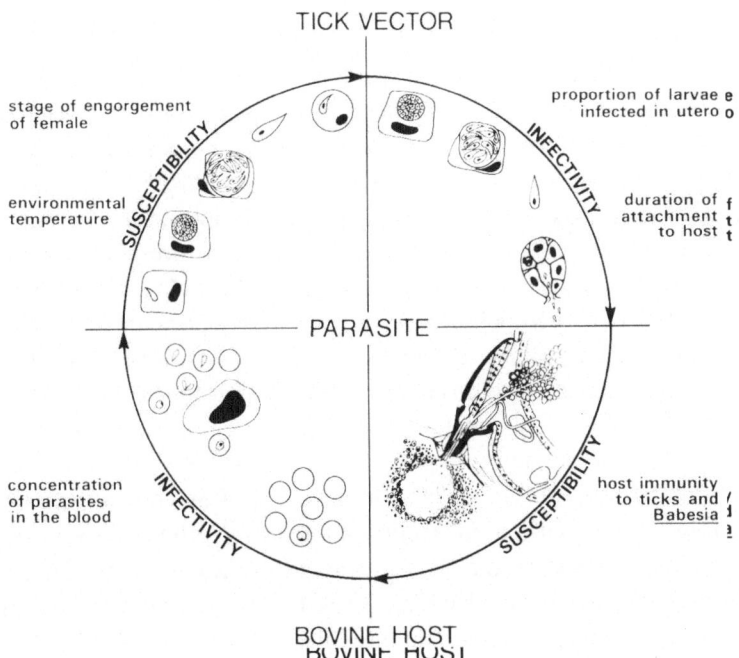

Figure 2. Factors affecting the *Babesia bovis* parasite transmission cycle. Reprinted with permission from Smith [22].

BASIC REPRODUCTION RATE

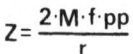

$$Z = \frac{2 \cdot M \cdot f \cdot pp}{r}$$

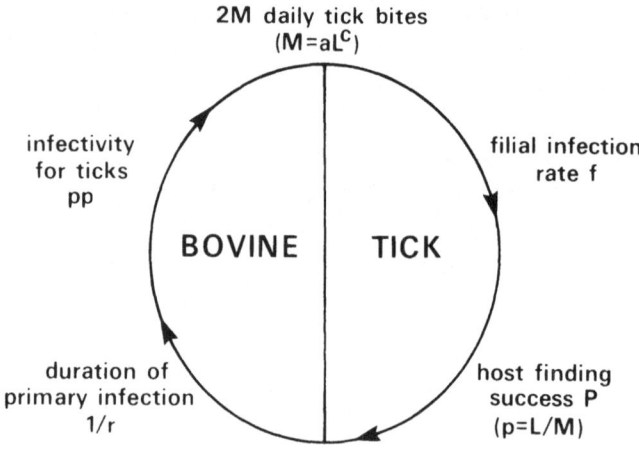

2M daily tick bites
$(M = aL^c)$

infectivity for ticks pp

filial infection rate f

BOVINE | **TICK**

duration of primary infection $1/r$

host finding success P $(p = L/M)$

Critical Level of Transmission
$(M_{z=1})$ =1.951212 tick bites/day

Figure 3. Estimation of the basic reproduction rate for *Babesia bovis* [for details see reference 22]. Reprinted with permission from Smith [22].

From the independent variables appearing in Figure 3, it is possible to estimate the basic reproduction rate (Z), or theoretical number of secondary infections which could be spread from a single primary case of babesiosis, assuming that no superinfections occur. Values of Z>1 reflect an expanding babesial population, whereas Z<1 reflects conditions favoring parasite eradication.

A basic reproduction rate of Z=1 reflects critical or threshold conditions for maintenance of babesiae in nature. Solving for M yields a critical value of approximately 2 engorged ticks (females) per day or approximately 4 tick bites/ day (assuming a 1:1 sex ratio). Below this level babesiae would cease to exist.

Under natural conditions parasite population expansion is limited by superinfection of animals already infected, and by recovery of the bovine host from infection. This phenomenon is depicted in Figure 4, the values for which were derived from the babesiosis model at equilibrium. Tick and bovine infection rates with *B. bovis* reach 'saturation' (represented as hyperbolic curves) despite a linear response of inoculation rates to increasing tick burdens. The 9-month serologic prevalence is included in Figure 4 as its value can be estimated relatively easily from field sampling. Note that all indices of babesial infection have their origin at 2 engorged ticks/day, as predicted above.

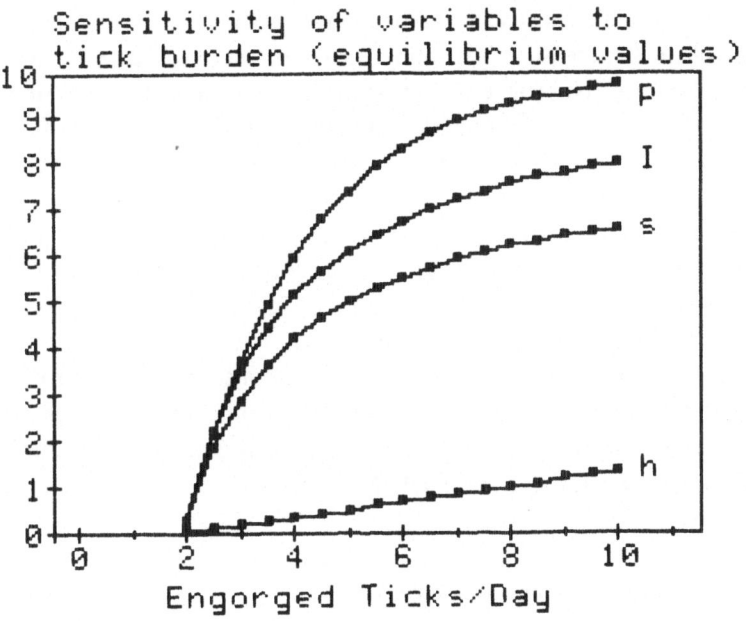

Figure 4. Sensitivity of state variables to tick burden at equilibrium. Abbreviations are (p) 9-month serologic prevalence. (I) herd infection rate. (s) tick infection rate and (h) inoculation rate.

4.4. *Sensitivity analysis*

Having defined the major independent and dependent variables in the *Bo microlus – B. bovis* cycle, it would be useful to see how the equilibrium numerical values for these parameters change over a range of inoculation rates. The range chosen in Table 3 corresponds to the zone of 'enzootic instability' which is described in detail in section 5. Its significance can be appreciated by noting the proportion of the herd in the 9–60 month age range which would experience a primary infection over this range of inoculation rates.

Table 3. Sensitivity analysis of model variables to changes in the *B. bovis* inoculation rate

Parameter	Inoculation rate		
	.0002	.0012	.005
9–60 month incidence	25.3%	61.1%	25.9%
9 month prevalence	5.2%	27.7%	74.1%
Host finding	6.13	6.56	7.73
Larvae/day	12.72	17.61	38.64
Tick infection rate	0.00005	0.00022	0.0005
Females/day	2.07	2.68	5.00

Estimates derived from Smith [22]

The inoculation rate is most sensitive to changes in the host-finding success over this range. A 26% increase in host-finding success results in a 25-fold increase in the inoculation rate. This suggests that slight changes in stocking rates or pasture management can have a major impact upon the rate of *B. bovis* transmission. It also suggests that transmission rates can vary considerably within a single region in response to small habitat changes.

The serologic prevalence of infection at weaning (approximately 9 months of age) is very sensitive (14-fold change) to the inoculation rate over the above range. The ease of sampling and epidemiologic significance of this index make it useful for predicting the risk of outbreaks.

The tick infection rate also shows a marked response (10-fold) over the above range of inoculation rates. However, statistically significant differences would be difficult to detect in field samples due to the precision and large sample sizes required to distinguish these extremely low values.

5. Outbreaks and the theory of control

5.1. *Age immunity*

A babesiosis outbreak may be defined as any infection in which one or more susceptible animals suffer clinical signs and symptoms of disease. In most cases losses attributed to babesiosis are due to upsets in the host-parasite balance, brought about either by introduction of highly susceptible animals into endemic areas or by husbandry practices which interfere with acquisition of infection prior to maturity [40]. In most areas where babesiosis is endemic it is highly desirable for animals to become infected early in life, while they are still protected by 'age immunity'. An exception to this rule may be *B. canis* infections as observed in the southern United States, where puppies appear to be more severely affected than adults [13]. Human infections are another obvious exception. As with other animal species, clinical illness may not provide an accurate indicator of the rate of *B. microti* transmission to man as subclinical infections may occur [74, 75].

Table 4 presents data representative of the degree of age immunity that can be expected in tick-borne *B. bovis* infections. Although all animals became infected, those greater than one year of age suffered more severe reactions and greater mortality than their 9-month old counterparts, which were exposed to the same tick-borne challenge.

Animals which recover from a primary babesial infection are usually refractory to subsequent reactions, even in the face of repeated superinfections. Experimental results depicting this phenomenon appear in Figure 5 where a group of 12 animals was divided into 2 groups following recovery from a primary *B. bovis* infection. No difference could be detected between control cattle and those reexposed on two separate occasions to tick-borne infection.

Table 4. Effect of age upon severity of tick-borne bovine babesiosis [54].

Age of cattle	No. of cattle	Morbidity (%)	Mortality (%)	Incubation period (days)	Febrile days	Daily temp. rise (C)	Maximum PCV reduction (%)
6–9 Months	10	100	10.0	8.50	7.00	1.69	65.78
12–15 Months	15	100	46.7*	11.07	4.38	1.82	42.23

* Treated to avoid higher mortality.

Thus, a balanced host-parasite relationship is one in which most animals are exposed to infection early in life, while age resistance is still operative. Following recovery from the usually mild reaction animals may be considered immune indefinitely [40, 63, 76]. The carrier state does not appear to affect recovered animals adversely.

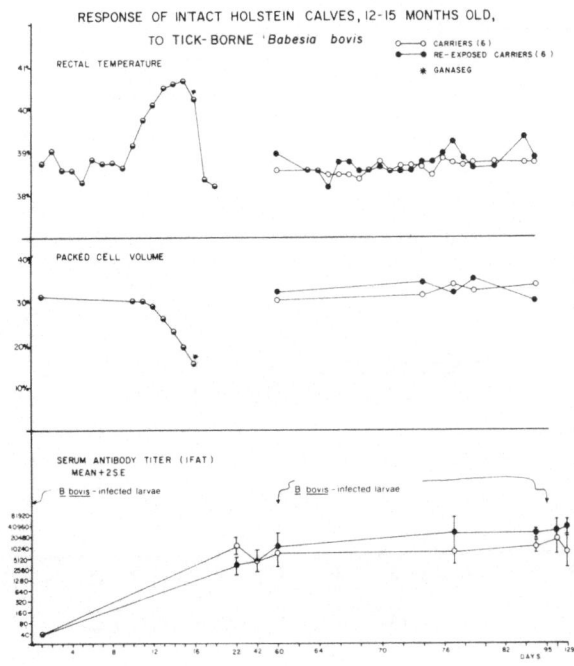

Figure 5. Response of cattle following primary and secondary exposures to tick-borne *Babesia bovis* infections.

5.2. *Enzootic stability and instability*

Enzootic stability and instability [67] are terms which have been used to describe the host-parasite balance in herds residing in babesia-endemic regions. The parasite inoculation rate is the major determinant of whether an area is enzootically unstable or stable ('marginal' or 'enzootic') [4, 23, 68]. If 'enzootic instability' is defined in terms of outbreaks we find that the greatest risk of outbreaks falls within the range of inoculation rates depicted in Figure 6.

If the incidence of primary babesial infections is evaluated in animals >9 months of age, the greatest incidence of disease outbreaks (=) 25% of susceptible cattle) occurs at inoculation rates between 0.0002 and 0.005. Since this age group is more likely to suffer severe reactions to infection (see Table 4), greater losses may be expected to occur when compared with comparable rates of infection in younger animals.

The above range of inoculation rates corresponds to approximately 2 to 5 engored ticks/day. Tick burdens and tick infection rates are very unstable over this range, contributing to the risk of outbreaks. Thus, enzootic instability may be defined as 'that range of babesial inoculation rates over which the greatest immunological and ecological instability occurs' [22]. Lower inoculation rates result in low (stable) rates of transmission to a relatively small proportion of the

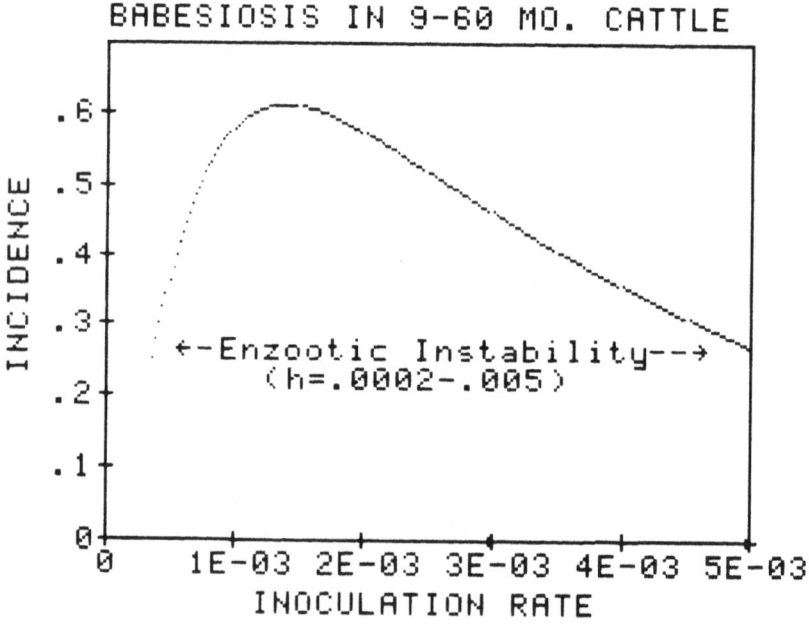

Figure 6. Relationship between inoculation rate and enzootic instability. Enzootic instability is defined to occur whenever >25% of cattle cattle experience a primary *Babesia* infection between the ages of 9 months and 5 years. Inoculation rates of 1E-03 = .001, 2E-03 = .002, etc.

population at risk. Higher inoculation rates result in high (stable) rates of transmission to relatively resistant animals (calves). Although tick transmission of babesiae occurs at both extremes, the risk of outbreaks among older animals is reduced, resulting in enzootic stability.

5.3. *Economic thresholds and tick control strategies*

As discussed in the previous section, a herd exposed to a greater tick burden may be at less risk of a babesiosis outbreak than a comparable herd where tick control measures may have reduced the tick population significantly. There is, however, an upper limit for tick burdens which is unrelated to the risk of babesiosis outbreaks. An inverse linear relationship between average daily tick burden and reduction in weight gain is reported to occur when infestations exceed approximately 20 engorged ticks/day, presumably the result of physiologic stress from tick feeding. Reductions in weight gain of from 0.26 and 0.28 kg/engorged tick/year [20, 77] to 1.18 kg/tick/year [78] have been reported over a range of daily tick burdens of from 20 to 200 engorged ticks.

Estimates of the effect of tick burden upon weight gain and babesiosis incidence are combined in Figure 7 to depict the limits of the economic threshold for tick burdens.

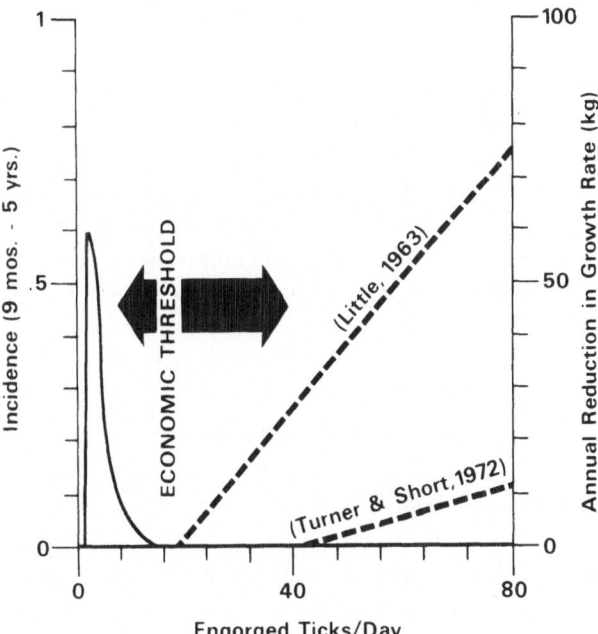

Figure 7. Relationship of tick burden to economic thresholds for *Babesia bovis* incidence and reduction in weight gain. Reprinted with permission from Smith [22].

There would appear to be two economic thresholds for tick infestations. The lower limit is approximately 8 to 9 engorged ticks/day. Below this range the risk of babesiosis outbreaks is significantly increased due to enzootic instability (down to approximatley 2 engorged ticks/day). The upper limit is approximately 30 engorged ticks/ day. Above this range there is little chance of babesiosis outbreaks among native cattle, but they are then subjected to physiologic stress due to tick feeding per se.

The point at which reduced gains justify tick control measures is dictated largely by economic considerations which, in turn, have given rise to different approaches to tick control (dipping) strategies [20, 21, 71]. 'Economic threshold dipping' is practiced where tick populations fluctuate seasonally, sometimes dropping below levels required to maintain enzootic stability. Here the objective is to avoid interfering with naturally acquired calfhood immunity to babesiosis by dipping cattle only when tick numbers exceed an arbitrarily determined level. This is usually based on the producer's perception of what level of infestation is economically important and, as such, is subject to considerable variability.

The philosophy behind 'planned dipping' is similar but dippings are carried out based upon knowledge of seasonal tick patterns or is integrated into pasture spelling schemes. In this way cattle roundups can be planned for certain times of the year without having to monitor tick burdens closely.

'Strategic dipping' [79, 80] is a relatively new approach to tick control based upon detailed knowledge of the time of emergence of overwintering non-parasitic stages. The objective is to reduce the need for periodic dippings throughout the year by intensive control of the first overwintering parasitic generation.

The effect of the above tick control strategies upon babesial transmission has been studied [71, 79]. Since strategic dipping creates conditions favorable for enzootic instability, it should not be practiced in the absence of immunoprophylactic measures in the herd [79]. Along this line, Norval [81] describes the resurgence of bovine babesiosis and other tick-borne diseases of cattle in Zimbabwe Rhodesia following a breakdown of compulsory dipping. The severity of outbreaks was exacerbated by the low level of herd immunity created by years of efficient tick control.

6. Indicators for forecasting babesiosis outbreaks

6.1. *Statistical validity of sampling*

In section 5.2. the epidemiologic significance of the inoculation rate was discussed in terms of the incidence of infections in an age group likely to suffer severe reactions to infection. Modeling has provided numerical estimates for several parameters in the babesial life cycle, some of which can be used to estimate the inoculation rate. These include tick infection rate, tick burden, and serologic prevalence [4, 22].

6.2. *Tick infection rate*

Although the tick infection rate provides a reasonable estimate of the inoculation rate at equilibrium conditions, manual collection and microscopic examination of ticks for this purpose is impractical under field conditions. Aside from the tedious nature of larval collection from cattle [60], sample sizes of between 6000 and 29000 would be required for any sort of statistical accuracy (see Table 5). Furthermore, the environmental history of field collected ticks will directly affect measurable infection rates [37, 50, 51].

Table 5 depicts the number of field-collected larvae that would have to be examined to estimate the tick infection rate (and indirectly the inoculation rate) with a given level of precision. The actual accuracy of these estimates would be somewhat less as the ability to detect babesiae in infected ticks is less than 100%.

Field sampling of multi-host ticks may be more feasible for predictive purposes, although the quantitative relationship between tick numbers, tick infection rate and disease risk needs further clarification [82, 83].

Table 5. Sample size vs confidence interval for estimating *Boophilus microplus* tick infection rates (s) with *Babesia bovis* [22]

Sample size	Mean (s)	95% c.i.	
18,000	.00022	0	−.00044
36,000	.00022	.000064–	.00037
72,000	.00022	.00011	−.00033
8,000	.0005	0	−.001

6.3. *Tick burden*

Routine monitoring of engorged tick burdens provides a possibly more accessible sampling parameter. However, the probability of ticks being present on predilection sites is too low to be statistically valid at infestation levels associated with the zone of enzootic instability (2–5 females/day), even when large numbers of cattle are examined [22, 60].

6.4. *Serologic prevalence*

Serologic testing of calves at weaning (8–9 months of age) is probably the most readily accessible and accurate method for determining risk. This procedure not only provides a direct estimate of the size of the population at risk, but also provides a retrospective estimation of the inoculation rate (Table 3). Actual risk would depend upon projected size and seasonal fluctuations of the vector population. Since antibody titers to *Babesia* are known to decline over time, compensation for this decline must be made in assessing prevalence among older age groups [72, 84].

7. Conclusion

Mathematical models have been referred to as 'epidemiological hypotheses' [85], whose predictions may be used in the elaboration of experimental protocols and in planning data collection. Furthermore, 'risk forcasting' would be of practical importance in the design of appropriate disease control strategies. Unfortunately, our knowledge of the natural history of many economically important babesial species is too fragmentary to construct more than rudimentary models. However, during the course of constructing even the simplest models one becomes aware of epidemiologic data which is lacking. Hopefully the emphasis of this chapter upon dynamic aspects of *B. bovis* transmission will encourage others to seek similar information on other babesial parasites.

Summary

Our knowledge of the epidemiology of infections caused by the approximately 71 species of *Babesia* is limited to diseases in a few economically important host species and man. In some cases losses attributed to babesiosis are inseparable from those caused by the tick vector alone. Infections are common in temporate as well as tropical regions and, except for one *Babesia* – argasid tick system, all of the known vectors are ixodid ticks.

The life cycle, mode of transmission and host spectrum of several of the babesiae has been elucidated, but quantitative data on tick and vertebrate host infection rates, recovery rates, vector efficiency and survival of non-parasitic stages are not available for most babesial species. Furthermore, our understanding of the way in which these variables interact to create conditions favorable for disease outbreaks is limited.

In this chapter a computer simulation model of the *Babesia bovis – Boophilus microplus* system is developed to identify limiting factors for babesial transmission. Numerical values for system variables are estimated and related to economic thresholds for tick burdens and the theory of control. Sensitivity analysis of modeling parameters is used to determine optimal field sampling strategies for predicting the risk of babesiosis outbreaks.

Simulation modeling of other babesial vector-parasite-host systems is hindered by a lack of quantitative data on the natural history of parasite transmission. Future studies should facilitate collection of epidemiologically-relevant data which can be used for predictive purposes.

References

1. Levine ND: Taxonomy of the piroplasms. Trans Amer Micros Soc 90(1):2–33, 1971.
2. Neitz WO: Classification, transmission, and biology of piroplasms of domestic animals. Ann NY Acad Sci 64(2):56–111, 1956.
3. Neitz WO: A consolidation of our knowledge of the transmission of tick-borne diseases. Onderstepoort J Vet Res 27(2):115–163, 1956.
4. Friedhoff KT, Smith RD: Transmission of *Babesia* by ticks. In: Babesiosis, Ristic M, Kreier JP (eds), New York, Academic Press, 1981, p 267–321.
5. Zwart D, Brocklesby DW: Babesiosis: non-specific resistance, immunological factors and pathogenesis. In: Advances in Parasitology, Lumsden WHR, Muller R, Baker JR (eds), New York, Academic Press, 17, 1979, p 49–113.
6. Purnell RE: Babesiosis in various hosts. In: Babesiosis, Ristic M, Kreier JP (eds), New York, Academic Press, 1981, p 25–63.
7. Nikolskii SN, Nikiforenko VI, Posov SA: Epidemiology of piroplasmosis in Siberia. Veterinariya (Moscow) 4:71–75, 1977.
8. Minami T, Ishirara T: *Babesia ovata* sp. n. isolated from cattle in Japan. Nat Inst Anim Hlth Quart 20(3):101–113, 1980.
9. Gray JS, De Vos AJ: Studies on a bovine babesia transmitted by *Hyalomma marginatum* rufipes Koch, 1844. Onderstepoot J Vet Res 48:215–223, 1981.
10. Killick-Kendrick R: Parasitic protozoa of the blood of rodents. II. Haemogregarines, malaria parasites and piroplasms of rodents: an annotated checklist and host index. Acta Tropica 31(1):28–69, 1974.
11. Anonymous: Animal health yearbook. Rome, FAO-WHO-OIE, 1981.
12. Knowles RC, Hourrigan JL, Holbrook AA: Equine piroplasmosis. Equine Practice. 2(1):10–14, 1980.
13. Breitschwerdt EB, Malone JB, MacWilliams P, Levy MG, Qualis CW Jr, Prudich MJ: Babesiosis in the greyhound. Am J Vet Res 182(9):978–982, 1983.
14. Purnell RE: Tick-borne diseases of British livestock. Vet Med Rev 1:58–69, 1981.
15. Taylor SM, Kenny J, Strain A: The distribution of *Babesia divergens* infection within the cattle population of Northern Ireland. Brit Vet J 138(5):384–392, 1982.
16. Uilenberg G, Rombach MC, Perie NM, Zwart D: Blood parasites of sheep in the Netherlands. II. *Babesia motasi* (Sporozoa, Babesiidae). Vet Quarterly 2(1):3–14, 1980.
17. Gern L, Brossard M, Aeschlimann A, Broquet CA, Quenet G, Stucki JP, Ackermann J: Piroplasmose bovine dans le Clos-du-Doube (Jura, Suisse): observations pr eliminaires. Schweiz Arch Tierheilk 124:549–556, 1982.
18. Gee GF: The economic importance of the cattle tick in Australia. Canberra, Bureau of Agricultural Economics, 1959.
19. Lombardo RA: Socioeconomic importance of the tick problem in the Americas. PAHO Scientific Publ. No. 316:79–89, 1976.
20. Sutherst RW, Norton GA, Barlow ND, Conway GR, Birley M, Comins HN: An analysis of management strategies for cattle tick (*Boophilus microplus*) control in Australia. J Appl Ecol 16:359–382, 1979.
21. Sutherst RW, Norton GA, Maywald GF: Analysis of control strategies for cattle tick on Zebu X British cattle. Proc 56th Annu Conf Aust Vet Assoc: 46–51, 1979.
22. Smith RD: *Babesia bovis*: computer simulation of the relationship between the tick vector, parasite, and bovine host. Exptl Parasitol 56:27–40, 1983.
23. Joyner LP, Donnelly J: The epidemiology of babesial infections. In: Adv Parasitol, Lumsden WHR, Muller R, Baker JR (eds), New York, Acad Press, 1979, p 115–140.
24. Friedhoff KT: Morphologic aspects of babesia in the tick. In: Babesiosis, Ristic M, Kreier JP (eds), New York, Academic Press, 1981, p 143–169.

230

25. Burgdorfer W, Varma MGR: Trans-stadial and transovarial development of disease agents in arthropods. Ann Rev Entomol 12:347–376, 1967.
26. Buscher G, Friedhoff KT, Yossef LSEA: Transmission of *Babesia bigemina* by *Boophilus* spp. and *Rhipicephalus evertsi* 2nd Intern Conf Malaria & Babesiosis Sept 19–22, Annecy, France, 1983.
27. Dalgliesh RJ, Stewart NP, Callow LL: Transmission of *Babesia bigemina* by transfer of adult male *Boophilus microplus*. Aust Vet J 54:205–206, 1978.
28. Gray JS, Potgieter FT: Studies on the infectivity of *Boophilus decoloratus* males and larvae infected with *Babesia bigemina*. Onderstepoort J Vet Res 49:1–2, 1982.
29. Abramov IV: A new type of transmission of *Nuttallia equi* by tick vectors. (In Russian). Veterinariya (Moscow) 32(8):43–45, 1955.
30. Stiller D, Frerichs WM: Experimental transmission of *Babesia caballi* to equids by different stages of the tropical horse tick, *Anocentor nitens* (Neumann). In: Recent advances in acarology. Vol. II, Rodriguez JG (ed), New York, Academic Press, 1979, p 263–269.
31. Mason CA, Norval RAI: The transfer of *Boophilus microplus* (Acarina: Ixodidae) from infested to uninfested cattle under field conditions. Vet Parasitol 8(2):185–188, 1981.
32. Gray JS, Potgieter FT: The retention of *Babesia bigemina* infection by *Boophilus decoloratus* exposed to imidocarb dipropionate during engorgement. Onderstepoort J Vet Res 48:225–227, 1981.
33. Mahoney DF, Mirre GB: A note on the transmission of *Babesia bovis* (syn *B. argentina*) by the one-host tick, *Boophilus microplus* Res Vet Sci 26:253–254, 1979.
34. Lewis D, Young ER: The transmission of a human strain of *Babesia divergens* by *Ixodes ricinus* ticks. J Parasitol 66(2):359–360, 1980.
35. Oliveira MR, Kreier JP: Transmission of *Babesia microti* using various species of ticks as vectors. J Parasitol 65(5):816–817, 1979.
36. Spielman A: Human babesiosis on Nantucket Island: transmission by nymphal *Ixodes* ticks. Am J Trop Med Hyg 25(6):784–787, 1976.
37. Piesman J, Spielman A: Human babesiosis on Nantucket Island: prevalence of *Babesia microti* in ticks. Am J Trop Med Hyg 29(5):742–746, 1980.
38. Walter G, Weber G: A study on the transmission (transstadial, transovarial) of *Babesia microti*, strain 'Hannover I', in its tick vector, *Ixodes ricinus*. Tropenmed Parasit 32:228–230, 1981.
39. Genga UE, Kreier JP: Transmission experiments with *Babesia microti* (Gray strain) using *Dermacentor andersoni*. Stiles as a vector. Ohio J Sci 76(4):188–189, 1976.
40. Callow LL, Dalgliesh RJ: Immunity and immunopathology in babesiosis. In: Immunology of parasitic infections, Cohen S, Warren KS (eds), Boston, Blackwell, 1982, p 475–526.
41. Ristic M, Lewis GE Jr: *Babesia* in man and wild and laboratory-adapted mammals. In: Parasitic Protozoa, Kreier JP (ed), New York, Academic Press, 1977, IV, p 53–76.
42. Marshall CM, Seaman GA, Hayes FA: A critique on the tropical cattle fever tick controversy and its relationship to white-tailed deer. Trans. twenty-eighth North American Wildlife and Natural Resources Conference, March 4–6, 1963, p 225–232.
43. Hourrigan JL: Epizootiology of bovine babesiosis and the current status of *Boophilus* eradication in Texas. Ann NY Entomol Soc LXXXV (4):217–220, 1977.
44. Piesman J, Spielman A, Etkind P, Reubush TK II, Juranek DD: Role of deer in the epizootiology of *Babesia microti* in Massachusetts, USA J Med Entomol 15(5–6):537–540, 1979.
45. Healy GR, Spielman A, Gleason N: Human babesiosis: reservoir of infection on Nantucket Island. Science 192:479–480, 1976.
46. Spielman A, Etkind P, Piesman J, Ruebush TK II, Juranek DD, Jacobs MS: Reservoir hosts of human babesiosis on Nantucket Island. Am J Trop Med Hyg 30(3):560–565, 1981.
47. Spielman A, Clifford CM, Piesman J, Corwin MD: Human babesiosis on Nantucket Island, USA: description of the vector, *Ixodes (Ixodes) dammini*. N. Sp. (acarina: ixodidae). J Med Entomol 15(3):218–234, 1979.

48. Hussein HS: *Ixodes trianugliceps:* seasonal abundance and role in the epidemiology of *Babesia microti* infection in north-western England. Ann Trop Med Parasitol 74(5):531–539, 1980.

49. Utech KBW, Sutherst RW, Dallwitz MJ, Wharton RH, Maywald GF, Sutherland ID: A model of the survival of larvae of the cattle tick, *Boophilus microplus* on pasture. Aust J Agric Res 34:63–72, 1983.

50. Dalgliesh RJ, Stewart NP: Some effects of time, temperature and feeding on infection rates with *Babesia bovis* and *Babesia bigemina* in *Boophilus microplus* larvae. Int J Parasitol 12(4)323–326, 1982.

51. Dalgliesh RJ, Stewart NP: Observations on the morphology and infectivity for cattle of *Babesia bovis* parasites in unfed *Boophilus microplus* larvae after incubation at various temperatures. Int J Parasitol 9:115–120, 1979.

52. Gray JS: The effects of the piroplasm *Babesia bigemina* on the survival and reproduction of the blue tick, *Boophilus decoloratus.* J Invertebr Pathol 39:413–415, 1982.

53. Mahoney DF, Mirre GB: Bovine babesiosis: estimation of infection rates in the tick vector *Boophilus microplus* (Canestrini). Ann Trop Med Parasitol 65(3):309–317, 1971.

54. Smith RD, Osorno BM, Brener J, De La Rosa R, Ristic M: Bovine babesiosis: severity and reproducibility of *Babesia bovis* infections induced by *Boophilus microplus* under laboratory conditions. Res Vet Sci 24:287–292, 1978.

55. Mahoney DF, Mirre GB: The selection of larvae of *Boophilus microplus* infected with *Babesia bovis* (syn *B. argentina*). Res Vet Sci 23:126–127, 1977.

56. Riek RF: The life cycle of *Babesia bigemina* (Smith & Kilborne, 1893) in the tick vector *Boophilus microplus* (Canestrini). Aust J Agr Res 15(5):802–821, 1964.

57. Riek RF: The life cycle of *Babesia argentina* (Lignieres, 1903) (Sporozoa: Piroplasmidea) in the tick vector *Boophilus microplus* (Canestrini). Aust J Agr Res 17:247–254, 1966.

58. Dalgliesh RJ, Stewart NP: Stimulation of the development of infective *Babesia bovis* (= *B. argentina*) in unfed *Boophilus microplus* larvae. Aust Vet J 52:543, 1976.

59. Dalgliesh RJ, Stewart NP: The extraction of infective *Babesia bovis* and *Babesia bigemina* from tick eggs and *B. bigemina* from unfed larval ticks. Aust Vet J 54:453–454, 1978.

60. Palmer WA, Treverrow NL, O'Neill GH: Factors affecting the detection of infestations of *Boophilus microplus* in tick control programs. Aust Vet J 52:321–324, 1976.

61. Roberts JA: Resistance of cattle to the tick *Boophilus microplus* (Canestrini). II. Stages of the life cycle of the parasite against which resistance is manifest. J Parasitol 54:667–673, 1968.

62. Mahoney DF: Bovine babesiosis: a study of factors concerned in transmission. Ann Trop Med Parasitol 63(1):1–14, 1969.

63. Mahoney DF, Wright IG, Mirre GB: Bovine babesiasis: the persistence of immunity to *Babesia argentina* and *B. bigemina* in calves (*Bos taurus*) after naturally acquired infection. Ann Trop Med Parasitol 67:197–203, 1973.

64. Johnston LAY, Leatch G, Jones PN: The duration of latent infection and functional immunity in droughtmaster and hereford cattle following natural infection with *Babesia argentina* and *Babesia bigemina.* Aust Vet J 54:114–118, 1978.

65. Ross DR, Mahoney DF: Bovine babesiasis: computer simulation of *Babesia argentina* parasite rates in *Bos taurus* cattle. Ann Trop Med Parasitol 68:385–392, 1974.

66. Mahoney DF: The epidemiology of babesiosis in cattle. Aust J Sci 24:310–313, 1962.

67. Mahoney DF, Ross DR: Epizootiological factors in the control of bovine babesiosis. Aust Vet J 48:292–298, 1972.

68. Mahoney DF: *Babesia* of domestic animals. In: Parasitic Protozoa, Kreier JP (ed), New York, Academic Press, 1977. IV. p 1–52.

69. Mahoney DF: The epidemiology of babesiasis. Proc 56th Annu Conf Aust Vet Assoc: 9–11, 1979.

70. Mahoney DF: The epidemiology of babesiosis in cattle with special reference to the *Babesia bovis/Boophilus microplus* system. In: Haemoprotozoan Diseases of Domestic Animals, Gautam OP, Sharma RD, Dhar. S (eds). Hissar (Haryana) India, Haryana Agricultural University, 1980, p 103–106.

232

71. Mahoney DF, Wright IG, Goodger BV, Mirre GB, Sutherst RW, Utech KBW: The transmission of *Babesia bovis* in herds of European and zebu X European cattle infested with the tick, *Boophilus microplus*. Aust Vet J 57(10):461–469, 1981.

72. Blewett DA, Beasley SJ, Campbell JA, Turnbull DMcD: A simple model for the interpretation of serological data for tick-borne diseases. In: Tick-borne diseases and their vectors. Proceedings of an international conference, Edinburgh 1976, Wilde JKH (ed). Edinburgh, Centre for Tropical Veterinary Medicine, 1978, p 130–131.

73. MacDonald G: Epidemiologic models in studies of vector-borne diseases. Public Health Reports 76(9):753–764, 1961.

74. Ruebush TK, II, Juranek DD, Chisholm ES, Snow PC, Healy GR, Sulzer AJ: Human babesiosis on Nantucket Island. Evidence for self-limited and subclinical infections. N Eng J Med 297:825–827, 1977.

75. Filstein MR, Benach JL, White DF, Brody BA, Goldman WD, Bakal CW, Schwartz RS: Serosurvey for human babesiosis in New York. J Inf Dis 141(4):518–521, 1980.

76. Mahoney DF, Wright IG, Goodger BV: Immunity in cattle to *Babesia bovis* after single infections with parasites of various origin. Aust Vet J 55(1):10–12, 1979.

77. Turner HG, Short AJ: Effects of field infestations of gastrointestinal helminths and of the cattle tick (*Boophilus microplus*) on growth of three breeds of cattle. Aust J Agric Res 23:177–193, 1972.

78. Little DA: The effect of cattle tick infestations on the growth rate of cattle. Aust Vet J 39:6–10, 1963.

79. Johnston LAY, Haydock KP, Leatch G: The effect of two systems of cattle tick (*Boophilus microplus*) control on tick populations, transmission of *Babesia* spp. and *Anaplasma* spp. and production of Brahman crossbred cattle in the dry tropics. Aust J Exp Agric Anim Husb 21:256–267, 1981.

80. Ralph W: Strategic dipping for tick control in northern Australia. Rural Res 116:12–14, 1982.

81. Norval RAI: Tick infestations and tick-borne diseases in Zimbabwe Rhodesia. J S African Vet Assoc 50(4):289–292, 1979.

82. Gray JS: Studies on the activity of *Ixodes ricinus* in relation to the epidemiology of babesiosis in Co. Meath, Ireland. Brit Vet J 136(5):427–436, 1980.

83. Gray JS, Lohan G: The development of a sampling method for the tick *Ixodes ricinus* and its use in a redwater fever area. Ann Appl Biol 101(3):421–427, 1982.

84. Ruebush TK, II, Chisholm ES, Sulzer AJ, Healy GR: Development and persistence of antibody in persons infected with *Babesia microti*. Am J Trop Med Hyg 30(1):291–292, 1981.

85. Fine PEM, Lehman JS Jr: Mathematical models of schistosomiasis: report of a workshop. Am J Trop Med

14. Malaria control

PIERRE AMBROISE-THOMAS
in collaboration with DOMINIQUE BAUDON, PIERRE CARNEVALE,
JEAN MOUCHET AND JEAN ROUX

Universite Scientifique et Medicale de Grenoble, Faculte de Medecine, Laboratoire de Parasitologie, Domaine de la Merci, 38700 La Tronche, France.

> The history of malaria is a great lesson for mankind: we should be more scientific in the way we think and more practical in the way in which we act. The fact of having neglected this lesson has already cost great losses in human life and prosperity in many countries.
>
> Sir Ronald Ross (1911)

Introduction

Malaria either affects or threatens several hundred million people. Each year, it causes more than a million deaths [1, 2]. It has considerable socioeconomic consequences and impedes the development of many thirdworld countries [3]. Malaria is undoubtedly the main disease affecting mankind and also one of the oldest since there are various indications that it appeared, possibly in East Africa, at about the same time as man himself.

The history of malaria is closely linked to that of the various civilizations with their vicissitudes, their periods of poverty or, conversely, their phases of expansion, wellbeing and progress. Our present knowledge of this disease has been largely acquired as the result of the technical improvements of various epochs, socioeconomic pressures and even military requirements. It is scarcely three and a half century since malaria was distinguished from other fevers on the basis of its particular responsiveness to certain types of treatment. During the last two centuries our knowledge has increased very rapidly with the discovery of the causative parasites, the agents by which they are transmitted, and new means of diagnosis, treatment and prevention.

All this progress generated a deep current of enthusiasm immediately after the Second World War that found expression at the Eight World Health Assembly in the decision to eradicate malaria, i.e. to bring about the total disappearance of this disease from the face of the globe. At the time this objective seemed within

Ristic, M. et al. (eds.) *Malaria and babesiosis.*
© 1984, Martinus Nijhoff Publishers, Dordrecht/Boston/Lancaster.

reach. Subsequent events showed that this was unfortunately not the case. Since then the situation has improved in certain respects, but in others it has, on the contrary, deteriorated considerably as some of our principal means of control have lost their effectiveness. In recent years a considerable research effort has been instigated both by international organizations (WHO) and, in certain countries, by national bodies [4]. Great hopes have been aroused by some recent advances. However, unless we guard against it, there is the danger that these discoveries will lead us to forget that the ultimate aim is not malaria research but the control of the disease. Malaria is a very ancient scourge of mankind, the prevention of which undoubtedly calls for new research. What is required above all is that those responsible for prevention should adopt a humble and pragmatic approach, and be prepared to adapt necessarily theoretical general concepts to the local needs in each epidemiological situation.

We shall now consider the means at our disposal, the improvements being made, what needs to be done, what hopes have been aroused by research and, last but not least, the optimal application of the available methods of control and the current principles of malaria control.

1. Currently available means of control

Since malaria arises from the transmission of various *Plasmodium* species to man through the bites of certain mosquitos, there are three obvious approaches to the prevention of the disease:
1 Avoiding the risk of being bitten by the insect vector;
2 Destroying this vector in one of its various development stages, and
3 Eliminating plasmodia when present in man before they give rise to clinical manifestations, when clinical signs become apparent, or before the parasites become infective for the anopheline mosquitos concerned and capable of transmission to other subjects.

1.1. *Protection of man against infecting bites*

Protection is based on a set of simple means, which have to be employed strictly and with perseverance. Some of these preventive measures, which have long been known for the most part, are as valuable as ever in cutting down the risk of transmission. This is especially so of the use of *mosquito nets* to cover beds (possibly with the important refinement that the netting be impregnated with insecticides) and the fitting of fine screens to windows and other openings in dwellings. These procedures, which were long neglected in favour of more spectacular means of control, are relatively cheap and useful additional methods, but they are obviously applicable only to protection against endophilous anopheline species. Furthermore, they require people to remain inside protected dwellings throughout the times of day when the mosquitos bite, i.e. generally between sunset and sunrise.

Other more restricting and costly measures are applicable to exophilous anopheline mosquitos, including the wearing of special clothing and the application of various repellents to uncovered parts of the body. The repellents remain effective for only a fairly short time, due to the action of perspiration. In practice, these means of prevention are of use only for individual staying for a very brief period in an endemic zone (e.g. tourists).

1.2. *Vector control*

1.2.1. *Larval control* [5, 6]
Control is possible in various ways: by modifying the environment, by the use of physico-chemical means or biological procedures.

a *Modification of the environment.* This is undoubtedly the oldest known means of prevention, since Hippocrates had already noted in his day that the people were in good health where rivers carried away stagnant water or rain water. In many temperate countries, where the level of transmission is admittedly low, malaria has been eliminated through environmental measures. Such was the case in the famous example of the Pontine marshes around Rome or the less well known example of the Brooklyn marshes where control measures were carried out in 1905. The *draining of marshy zones* may be supplemented or replaced by the planting of certain trees (*Eucalyptus*). The measures employed where standing water has to be maintained (irrigation) are weed clearance and above all periodic draining. The choice of method is, of course, dependent on local conditions, but also on precise knowledge of the biology of the anopheline vector species. Water bodies whose distance from villages is within the flight range of the insect vector (about 1.6 km) must obviously be given priority treatment.

Even when only partly effective, these preventive measures remain as relevant as ever. They enable transmission to be reduced and, above all, they have the considerable merit of directly involving the people in malaria control. In some respects they are, moreover, techniques with a future since they have to be employed systematically to prevent or limit the occurrence or spread of new man-made foci of malaria whenever the environment is modified in any way (dam, irrigation system).

Furthermore, this type of preventive measure does not necessarily involve a great deal of work. Simple changes of local customs may be sufficient. Thus, for example, in some regions of Africa it is the custom to keep drinking water in jars close to or inside dwellings and these jars are in many cases breeding grounds for anopheline mosquitos within the home.

b *Physico-chemical means*. The *spreading* of mineral oil over the surface of stagnant water is sufficient to kill all larvae by asphyxia. The oil has to form a perfectly regular film, and this is dependent on the characteristics of the particular oil. The procedure, although very simple, has to be repeated regularly because hydrocarbons evaporate rapidly or form a deposit along the sides of water bodies. There is the further possibility of combining this physical procedure with chemical control by mixing 1% of an insecticide such as DDT with the oil for spreading. Vegetable oils or liquid paraffin are used to treat drinking water (water tanks).

A great number of *larvicides* has been used for *chemical control*. Paris green, which is the oldest known (1921), has various disadvantages in use. Dieldrin or DDT, the products most frequently employed after the Second World War, are avoided nowadays because they exert considerable pressure on the biological evolution of anopheline populations and accelerate the development of insecticide resistance.

The use of other larvicides remains relatively restricted, despite some interesting results, in particular against *Anopheles stephensi*, because the non-target aquatic fauna may adversely be affected by the products released, and above all, because of the cost of larviciding operations and the restrictions that they impose. Nevertheless, these larvicides have been shown to be effective in some regions (Réunion) and in periurban areas.

c *Biological control*. Strictly speaking, the planting of trees or other plants to create shady conditions and impede the proliferation of mosquito larvae could be included among biological control procedures. In practice, biological control refers exclusively to the use of predators or microorganisms that destroy larvae. Among the predators, little use is made of larvivorous fish (*Gambusia*, *Nothobranchius*), which are justified only in permanent breeding grounds. Protozoa (*Nosema*), microscopic fungi (*Celomomyces*) and some nematodes have been used, but only briefly and on a very limited scale. On the other hand, *Bacillus thuringiensis* serotype H14, or its *israelensis* variety, a bacterium that forms microcrystals of a toxic protein causing fatal lesions in anopheline larvae, seems more promising.

1.2.2. *Control of the adult stage* [6]

a *Biological means*. (the release of sterile males) have in practice been used only on an experimental scale. On the other hand, *insecticides* active against adults (imagocides) have been and are still widely employed. One of them, DDT, even appeared so promising after the end of the Second World War that the malaria eradication programme put forward by WHO was exclusively based on vector control. The various imagocides that are available belong in practice to four groups:

1 Natural pyrethrins (extracts produced from plants related to chrysanthemums) or synthetic pyrethrin (pyrethroids) such as decamethrin;
2 Chlorinated hydrocarbons (DDT, HCH, dieldrin);
3 Organophosphorus compounds (malathion, fenthion, fenitrothion, dichlorvos); and
4 Carbamates (carbaryl, landrin).

These insecticides act in various ways: through ingestion, inhalation and contact.

The considerations that influence the choice of product are effectiveness against the target insect, the duration of the residual action (which is related to the substrate on which it is sprayed), ease of application, low toxicity to man and domestic or wild animals, and, lastly, cost.

Insecticide spraying on the inner walls of houses yields excellent results in regions in which the anopheline vectors of malaria are endophagous and endophilous, i.e. to be found inside dwellings or cattle sheds. Knowledge of the biology of local vectors is therefore an essential prerequisite to a spraying operation. Without such knowledge, the measures may fail as, for example, in Venezuela in the control of *A. nuñeztovari*, which does not enter houses and consequently escapes house-spraying.

The effectiveness of an insecticide may also be decreased by its irritant effect which causes the mosquito to take flight before receiving a lethal dose. This vector behaviour pattern may vary with the species or the biotope. The irritant nature of the insecticide is dependent on its composition, its concentration and its mode of application. This is why much research has been devoted for several years to the development of tests for assessment of the effectiveness of various categories of compounds.

b   The problem is further complicated by the existence of *insecticide resistance*, which has developed very rapidly. In 1946, there were only two *Anopheles* species known to be resistant to DDT, whereas now there are some 50 species resistant to one or more insecticides.

Resistance is to be found mainly in West Africa and the Sudan, where *A. gambiae* is resistant to DDT and dieldrin, in Central America, where *A. albimanus* is resistant to chlorinated hydrocarbons and malathion, in several of the countries of South-East Asia, where *A. stephensi* and *A. culicifacies* are resistant to chlorinated hydrocarbons, and lastly in the Near East, especially Turkey, where *A. sacharovi* has developed resistance to the most widely employed insecticides.

Resistance results not from progressive adaptation but rather from the selection of individuals within an anopheline population who possess from the outset genes that enable them to escape the action of the insecticide, either through the production of enzymes that break it down, or through other mechanisms that, for example, reduce its penetration. When resistance is *monogenic,* only one insecticide (DDT, for example) or a group of insecticides (HCH and dieldrin, for example) is involved. Resistance that is dependent on *several genes* enables the insect to escape from several insecticides (for example, *A. albimanus* is resistant to DDT, HCH, dieldrin, organophosphorus insecticides and carbamates). The rate at which resistance appears and extends differs from case to case. Thus, combined HCH-dieldrin resistance is more prevalent than HCH resistance because the gene responsible is dominant in the first case and recessive in the second.

Resistance to imagocidal insecticides is one of the causes of the failure of the eradication campaign. It has led to *much recent research* in a race to find new insecticides, the most promising of which would appear to be pyrethroids (allethrin, resmethrin, tetramethrin, etc.) that are highly active against insects and of very low toxicity to man, and that have been made far more stable (with a residual action that may last for about six months). Other ways of using insecticides are also being examined: in Mali and Upper Volta, for example, mosquito nets impregnated with insecticides (decamethrin and permethrin) are in use.

1.3. *Plasmodial control*

1.3.1. *Antimalarials*

The use of quinine, the first known antimalarial drug, began to reveal the nature of malaria. Since 1650, the history of antimalarial drugs has been extremely colourful and graphic, and rich in anecdotal stories. One striking feature is the extent to which the recent history of these drugs is bound up with that of the various wars of the 20th century. It was largely the appalling mortality from malaria in some theatres of operations during the First World War (the Dardanelles) that prompted the first research on synthetic antimalarials and led to the development of pamaquine in 1924. During the Second World War, when the main cinchona plantations passed into the control of the Japanese armies, considerable efforts by the American chemical industry led to the synthesis of new drugs and their production in vast quantities. Some authors consider that these new drugs played as important a role in the Pacific War as did the large building programme of aircraft carriers. The next episode was one of resistance to synthetic antimalarials. The first known case appeared in Colombia in 1960. However, it was with a new conflict, the war in Viet Nam, that *Plasmodium falciparum* strains resistant to one or more drugs really began to multiply. Since that time these strains have spread from the initial focus and are now to be found in South-East Asia, and are beginning to appear in East Africa. As this has happened, intensive research has been undertaken on new antimalarials. Over a period of a few years more than 200 000 new formulations have been examined in the United States of

America alone. New and relatively promising drugs have been developed, but their limitations are beginning to become apparent.

1.3.2. *The antimalarials in current use and their mode of action*

There are two main categories of antimalarial drugs, depending on their activity against the different stages in the development of *Plasmodium* species. These are *schizontocides* which are active against all asexual forms, and *gametocytocides,* which destroy gametocytes present in the circulating blood and, at least to some extent, the intrahepatocytic stages. No drug effective against sporozoites is known at the present time.

a *Quinine.* Quinine remains the drug of choice in emergency treatment of *P. falciparum* cerebral malaria. This drug has the advantage of being extremely rapidly absorbed and of producing a high concentration in the blood. On the other hand, its half-life is short and renal elimination is practically complete within 24 hours. The benzene nucleus is said to be the active element of the molecule. The drug acts by penetrating the red cells and attaching to the RNA of *Plasmodium* at several levels, which accounts for the rarity of resistance. Quinine blocks the schizogonic cycle as the merozoites pass into the plasma or during the transformation of trophozoites within the erythrocytes into schizonts. True quinine resistance is unusual, but is known in the Far East and in Latin America.

b *4-aminoquinolines.* The synthesis of these compounds resulted from structural analysis of the quinine molecule and of the localization of antimalarial activity at the level of the oxyquinoline benzene nucleus. The best known of these drugs is chloroquine (Nivaquine*, Resochin*, Aralen*), which has excellent schizontocidal action and even now remains the most widely used antimalarial. Amodiaquine, synthesized in 1946, is similar to chloroquine even at the pharmacokinetic level. 4-aminoquinolines are schizontocides of the endoerythrocytic phase. They act by attaching to the nucleus of *Plasmodium* after penetrating the red cell and inserting into the double helix of the RNA, inhibiting its replication. These drugs have numerous advantages related to their effectiveness, their convenience and their low cost. Absorption, although rapid, is less than for quinine. On the other hand, urinary elimination is far more protracted, and this explains their use in chemoprophylaxis.

Unfortunately, many instances of *P. falciparum* resistance have appeared in various countries. The mechanism of such resistance is probably to be found in a membrane phenomenon involving the penetration of the drug.

c *Folic acid antagonists.* This category of drugs includes the sulfonamides and the sulfones. Although their schizontocidal activity has long been known (1940) it

---

* Registered trade-mark.

is so slow and slight that they were kept in reserve for more than 30 years before they were used in association with other drugs. They act by the enzymatic inhibition of the dehydrofolic acid synthethase which is essential to the growth of *Plasmodium* and is produced by the parasites from para-aminobenzoic acid.

d *Folinic acid antagonists.* The mechanism of these drugs is very similar to that of folic acid antagonists, acting at the level of dehydrofolic acid reductase by preventing its transformation to tetrahydrofolic acid. This group of drugs consists of the diguanides, more especially proguanil (Paludrine*) and above all the diaminopyridines, with pyrimethamine and trimethoprim, of which the latter is used primarily in association with other drugs.

e *Association of schizontocides.* The different way in which synthetic schizontocides act at the folic and folinic levels of the metabolism of para-aminobenzoic acid in *Plasmodium* have led to the grouping of this potential double activity in a single preparation, and to the association of two substances each possessing one of the desired properties. At the present time two combinations are widely used: sulfone-pyrimethamine (Maloprim*), which is not very effective in treatment but is, on the other hand, useful in prophylaxis by virtue of its prolonged action and, above all, sulfadoxine-pyrimethamine (Fansidar*). The latter combination is rapidly absorbed, reaching an effective serum concentration in less than six hours. It is active against strains resistant to pyrimethamine and chloroquine. Because of its persistence in the organism, the sulfadoxine-pyrimethamine combination is used in chemoprophylaxis at a dose rate of one 500 mg tablet per week or two tablets every 15 days.

The chemoprophylaxic indications are, however, restricted in largescale practice by the classical contraindications against the use of sulfonamides and the possible appearance of side-effects. Furthermore, there have been many cases of resistance in South-East Asia, in Amazonia and more recently in East Africa.

The sulfamethoxazole-trimethoprim or co-trimoxazole association (Bactrim*, Eusaprim*) acts as a folic acid and folinic acid antagonist at the level of the *Plasmodium*, just as does the sulfadoxine-pyrimethamine combination. It is, however, slow-acting and less effective, but it can be used after treatment with quinine.

f *Antibiotics.* Tetracycline, minocycline and doxycycline have proved to be active against chloroquine-resistant strains of *P. falciparum*. Parasitaemia is, however, very slow to disappear (eight to ten days) and they are therefore schizontocides of limited use, except for treatment in areas in which polyresistant strains predominate.

---

* Registered trade-mark.

g *8-aminoquinolines.* These products and their derivatives are gametocytocides, the best known of which is primaquine, synthesized in 1946. They act upon the gametocytes present in human blood, inhibiting their transformation to gametes in *Anopheles*, thus blocking sporogonic transmission. They also have some slight activity against exoerythrocytic plasmodial forms (*P. vivax* and *P. ovale* hypnozoites). In association with a schizontocide they therefore normally effect radical cure of malaria caused by these two *Plasmodium* species.

1.3.2. *Resistance to antimalarial drugs* [7, 8, 9]

Resistance to antimalarial drugs is defined as 'the ability of a strain of malaria parasite to survive or to reproduce itself despite the administration and absorption of a drug used in doses equal to or greater than the ordinarily recommended doses, and within the limits of tolerance of the individual' (WHO, 1955).

a *The detection of resistance.* In practice, this definition applies above all to the resistance of *P. falciparum* to schizontocides. There is a series of transitions between complete sensitivity and total resistance for which WHO has proposed a classification based on the evolution of the parasitaemia rather than of the clinical symptoms. These three stages (RI, RII, RIII) reflect the chloroquine resistance of *P. falciparum* strains at normally recommended doses (25 mg/kg, three days in succession) [10].

These criteria are simple but relatively imprecise and they require long-term surveillance, which is not always possible [11]. *In vitro* tests have therefore become the only recognized procedure for the detection and measurement of the resistance of *P. falciparum*. There are currently two methods that can be used even in poorly equipped laboratories [12]. The macrotest (WHO standard test, 1968) and the microtest examine the inhibition in the maturation of trophozoites by increasing concentrations of the antimalarial drug in comparison with control samples. The macrotechnique, which may be used for 4-aminoquinolines and mefloquine, requires a 10 ml blood sample. The microtest can be carried out with 0.1 ml of blood and is also applicable to quinine. Another method, which is based on the *in vitro* culture technique developed by Trager, measures the inhibition in parasite multiplication or the disappearance of the parasite under the influence of increasing concentrations of the antimalarial drug under investigation. The test is theoretically more precise than the previous ones but there are various sources of error, particularly related to reproducibility.

In general, at least in the developing countries, *in vitro* tests cannot be used in the field outside urban areas. These tests require a minimum of facilities and laboratory equipment, and also skilled technicians. On the other hand, *in vitro* tests are essential in an urban hospital environment whenever resistance to antimalarials is suspected. They provide confirmation of such resistance and they are the basis for estimation of its degree and for decisions on the modification of treatment.

b *The mechanisms of chemoresistance.* Recent research has gone a long way towards elucidating the biochemical mechanisms of resistance to synthetic anti-malarials. Blood schizontocides such as 4-aminoquinolines, mefloquine and quinine attach themselves to membrane receptors of the red blood cells induced by the intraerythrocytic development of plasmodia. Mefloquine and quinine have a receptor that is the same as that of chloroquine and also receptors of their own. These drugs, especially chloroquine, are strongly concentrated inside the red blood cell, and consequently within the parasite, and attach themselves to the DNA, blocking its replication and also inhibiting various enzymes. Chloroquine blocks the acid proteases and peptidases in parasite phagosomes and thus pro-duces amino acid deficiency. The mechanism of action of quinine and mefloquine have not been fully elucidated. Chemoresistance comes from a reduction in the affinity of the drug for the erythrocyte receptors and above all a reduction in the concentration mechanisms or an alteration in the parasite enzymes. High degrees of resistance occur when more than one of these mechanisms act together. Folinic acid antagonists inhibit dihydrofolate reductase and, consequently, nucleotide biosynthesis. Folic acid antagonists compete with para-aminobenzoic acid. Here resistance is due, in general, to the presence of an isoenzyme having less affinity or none at all for the drug, and a single alteration can cause high resistance. There is no cross resistance between antimetabolites (folic acid and folinic acid antago-nists) and other schizontocides. In this latter group, strains that are highly resistant to chloroquine are less sensitive to mefloquine and quinine. Strains that are resistant to quinine are also resistant to chloroquine. Chloroquine resistance has not yet been described for plasmodial species other than *P. falciparum*. On the other hand *P. vivax* is known to respond only very weakly to dihydropteroate synthetase inhibitors. Folinic acid inhibitors are the only antimalarials for which resistance has been reported among various human plasmodial species.

c *Conditions under which resistance appears* [13]. There has been intensive research on the genetics of chemoresistance resulting from a mutation that appears as a spontaneous chance phenomenon unconnected with any given antimalarial agent. Resistance, which is of stable chromosome type, may appear suddenly, and may be weak or strong, depending on the drug. Thus, a single mutation may give rise to resistance of variable intensity in the case of pyrimetha-mine, whereas for chloroquine strong resistance is invariably due to several successive, mutually independent mutations. The hematozoa are genetically isolated in man so that exchanges of genetic material occur only during the sporogonic cycle in the insect.

Furthermore, the factors involved in the emergence and diffusion of resistant mutants are many and varied: drug pressure, the immune level of the population and certain non-immunological human factors, as well as characteristics related to the vector. *Drug pressure* is the essential factor in the selection of mutants. In general, chloroquine resistance appears only slowly and by successive degrees whereas, on the contrary, the massive use of pyrimethamine leads to the rapid appearance of resistance within a few months. Although chloroquine resistance is often found in countries in which the drug has been used extensively for chemoprophylaxis, this is not always the case (Latin America) and it does not appear that its use in medical treatment exerts selective pressure.

The *immune level of the population* may favour selection and consequently the speed with which resistant strains spread. In hyperendemic regions or in areas in which malaria transmission is continuous, the specific immunity level is high and there is little risk of the selection of resistant strains. Conversely, resistance may appear and extend more rapidly in populations in which immunity is weak or unstable. This is the case, in particular, of individuals coming from non-endemic areas or of young children who are not yet immune among whom extensive chemoprophylaxis tends to select the resistant strains and promote their spread.

The *vector capacity* of a given anopheline species plays a considerable role in the extension of resistant strains. Thus, it has been possible to establish a direct relationship in South-East Asia between the general spread of chloroquine-resistant strains of *P. falciparum* and the presence of *A. balabacensis,* an excellent vector that is anthropophilous and exophilous, and is therefore difficult to combat effectively in a vector control campaign.

Lastly, *individual human factors* may be responsible for pseudoresistance. This may sometimes be due to disorders that decrease absorption of the drug (defective intestinal absorption, vomiting, diarrhoea), or to enzyme deficiencies upsetting the metabolism of a normally absorbed antimalarial agent, which although attaining a normally effective concentration in the plasma, is present in an ineffective form. In both cases, what is involved is not true *Plasmodium resistance* but a quantitative or qualitative lack of the antimalarial agent.

d   *Areas of resistance.* The essential condition for the appearance of chemoresistance is the presence of resistant mutants. Resistance to 4-aminoquinolines is especially prevalent in South-East Asia and South America. Despite considerable use of these antimalarials in Africa, it is fortunately the case that resistance is rare and is confined to East Africa (Tanzania, Ethiopia, Kenya, Madagascar). Until September 1982, only 26 confirmed cases of resistant *P. falciparum* malaria fever had been described in nonimmune travellers. Clinical resistance was of the retarded RI type in all of these cases, with recrudescence on the 20th day after treatment. Systematic field epidemiological studies on semi-immune populations have revealed only extremely rare cases of resistance. On the other hand, reduction of the sensitivity of *P. falciparum* strains is found in north-eastern Tanzania where chloroquine-based medicinal salts have been widely used for several years for extensive chemoprophylaxis. Resistance to folinic acid antagonists is developing rapidly wherever they are used on a large scale. Resistance to the pyrimethamine-sulfadoxine combination was discovered in and after 1968 in the Indo-Chinese peninsula. This resistance is currently extending in South-East

Asia and has also been reported in South America and East Africa (eight cases). Lastly, polyresistant strains of *P. falciparum* have been described both in South-East Asia and in some areas of Latin America, and would appear to be extending (resistance to chloroquine and quinine, to the sulfadoxine-pyrimethamine combination and, sometimes, to mefloquine).

2. The progress that is needed and the encouragement provided by research

2.1. *Epidemiological evaluation*

Before proceeding to control malaria in a given area, it is obviously essential to determine the incidence of the disease and its epidemiological features.

2.1.1. *In endemic areas*

For several decades there was practically no improvement in the techniques for measuring the amount of malaria (spleen rate, parasite rate, sporozoite rate). During the last few years immunology has made various spectacular contributions.

The indications and the limitations of serology (indirect immuno-fluorescence, haemagglutination, ELISA test) are now well known. These methods provide an account, in schematic form, of the whole of the past malarial history of the individuals examined and they yield information comparable to that supplied by the spleen rate. Use of serology is justified above all in areas where transmission is low or incidence is below 0.1% [14]. It may give some indication of the immune status of the populations investigated with, in particular, the changes arising as a result of intensive chemoprophylaxis [15]. The main limitation of serology is the persistence of circulating antibodies for some months or even years after the end of the parasitism [16, 17, 18]. This limitation may be avoided by the serological study of very young children but above all by the detection of plasmodial antigens present in microsamples of parasitized blood. Such detection has been carried out using various methods (radioimmunology, the ELISA test [19]. It is possible to detect very low levels of parasitaemia (between 10 and 500 plasmodia/μl) and above all to perform rapid analysis of a great many samples (300–500 per technician per day). These methods are still under investigation and must be improved, particularly in terms of reproducibility and application to microsamples of blood dried on filter paper. The next step will be to determine their practical value in endemic areas in which the essential point is not so much the sensitivity of the method (very low levels of parasitaemia, below 50/μl, are not of great importance in terms of transmission) as technical simplicity so that microsamples taken in the field can be examined in decentralized laboratories.

It is therefore probable that in the more or less immediate future the parasite rate will no longer be determined solely by microscopic examination of stained blood smears, as it has been for more than a century. Further progress is however still essential before malariologists will be prepared to abandon such a well-tried means of evaluation and to replace the microscope by serological microtitration plates. Lastly, the specific detection of gametocytes present in a blood microsample may one day be possible by immunological means with greatly improved sensitivity and, above all, speed. This could be a decisive advance in epidemiological evaluation.

Such progress has already been achieved in determination of the sporozoite rate, thanks to the research of Professor R. Nussenzweig and her colleagues in New York. Due to the remarkable species specificity of sporozoite antigens, sporozoites can be identified serologically in the salivary glands of infested mosquitos using polyclonal or monoclonal antibodies [20, 21]. Detection is highly sensitive and species-specific. The first trials were carried out using a radioimmunoassay, which is now being adapted to immuno-enzymology, which should facilitate application of this method in the field. Evaluation is now in progress in West Africa.

While the conditions for the collection of basic data may be improved in the very near future, the interpretation of results has already been improved, particularly due to the development or refinement of various *mathematical models*, such as that resulting from the Garki project.

2.1.2. *In non-endemic areas*
The essential task is to detect imported cases that may give rise to local resumption of transmission (should an adapted vector persist) or result in post-transfusion malaria. The detection of small epidemics caused by the introduction of infested vectors ('airport malaria') also comes under the same heading. In order to prevent these accidents, it is essential to be able to detect very low levels of parasitaemia (asymptomatic carriers) and to examine rapidly large numbers of blood samples. It is probably in this area that immunological detection will be most indicated [18].

2.2. *Vector control*

The hope of discovering the miracle insecticide that would, alone, eliminate malaria has clearly been abandoned since the halting of the eradication programme. Although no longer aspiring to such an utopian objective, vector control remains as valuable as ever [22, 23]. Unfortunately, it is tending to be neglected and this is undoubtedly the field in which progress has been the less significant over the last few years. There are many reasons for this: resistance to the various insecticides, especially DDT, the rising cost of petroleum derivatives, and refusal of populations to take part.

Nevertheless, better understanding of the mechanisms of insecticide resistance has led to precise definition of the indications for the use of the various products and to improvement in their application in relation to the biology of the vectors in each epidemiological situation.

In addition, there has been research on biological control, especially control based on *Bacillus thuringiensis* or serotype H14. Although some interesting experimental results have been obtained, unfortunately they have no practical application in the field.

2.3. *Antimalarial drugs*

2.3.1. *New products*
The rapid extension of areas in which chloroquine-resistant *P. falciparum* predominates, followed by the appearance of multiple chemoresistance, has stimulated the search for new antimalarials. From among the new drugs that are currently available or still under investigation, we should mention essentially:
– the compounds investigated by the Walter Reed Army Institute of Research (the WR series of compounds) under the research programme coordinated in the United States by the Agency for International Development (AID): quinoline-methanols (including mefloquine) and phenanthrene-methanols (including halofantrine);
– Quinghaosu.

a *Mefloquine.* Mefloquine (WR 142,490), which belongs to the quinoline-methanol family, is the best known of the new antimalarials. Chemically and in mode of action it is similar to quinine. Pharmacokinetic studies carried out in man have shown rapid and almost total absorption in 36 hours, a mean half-life of 15 days, varying with the individual between 8 and 23 days, and an activity against *P. falciparum* strains resistant to chloroquine and pyrimethamine. Tolerance is fairly good, although this drug does give rise to various side-effects. The essential problem is to limit the multiplication of the resistant or partly resistant strains already known; for this purpose the dose rate has to be increased, which increases the risk of side-effects. The answer may be a combination with other antimalarials with different modes of action.

b *Halofantrine.* Halofantrine (WR 171,669) is one of the most promising of the phenanthrene-methanols. It is a very well tolerated and potent schizontocide which is effective against *P. falciparum* strains resistant to chloroquine.

c *Qinghaosu.* Qinghaosu or Artemisinine is the active principle of the Qing Hao plant (*Artemisia annua*), which has been known since ancient times in China for the treatment of fevers. Qinghaosu was isolated in 1972 and has been shown biochemically to be a new type of sesquiterpene-lactone containing a peroxide radical with the chemical formula $C_{15}H_{22}O_5$. Qinghaosu is rapidly and fully absorbed *per os,* but plasma concentration is low, 80% of the dose being eliminated in 24 hours, and the half-life is of the order of four hours. In parenteral administration, tissue diffusion is very extensive but elimination is equally rapid. Relatively high dose rates are therefore required. Qinghaosu and its derivatives are active at the level of the parasite membrane from the eight hour onward. Only asexual blood forms are affected and there is no action against gametocytes. The drug is equally active against chloroquine-sensitive and chloroquine-resistant *P. falciparum* strains. Clinical studies have been carried out in China on more than 2000 cases. The drug would appear to be effective against both simple and complicated infections, but must be given by parenteral administration (daily intramuscular injections of 0.3 g). Much research is still needed to analyse the pharmacology and toxicology of Qinghaosu and its derivatives.

Despite a great deal of research, very few compounds have been found in the last 15 years. The new drugs have interesting characteristics, but we should guard against over-optimism, in view of the rapid appearance of resistant strains, in some cases at least. Furthermore, current research concentrates essentially on schizontocides, and no new gametocytocide has been developed that is both active against hypnozoites and non-toxic. The successful *in vitro* cultivation of exoerythrocytic forms of various plasmodial species may facilitate future research in this area. Lastly, it should be emphasized that no sporozontocidal drug, which would be an elegant chemoprophylactic solution, has as yet been identified.

2.3.2. *Surveillance and prevention of chemoresistance*
The development of methods for the surveillance and prevention of chemoresistance is justified by the scarcity of new antimalarials and the scale of the current extension in resistance to drugs.

Surveillance. This is of key importance for the rapid detection of the appearance of chemoresistance or even of a reduction in sensitivity to an antimalarial drug. Such surveillance is carried out in the first instance by means of *in vivo* tests which require simple protocols subject to certain errors in interpretation. Thus, for example, the treatment of simple attacks of malaria with chloroquine is carried out in France by giving a dose of 35 mg/kg over a period of five days: this may lead to the classification of *P. falciparum* strains as sensitive, whereas according to WHO standards they would be regarded as of the resistant RI type. Detection of a case of resistance should of course trigger a systematic investigation in the patient's environment or in the country where the infection originated, supplemented if possible by *in vitro* tests.

It is essential to centralize results at country level and on an international scale (WHO and Africa, OCCGE, OCEAC[1], etc). Conversely, good surveillance

[1] Respectively 'Body for Cooperation and Coordination of the Control of Major Epidemics' and 'Organization for Coordination in the Control of Endemic Diseases in Central Africa'.

necessitates full information to practitioners who must be informed regularly of the position regarding the chemosensitivity of *P. falciparum* in the various countries.

Action to counter the appearance of a focus of resistance. Whenever a new focus of resistance appears urgent steps must be taken to limit its extension and to eradicate it as far as possible. The antimalarial drug concerned must no longer be distributed. Patients must be treated with other schizontocides, if possible in association with a Gametocytocide such as primaquine, in order to eliminate the resistant strains. Vector control adapted to the local vectors must be carried out on a wide scale to halt or temporarily to limit transmission. It is not always possible to carry out all these measures in the field and to do so is extremely costly. Efforts must therefore be concentrated on the prevention of new chemo-resistance. We know that drug pressure is the essential factor in the emergence of resistant strains. The large-scale and continuous use of an antimalarial agent as carried out in mass chemoprophylaxis must therefore be prohibited, since it leads almost inevitably to the appearance of resistance sooner or later. Rules that are simple, precise and restrictive enable to define the optimal use of the various available antimalarials for treatment and for chemoprophylaxis.

2.4. *Vaccine(s)*

This is undoubtedly the field in which the struggle against malaria has made the most spectacular progress in recent years, thanks to the development of the first *in vitro* cultures (Trager & Jensen, 1976) [24] the contribution made by various techniques for purification and characterization of antigens (chromatography, affinity chromatography, electrofocalization, HPLC, autoradiography, etc.), and lastly the discovery or better knowledge of laboratory animals suitable for use in the study of human malaria (*Aotus trivirgatus griseimembra, Saimiri sciureus*) [25, 26].

2.4.1. *Vaccines currently under investigation*
Theoretically vaccines may have potentially four main points of impact on the developmental cycle of *Plasmodium* species: sporozoites, exoerythrocytic forms, asexual blood forms, and gametocytes. In practice, the main results are primarily concerned with sporozoites and asexual blood forms [27, 28].

a At the present time, research on a vaccine against sporozoites is the most advanced, largely due to the work of R. and V. Nussenzweig. These scientists have succeeded in isolating various circum-sporozoite antigens (CS antigens) from rodents, monkeys and man *Plasmodium* parasites (*P. berghei, P. knowlesi, P. falciparum* and *P. vivax* respectively). These CS antigens are polypeptides with molecular weights of between 44 and 58 kilodaltons (kd) [29, 30]. Following trypsin digestion, polypeptide mapping was carried out for the main CS polypeptides, as the first stage in synthesis of these sporozoite antigens which have also been produced by recombinant DNA techniques. In the case of anti-sporozoite vaccines, thorough biochemical analysis and the various sophisticated production techniques are absolutely essential. Sporozoites obtained by the dissection of infected *Anopheles* obviously yield negligibly small amounts of antigens. This biological material, obtained at great cost, has been insufficient for anything other than preliminary investigations, but experimental trials on animal call for a scale of production that requires chemical or genetic synthesis.

Sporozoite antigens, which are of relatively low molecular weight, must necessarily be administered along with an adjuvant, which may be another vaccine (diphtheria or hepatitis vaccine). The first vaccination trials on laboratory animals (chimpanzees, *Aotus trivirgatus*) have been encouraging. However, it would appear that the immunity obtained may be of quite short duration (six to eight months) and the degree of protection afforded against plasmodial strains of different geographic origin still has to be established.

In principle, an anti-sporozoite vaccine has the merit of providing very early protection, because it prevents infection. It is, therefore, first and foremost a vaccine for tourists or armed forces and, more generally, for individuals visiting areas of endemic malaria for the first time. Furthermore, it will undoubtedly be of only limited interest for the population of areas of transmission who are already infected. In these areas its administration to young children who have not yet been exposed may even be contraindicated because it would prevent the subsequent natural acquisition of protective immunity, and when post-vaccinal immunity disappears it would leave the children completely susceptible. Moreover, as its point of impact is right at the beginning of plasmodial development in man, the anti-sporozoite vaccine would have to be 100% effective. It would lose all its protective role if a few sporozoites, even an infinitely small proportion, escaped its effects.

b   The vaccine against asexual blood forms has been the subject of many more studies [31]. This research has benefited directly from *in vitro* culture methods, from the various technical improvements made to them, and from all the knowledge acquired during the last few years on the biology of *Plasmodium* species and on the interactions between these parasites and the red blood cells of the host. From among the various developmental stages in the blood, merozoites are the target of choice. Most of the vaccines currently under investigation inhibit their penetration into erythrocytes and consequently their intracellular development. Generally speaking, the antigens employed originate from two main sources: *somatic antigens* extracted from merozoites previously isolated from cultures, and *metabolic antigens* or *exo-antigens* from the supernatant of cultures [32]. Highly purified fractions have been isolated and characterized thanks to the various purification techniques and analytical techniques available. Their performance as vaccines is under investigation in different laboratory animals and with several adjuvants. The need for adjuvants may pose a problem in relation to somatic antigens; some experimental results have been obtained with adjuvants that cannot be used in man (Freund's complete adjuvant). On the other hand, it would appear that exo-antigens can be used with adjuvants that are already widely employed in other human vaccines.

Because of its point of impact, a vaccine effective against merozoites could be used both for prevention and for immunotherapy. Its spectrum of activity would therefore be comparable in certain respects to that of schizontocides such as chloroquine that are used both for chemoprophylaxis and for chemotherapy. This is a considerable advantage because such a vaccine could be used equally for 'new individuals' entering an endemic area for the first time and for certain categories in the local population (children, pregnant women and socioeconomic groups of particular importance). Furthermore, even if this type of vaccine does not act against 100% of merozoites but allows a proportion to develop, it will be effective provided parasitaemia is maintained at a sufficiently low level. Here again, the analogy with schizontocides is obvious. These potential advantages apart, vaccines active against merozites have the disadvantage that they may possibly give rise to immunopathological effects. The administration of plasmodial antigens and powerful adjuvants to individuals already infected by malaria may conceivably increase the risk of haemolytic anaemia, renal complications and, more generally, disorders connected with the presence of circulating immune complexes. There is as yet no experimental evidence to confirm such fears, which are based on theoretical considerations but which obviously make it essential that there should be rigorous control in laboratory animals before such vaccines are used in man.

2.4.2. *Problems to be solved*

For each of the main types of vaccine currently envisaged, the immunogenic properties of each isolated fraction are at present based only on very preliminary investigations. In each case it is essential to assemble sufficient batches of antigens to carry out all the control tests of effectiveness and tolerance. In the case of sporozoite antigens, such batches can be prepared only by means of chemical synthesis or genetic recombination. In the case of merozoite antigens, it may be possible to produce batches for preliminary investigation from cultures. On the other hand, such cultures are clearly unusable for possible subsequent production because of their very low yield despite certain recent improvements, their cost, and the difficulty of removing additional contaminants (originating in the blood) that they may introduce into the vaccine.

Various antigen fractions that have been isolated so far are effective only with powerful immuno-stimulants. In most cases further research is still needed to establish the best type of adjuvant and the most effective immunization conditions (the number and timing of the injections).

In these vaccine trials, the crucial problem in fact remains that of laboratory animals. *In vitro* tests (circum-sporozoite precipitation, inhibition or serum neutralization tests carried out with the sera of immunized animals or with monoclonal antibodies) give only a very approximative idea of the possible immunizing properties of an antigen fraction. It is therefore essential to carry out tests in animals, but few species are susceptible to the *Plasmodium* species of human malaria. Apart from chimpanzees, the experimental use of which is obviously very restricted, only a few small monkeys can be infected by *P. falciparum* (*Aotus trivirgatus griseimembra, Saimiri sciureus*). Intensive and perhaps thoughtless use of these monkey species as laboratory animals has threatened their survival and is making it increasingly difficult to obtain them, although they are absolutely essential for some stages of pre-clinical trials. Before being used in man, vaccines will have to be proved harmless to these monkeys (especially the absence of immunopathological effects in the case of merozoite vaccines) and proved effective against different strains of *P. falciparum*, and possibly, against other human plasmodial species.

In view of all these indispensable controls, it is extremely difficult to estimate how long it will be before a malaria vaccine becomes available. Scientific progress is irregular and phases in which the work progresses rapidly are sometimes followed by slack periods in which research makes no obvious headway. In this respect, it is interesting to note that there has been no follow-up of certain results that seemed very promising four years ago at the time of the First International Conference on Malaria and Babesiosis. Furthermore, apart from these scientific difficulties or imponderables, various considerations, especially of a commercial or military nature (a malaria vaccine can in certain circumstances be truly a strategic product), lead to certain results being presented in a deliberately optimistic manner (attempted bluff) or, on the contrary, being just as systematically played down or even passed over in silence (desire for secrecy).

Even on the most favourable estimate that pre-clinical trials might be carried out in the course of the next three years, a malaria vaccine would not be available for a further five to six years because of the numerous constraints related to controls and production. In addition, the product must be economically within the reach of the populations who should benefit from it. In this context, an interesting estimate has been made. In view of packaging costs for vaccines, to 'cold chain' transport costs, and to administration in one or, especially, in several injections, a malaria vaccine could only be made available to the third world if the cost price of an immunizing dose is, on the present basis, less than French Francs 2.—.

Even if a vaccine became available in the short term and under economically acceptable conditions, it could not in itself lead to the eradication of malaria. We must be fully on our guard against undue optimism and we must not repeat the error previously made over vector control. At best a vaccine will do no more than replace chemoprophylaxis which could be carried out previously (before the appearance of resistant strains) with drugs that were cheap and easy to administer. Despite these advantages, chemoprophylaxis yielded useful results only at the individual level and never offered any serious prospect of eradication (irrespective of the problem of chemoresistance). Even when effective and reasonably cheap, immunization is never more than one of several means of prevention. This is well illustrated by measles vaccination. We are aware of the seriousness of measles in Africa and we have vaccines to deal with it that are active, well tried and relatively cheap. Despite that, vaccine coverage is still very inadequate and infant mortality, by and large, has been only slightly reduced. To sum up, malaria immunization is now an objective that is attainable, probably in the fairly near future. Experimental results indicate that several types of immunization can be envisaged. Two complementary vaccines would be active on the one hand against sporozoites, thus putting a stop to infection in its very first stage, and on the other hand against the blood forms, thus simultaneously ensuring immunoprophylaxis and immunotherapy. The individual prevention of malaria will undoubtedly be considerably simplified by these vaccines, particularly for traveller entering an endemic area. On the other hand, it will be difficult to apply immunization to all the people inhabiting areas of transmission, in which priority will be given to children or other population groups especially at risk.

2.5. *The training of malariologists and specially equipped malaria control team*

A number of authors have taken pleasure in pointing out with bitter irony that even if the eradication campaign did not enable malaria to be eliminated, it did at least do away with malariologists [33]. What in fact has occurred has not been elimination, but non replacement. Over the years malariologists who were trained, very often on the job, during or immediately after the last world war have gradually retired. Unfortunately, practically none of them were replaced as it seemed pointless to train new specialists when there was the prospect of eradication based on the strict application of very precisely defined control measures.

Nowadays, training of malariologists should be regarded as a most urgent issue. Malaria control will obviously not be brought about by the appearance of some miracle procedure. The results of vector control or *Plasmodium* control research, which have proved in the end to be limited or disappointing, are instructive in this respect, as are the forseeable limitations of immunization. Consequently, progress is possible only by the better use of the available means in each particular context [34]. This calls for ability at very differing, completely complementary levels: extensive knowledge of the epidemiology of malaria and mastery of the various techniques of evaluation and prevention at the general level; intimate knowledge of the various facets of malaria epidemiology, with its medical, parasitological, entomological, socioeconomic and other aspects, at the local level. These abilities obviously call for extensive initial training as well as continuous careful activity in the field [35]. In addition, it is essential to build-up a team around each malariologist. It is the malariologist who should be responsible for local recruitment and, at least in part, for the training of the various collaborators required. On the other hand, it is probably only internationally that senior malariologists can be selected and trained.

3. Current principles of malaria control

3.1. *Results and lessons of the eradication campaign*

Substantial progress was made as a result of the eradication campaign decided upon in 1955 at the Eighth World Health Assembly. Malaria was eliminated from many countries, and hundreds of millions of people previously exposed to the disease were completely freed from risk. Nevertheless, this success was achieved mainly in favourable areas where malaria was hypoendemic, ecologically unstable, and transmitted by endophilous and anthropophilous anophelines in countries or regions in which there were geographical barriers to reinforce the control operations, as well as improvements of living conditions and of the nutritional level of the people. The successes have become progressively less frequent. Malaria has reappeared in some countries from which it had been eliminated, and has sometimes reached a level of transmission and severity that were previously unknown. During the decade 1970–1980, it could be considered that, on a very rough estimate, the number of sufferers from malaria was two and a half greater than before the eradication campaign, and even this figure was probably underestimated.

The many causes of these set-backs have often been analyzed and merit examination not in any spirit of masochism but in order to draw the appropriate lessons from them. It has been above all various technical difficulties (spontaneous or induced exophily of *Anopheles* species, insecticide resistance of the vectors) or administrative difficulties (delay in the course of campaigns, lack of qualified personnel, lack of financial support or its discontinuation, the energy crisis) that have been invoked to explain the failures of the world eradication campaign.

All these reasons are valid but do not provide a complete explanation. Human factors also played an important role. The world eradication campaign was planned as a military operation, as is very well illustrated by the terminology employed, which could be applied to an army in the field, a point made by several authors including Ramakrishnan. Although a clear strategy is certainly essential to the winning of a war, it is impossible to imagine staff officers defining a strategy for use in all the world's battlefields by troops differing greatly and fighting against adversaries who are never the same. This was, however, the case in the attempt to eradicate malaria which, for many reasons, is never completely the same. There is in fact not one malaria, but several forms of human malaria. It is a local disease that requires local solutions. It is obvious that no strategy on the world-scale could take account of this essential fact. Lack of flexibility is probably one of the principal causes for the failure [35]. Furthermore, the success of a military campaign is dependent either on the absolute commitment or the blind obedience of the troops. The latter option obviously could not be envisaged for the peoples and states who were to benefit from the eradication campaign but who were completely unwilling to relinquish their free will in any respect. In as far as voluntary participation is concerned, it has only rarely been obtained, the eradication services being too often divorced from the health services of the countries concerned. Furthermore, by definition, eradication presupposed practically simultaneous action in all countries affected by malaria. This action was readily accepted in countries in which the endemicity level made malaria the foremost health problem. The same did not apply in areas of moderate transmission or in countries in which other health priorities obscured the importance of malaria. Many set-backs are to be explained by lack of synchronism or by unequal determination in national eradication campaigns.

This situation became progressively worse with the appearance and subsequent extension of areas of chemoresistance. The relative failure of the eradication campaign was officially recognized in 1968 at the Teheran Congress. The World Health Organization modified its position at that time, defining malaria control as the main objective.

3.2. Malaria control

3.2.1. General principles [36, 37]
For some 15 years the eradication of malaria has been seen as an objective that unfortunately cannot be realized at least in the short term. The various countries concerned and the World Health Organization have therefore contented themselves with a more modest position, that of malaria control, the aim of which is to reduce malaria to a level acceptable to the population. The lack of precision of this definition is a good illustration of the confusion that followed the firm decisions and precise methodologies of the eradication campaign. There was a changeover from the concept of a world strategy to one of a series of local decisions in which each country organizes control in relation to its own malaria problem and its manpower and economic resources.

The Regional Assembly of WHO held in Accra in 1980 henceforward left states a large measure of initiative in the definition of their actions. There are three cardinal points to this new policy:

1 The working out of 'personalized control' by and for each country, in accordance with its needs and the availability of resources;
2 The use of all available methods for malaria control:
   – drugs, whether 'western' or 'traditional', while awaiting the vaccines that will possibly supplement them;
   – diversified vector control related to the biotope (town, village) and the vector (larval control for exophilous anophelines, control of the adult mosquitos in the home, etc.);
3 Integration of malaria control into horizontal systems of primary health care with the active participation of the communities [38].

There have therefore been profound changes that stress the special characteristics both of the parasites and their vectors and of the population exposed, the need for programme adaptability and feasibility, the indispensable participation of the peoples and countries concerned, and lastly the priority that should be given to protection of the individual relative to the protection of society as a whole.

It was on this general basis that a WHO Expert Committee defined four different activity levels (tactical variants) in 1979 with: (1) reduction of malaria mortality, an objective on which agreement was obviously reached; (2) control of morbidity in certain population groups; (3) reduction of incidence; and lastly (4) eradication.

3.2.2. *Reduction of mortality*
This is obviously the objective on which agreement is unanimous. It may be achieved by systematic chemotherapy of all attacks of fever. The action is one that can perfectly well be integrated into primary health care systems. It is feasible and has three main advantages:
– *clinically*, it avoids the occurrence of the complications of malaria, and particularly cerebral malaria.
– *immunologically*, it completely preserves the acquired immunity of treated individuals. The state of premunition is not in fact altered by curative treatment;
– *epidemiologically*, it involves little selective pressure towards the development of chloroquine resistance in P. *falciparum, unlike 'mass treatment' which tends to select strains resistant to the antimalarials in use (the appearance of such resistance in Africa clearly emphasizes the seriousness of this problem).*

In practice, this treatment must be carried out under conditions adapted to local requirements. In areas where there are no chloroquine-resistant strains (essentially Central and West Africa) an attack of malaria can be treated in semi-immune individuals by a dose of 4-aminoquinolines (10 mg/kg, per os). This dose may be prescribed on two consecutive days in East Africa where the sensitivity of P. *falciparum* to chloroquine is reduced, at least in some areas. Should malaria caused by a truly resistant strain occur in these regions, treatment would have to be modified. Moreover, the dose prescribed for nonimmune individuals is of the order of 30–35 mg/kg given over four to five days. In regions where chloroquine resistance is spreading rapidly, other antimalarials such as quinine, the sulfadoxine-pyrimethamine combination, and mefloquine when available are used in the treatment of uncomplicated malaria. It is now recognized that cases of chloroquine-resistant simple malaria call for treatment using an association of the type of quinine-sulfadoxine-pyrimethamine or mefloquine-sulfadoxine-pyrimethamine.

In social terms, this type of control of malaria morbidity has the obvious advantage of attracting the complete support of the populations treated. Participation by the primary health care services is also rapidly achieved.

From the economic point of view, the measures involved are not too expensive. The cost has been evaluated precisely (Bruce-Chwatt) and it is quite compatible with what is financially possible for affected states, possibly supplemented by international aid. However, chemotherapy does require the development of new drugs for areas in which there is resistance, or the definition of more suitable treatment schemes. Better knowledge and improvement of the ways in which medicaments are dispatched to the most remote rural areas are also indispensable. Worthy decisions taken by national or international bodies to treat every attack of malaria will remain in vain and even derisory if, in practice, it is impossible to give treatment to all patients in need. As regards immunization against bacteria or viruses, there have been detailed studies of the 'cold chain'. A similar effort is essential in order to improve the conditions under which antimalarial drugs are transported, stored and administered.

3.2.3. *Control of morbidity in the most vulnerable population groups*
Unlike the previous one, this measure is far from being unanimously accepted. It in fact raises many difficulties concerned with (1) the precise definition of vulnerable population groups; (2) the best conditions for chemotherapy: (3) cost and administrative constraints; and lastly (4) the consequences of chemoprophylaxis for the immune status of the individuals treated.

a The population groups that ought to benefit from chemotherapy include travellers coming from areas in which malaria transmission does not exist, children below the age of two, pregnant women and, lastly, socioprofessional groups essential to the life of the country. There is no dispute over the need for chemoprophylaxis for travellers. In chloroquine-sensitive areas it must be carried out by the administration of a 4-aminoquinoline at a rate of 600 mg/week for adults. It is essential to cover not only the whole of the stay in the endemic area, but also a period of at least 45 days, and if possible 60 days after return to nonmalarial area. For visit to areas of resistance, provided it not become widespread, chloroquine or amodiaquine remain justified, but it is essential to warn those for whom they are prescribed of the risk of possible infection by a resistant strain, which would necessitate treatment with the sulfadoxine-pyrimethamine combination or with a new antimalarial such as mefloquine (it is obviously preferable that travellers visiting isolated areas should acquire a stock of these medicaments in advance). The treatment of young children below the age of two, of schoolchildren and of some socioprofessional groups is far more open to dispute. The cost of the operation becomes rapidly prohibitive. Furthermore, if it is not possible to carry out chemoprophylaxis under perfect conditions, it becomes ineffective. Against chemoprophylaxis is the fact that it considerably increases the risk of the selection of resistant strains, especially where semi-immune subjects such as young children of school-age are concerned. Admittedly, children below the age of two are a group especially at risk. Nevertheless, the most effective protection for them is the rapid treatment (chemotherapy) of every attack of fever (for which it is essential to have the necessary drugs immediately available) rather than chemprophylaxis that would retard or hinder the natural acquisition of immunity that is ultimately the best protection from fatal malaria. A few years ago, the possibility of 'minimum-level chemoprophylaxis' was proposed, which would theoretically protect against attacks of malaria without hindering the gradual acquisition of immunity. This idea has not been put into practice and the room for manoeuvre is quite limited, especially in relation to what is actually done in the field rather than decisions taken in the 'health headquarters'.

Lastly, it is more difficult to weigh the advantages and disadvantages of suppressive chemoprophylaxis in pregnant women from the fourth month of pregnancy onward. The seriousness of malaria during pregnancy and its effects on the newborn child are one aspect of the problem. Suppressive chemoprophylaxis runs the risk of lowering the immune level of mothers-to-be and, consequently, the immunity passively transmitted to the fetus. It would therefore seem essential to carry out comparative studies.

b   Even selective chemoprophylaxis is a considerable expense for populations inhabiting endemic areas. The strain which it places on the various health services is considerable and there is above all the risk of far less popular support than in the case of chemotherapy.

c   Furthermore, the choice of prophylactic scheme is often difficult. The antimalarial employed in Africa for semi-immune populations must remain a 4-aminoquinoline at a daily dose rate of between 5–10 mg/kg body weight, per os. In countries in which chloroquine resistance is extensive, systematic chemoprophylaxis is practically impossible, especially among pregnant women, because of the toxicity risk with some antimalarials.

It is still very difficult to predict what the place of vaccines will be in the general framework of the control of morbidity. The answer will depend on the impact of each of the available products, but also on the duration of their action, and on the possibility of naturally acquired immunity gradually supplementing the immunity induced by immunization, etc. Nevertheless, it already seems probable that in any case these vaccines will be available only to certain groups particularly at risk. In contrast to the use of antimalarials, their use will not entail any risk of an increase in chemoresistance. On the other hand, on the economic and practical level, the administration of vaccines will undoubtedly be limited by their cost and by the various difficulties connected with their transportation and storage.

In the area of morbidity control, any dogmatic stand leading to excessively general conclusions should be avoided. The need for prophylaxis has to be considered in each particular instance in relation not only to what is possible locally, but also to the endemicity level and the type of transmission. Thus, for the time being, chemoprophylaxis would not be appropriate and would even be dangerous in holoendemic areas in which there is continuous transmission, but can on the other hand be fully justified in hypoendemic areas in which there is limited seasonal transmission.

3.2.4. *Reduction of incidence*

(a) *In endemic countries.* Reduction is based on vector control, possibly in association with treatment measures when the latter are possible. For vector control there are various procedures that can be envisaged at the present time:
– *House-spraying* of residual insecticides. This is the most effective method, one that destroys the epidemiologically dangerous part of the anopheline fauna (dangerous because it comes into contact with man) while leaving the equilibrium of the area concerned practically unaffected since the insecticide remains in the houses. However, the proliferation of resistance to DDT and many other insecticides is making the choice of product increasingly difficult, the more so because the cost of new compounds is some ten times more than the cost of DDT. Moreover, the choice of vector control method must be based on detailed knowledge of the biology of the vectors and on accurate assessment of the available financial resources. The effect of the abrupt interruption of insect control operation is to leave populations who have lost a part of their immune defences faced with a resumption of transmission and therefore exposed to increased risk of death from malaria.
– *Larval control* is the only means of vector control when house-spraying is ineffective or difficult. However, it presents considerable practical problems because it must be almost completely effective (about 99%) in order to affect the level of transmission. Larval control does not select the fraction of the anopheline population that is dangerous to man. Even so it may be considered as a temporary and local measure in arid regions where there are few larval breeding sites that are easy to locate and readily accessible, or in urban or peri-urban areas. In some very special epidemiological contexts it is an effective measure for combating the reintroduction of malaria (Réunion). Lastly, larval

control is obviously the last resort in areas where *P. falciparum* is resistant to various antimalarials and is transmitted by resolutely exophilous anophelines. On the whole, this approach to reduction in malaria morbidity cannot lead to more than a relative improvement, usually strictly confined to certain areas.

b *In non-endemic countries.* Prevention is a very different matter in non-endemic countries seeking to avoid the reintroduction of malaria or the occurrence of accidental cases (transfusion). Here the problem is one of very rapid detection of imported cases (clinical, active or passive detection, parasitological control which will perhaps be made easier by immunological methods, and serological controls) followed by immediate suppresive chemotherapy. Where epidemics are caused by the importation of infected vectors (airport malaria) prevention requires the regular disinsectization of airports and aircrafts. Should a few autochthonous cases of malaria appear, rapid epidemiological enquiries must be made so that curative treatment may be given to all patients and, possibly, so that localized vector control may be carried out. Lastly, in non-endemic countries, the frequency and potential seriousness of post-transfusional malaria should not be underestimated. This accident is one that is particularly difficult to prevent because it may be caused by the injection of blood which is so little parasitized that it does not cause any clinical manifestation in the donor ('healthy carrier'), and would be without danger under normal conditions of vector transmission. In view of this risk, several countries have adopted pragmatic measures prohibiting the transfusion of blood taken from individuals who have been in zones of endemic malaria in the previous three or five years (the five-year rule). This is a simple measure. However, it can be effective only against *P. falciparum* malaria. In addition, it has the serious disadvantage of being based solely on information obtained by questioning, a procedure with known difficulties and limitations. The systematic control of blood donors is therefore increasingly the practice. At the present time this control is carried out in many centres on the basis of serology, with many limitations and difficulties in interpretation. It is possible that the immunological detection of plasmodial antigens might make possible, in this case also, a spectacular improvement and the detection and treatment of all healthy carriers.

Conclusions

Such are the difficulties, the hopes and the requirements of malaria control. The hopes are essentially related to the discovery of new methods, but the training of many specialists capable of making more judicious use of these methods is also required and, above all, several changes of attitude.

In the set-backs hitherto encountered in the eradication of malaria, an important part is accorded to changes in the behaviour of *Plasmodium* species and their vectors. Man now has to change his habits in order to convert these set-backs into successess. The changes needed will have to concern individuals as well as public and private institutions, nations and international organizations. As regards individuals, there is a need for better integration into the basic health services and an improvement in health education to enable every individual personally to take part in the control of a crucial health problem. Better synergism is required between public and private bodies. It is essential for the development of anti-malarials, insecticides and vaccines that the effort should not be confined to public bodies, but that private companies should play an important part. It is also essential that private companies should be able to protect their discoveries and receive fair compensation for their efforts. Moreover, newly developed products must be manufactured where they will be best, cheapest and most readily avail-able. At the state level, there is an increased need for solidarity on the part of the rich countries. Furthermore, this effort must be adequate and continuous not only for considerations of international solidarity, but also because of the univer-sal nature of malaria which constitutes a not unimportant threat to the countries of the temperate zone through imported cases, the infection of tourists or travellers, and post-transfusion accidents. Third World countries must take on the effort of organization and above all the recruitment and training of high-level malariologists skilled in all available techniques but still perfectly able to adapt these techniques in a pragmatic way to the various local situations. It is in training that the main emergency probably exists. There are many research workers who have specialist training in malaria, but very few malariologists. We must cease to regard malaria solely as an experimental model; control of this disease must once again become an end in itself and one of the world health priorities. National and international bodies must play a decisive role in this training, a role that obviously does not rule out the current research effort but, on the contrary, will give it its true value.

These requirements are many and onerous. They may even seem utopian. Nevertheless, more than the discovery of some miraculous remedy, they are the prerequisite for the success of malaria control and, beyond that, for the achieve-ment of the exhilarating ideal of health for all.

References

1. Picq JJ: Epidemiologie du Paludisme, première endémie mondiale. Médecine Tropicale, 42:365–381, 1982.
2. Wernsdorfer WH: The importance of malaria in the world. In Malaria, Vol. 1, Academic Press Ed. New York, 1980.
3. Bruce-Chwatt LJ: Essential Malarialogy, William Heinemann Medical Books, Ltd. London Ed., 1980.
4. Kreier J: Malaria. Academic Press Ed. New York, 1980.
5. Russel PF, West LS. Manwell RD: Practical malariology. W.B. Saunders Ed, Philadelphia, 1946.

6. Mouchet J: Lutte contre les vecteurs et nuisances en Santé Publique. Encyclopédie Médico-chirurgicale, Paris, Maladies infectieuses et parasitaires, 8120 B 10, 1980.

7. Peters W: Antimalarial drug resistance: an increasing problem. British Medical Bulletin, 38:187–192, 1982.

8. Wernsdorfer WH, Kouznetzov RL: Drug resistant malaria. Occurence, control and surveillance. Bulletin of the World Health Organization, 3:342–352, 1980.

9. Onori E, Grab B, Ambroise-Thomas P, Thelu J: Incipient resistance of Plasmodium *falciparum* to chloroquine among a semi-immune population of the United Republic of Tanzania. Bulletin of the World Health Organization, 60:899–905, 1982.

10. Bruce-Chwatt LJ: La chimiothérapie anti-paludique cent ans après Laveran. Problèmes et perspectives. Médecine Tropicale, 40:651–656, 1980.

11. Cohen S: Malaria. Churchill Livingstone Ed. New York, 1982.

12. Wernsdorfer WH: Field evaluation of drug resistance in malaria. In vitro micro-test. Acta Tropica, 37:222–227, 1980.

13. Walliker D: Genetic variation in malaria parasites. British Medical Bulletin, 38:123–128, 1982.

14. Ambroise-Thomas P, Wernsdorfer W, Grab B, Cullen J, Bertagna P: Longitudinal sero-epidemiological studies on malaria in Tunisia. Bulletin of the World Health Organization, 54:355–367, 1976.

15. Fondation Merieux & OMS: Méthodes immunologiques en paludologie. Doc. O.M.S. WHO/MAL/81.948.972, 1981.

16. WHO: Immunology of malaria. Bulletin of the World Health Organization, 57:1–290 (suppl.), 1979.

17. Ambroise-Thomas P: L'immuno-fluorescence dans la sérologie du'paludisme. Doc OMS WHO/MAL/81.953.

18. Ambroise-Thomas P, Quilici M, Ranque PH: Réapparition du paludisme en Corse. Intérét du dépistage séro-épidémiologique. Bull Soc Path Exot 65:533–542, 1972.

19. Mackey L, MAC Gregor IA, Lambert PH: Diagnosis of Plasmodium *falciparum* infection using a solidphase radio immuno assay for the detection of malaria antigens. Bulletin of the World Health Organization, 58:439–444, 1980.

20. Zavala F, Gwadz R, Collins W, Nussenzweig R, Nussenzweig V: Monoclonal antibodies to circum sporozoite proteins identify the species of malaria parasite in infected mosquitoes. Nature, 299:737–738, 1982.

21. Ramsey JM, Beaudoin RL, Bawden MP, Espinal CA: Specific identification of *Plasmodium* sporozoïtes using an indirect fluorescent antibody method. Transactions of the Royal Society of Tropical Medicine and Hygiene, 77:378–381, 1983.

22. Molineaux L, Gramiccia G: Le projet Garki, recherche sur l'épidémiologie du paludisme et lutte antipaludique dans la savanne soudanienne de l'Afrique Occidentale. OMS Ed. 1980.

23. Davidson G: Developments in malaria vector control. British Medical Bulletin, 38:201–206, 1982.

24. Trager W, Jensen JB: Human malaria parasites in continous culture. Sciences, 193:673–675, 1976.

25. Gieman RM, Maegher MJ: Susceptibility of a new world monkey to Plasmodium *falciparum* from man. Nature, 215:437–439, 1967.

26. Gysin J, Fandeur T: *Saimiri sciureus* (karyotype 14-7) an alternative experimental model of *Plasmodium falciparum* infection. Am J Trop Med Hyg 32:461–467, 1983.

27. Ambroise-Thomas P: Vers une vaccination contre le paludisme. Bases théoriques et perspectives pratiques. Therapeutisch Umschan, 40:248–252, 1983.

28. WHO: Development of Malaria vaccines. Bulletin of the World Health Organization, 61:81–92, 1983.

29. Nussenzweig RS: Progress in malaria vaccine development: characterization of protective antigens. Scandinavian Journal of Infectious diseases, suppl. 36:40–45, 1982.

30. Gwadz RW, Cochrane AH, Nussenzweig V, Nussenzweig R: Preliminary studies vaccination of rhesus monkeys with irradiated sporozoïtes of *Plasmodium knowlesi* and characterization of surface antigens of these parasites. Bulletin of the world Health Organization, 57:165–173, 1979.

31. Cohen S: Progress in malaria vaccine development. British Medical Bulletin, 38:162–165, 1982.

32. Thelu J, Ambroise-Thomas P, Contat M, Kupka P: Antigènes excrétés-sécrétés par *Plasmodium falciparum* en cultures *in vitro*. Etude comparée avec les antigènes somatiques et les antigènes figurés. Bulletin de l'Organisation Mondiale de la Santé, 60:761–766, 1982.

33. Aldighieri R: Eradication ou lutte anti-paludique. Retour à la formation en malariologie. Bull Soc Path Exot 74, 76:5–9, 1983.

34. Bruce-Chwatt LJ, Pull JH: Paludisme. Quarante vérites premières ou/prétendues telles. La Nouvelle Presse Médicale, 9:1577–1580, 1980.

35. Janssens PG: Malaria quousque tandem? Cah ORSTOM, Sér Ent méd et Parasitol, 28:153–158, 1980.

36. Bruce-Chwatt LJ: La lutte contre le paludisme cent ans après Laveran. Cah. ORSTOM, sér Ent méd et parasitol, 28:149–153, 1980.

37. Pull JH, Lepes T, Wernsdorfer W: Développement scientifique depuis la découverte de Laveran. Situation actuelle de la lutte antipaludique dans le monde. Cah. ORSTOM, sér Ent Méd et Parasitol, 18:158–162, 1980.

38. OMS: Lutte anti-paludique et objectifs nationaux de santé. Organisation Mondiale de la Santé, Service des rapports techniques, no 680, 1982.

15. Control of bovine babesiosis

EUGENE PIPANO and ARIE HADANI

Veterinary Services & Animal Health, Kimron Veterinary Institute, Beit Dagan, Israel

1. Introduction

Bovine babesiosis occurs on all five continents, and is particularly devastating in the tropics and sub-tropics where most of the world's cattle population is concentrated.

Babesia bigemina and *B. bovis* are widespread in the *Boophilus* spp. infested zones, between the 32°S and 40°N latitudes. *B. major* and *B. divergens* transmitted by *Haemaphysalis punctata* and *Ixodes ricinus* respectively, are encountered in Western and Central Europe, while *B. major* has been reported also from North Africa, USSR and Japan [1, 2, 3].

Ticks comprising three families and about 800 species [4] are considered throughout the world as the single economically most important group of ecto-parasites. Cattle are mainly concerned with the so-called 'hard ticks', *Ixodidae,* of which by far the most important are the three *Boophilus* species (*B. microplus, B. annulatus* and *B. decoloratus*). The tremendous losses inflicted by ticks and tick fevers have stimulated intensive research in the USA and South Africa, later in North Africa, and during the last 30 years or so in Australia, East Africa, several European and Latin American countries, the USSR and Israel. Australia has even become a sort of a 'proving ground' for the research and implementation of tick and babesiosis control measures.

The eradication campaign of *B. annulatus* in the USA, which started in 1906 and terminated successfully in 1960, inspired other countries to devote resources and manpower to find a partial or radical solution to this problem. International organizations and particularly the FAO [3] have been substantially involved in assisting developing countries in their efforts towards controlling ticks and babesiosis.

Prevention of babesiosis [5, 6, 7, 8, 9, 10] and tick control [11, 12, 13, 14, 15, 16, 17] have been discussed in several reviews. This report deals with the present strategies and currently applied techniques for controlling bovine babesiosis and the vector ticks, particularly *Boophilus* spp. Future prospects for improved babesiosis and tick control measures are discussed as well.

Ristic, M. et al. (eds.) *Malaria and babesiosis.*
© 1984, Martinus Nijhoff Publishers, Dordrecht/Boston/Lancaster.

2. Economic importance of ticks and tick fevers

The damage caused by babesiosis can be expressed in terms of mortality, morbidity, loss of production, retardation in growth, cost of drugs, extra labour, as well as restrictions imposed on the movement of the animals. The detrimental effect of babesiosis on livestock development and improvement projects in developing countries is particularly important.

The economic impact of babesiosis and *Boophilus* spp. becomes particularly significant in areas where the tick has been introduced recently. The cases of *B. annulatus* in the USA and *B. microplus* in Latin America and Australia have been well documented [18]. In such instances outbreaks of babesiosis are to be expected and *Boophilus* ticks thrive on the highly susceptible cattle, lacking previous experience of infestation with this tick species. Ticks and babesiosis are much less harmful to indigenous cattle in endemic areas where the animals have developed resistance to local species of ticks through long years of close association. Enzootic stability, established under these conditions, prevents clinical outbreaks of the disease.

Relatively few precise analyses of the losses caused by ticks and tick borne diseases in livestock have been carried out. One encounters assessments in the range of '. . . thousands of millions of dollars . . .' [19] but as McCosker puts it [3]' . . . these losses have not been adequately and fully defined.' In 1977 the FAO Expert Consultation [20] recommended that 'FAO undertakes a comprehensive study of the economic impact of ticks and tick borne diseases on animal production'.

The available economic analysis is mostly related to beef cattle. Similar information with regard to dairy cattle is scarce. The only well studied case is the detailed prospective study carried out by the USDA as a result of the *B. annulatus* eradication campaign in the USA [21]. In this report the economic losses, during successive years following primary tick infestation, in an average sized dairy herd (200–400 animals) in an endemic area are estimated in terms of milk loss, beef loss, mortality losses, acaricide costs and extra labour. McCosker [3], having analyzed the document came up with an expected loss of $ 23.2 per animal for both beef and dairy cattle, of which $ 1.9 is attributable to babesiosis and $ 19.4 to the direct effect of ticks on production etc. Graham and Hourrigan [22] claimed direct and indirect losses caused by *B. annulatus* in the USA, to amount to $ 130,000,000 per year. Annual losses in Queensland and New South Wales are estimated at about $ 7.8 per head, of which only 7.3 cents are attributed to mortality caused by babesiosis and its control. In another study [15] losses due to *B. microplus* in Australia were estimated at $ A 4–5 per animal per year and $ A 12 per prime steer. The same authors claim that 33% of the 42 million $ A, spent annually on tick control in Australia, are accounted for in the cost of labour and acaricides.

Beltran in Mexico [23] referred to an annual loss amounting to 3587 million pesos of which 6.3% could be attributed to death, 83.6% to loss in meat production, 8.5% to loss in milk production and 1.6% to loss in hides.

In an extensive survey carried out by Elder [24] loss in production was found to be the main reason for tick control to be followed by tick worry, mortality due to ticks and tick fevers and finally damage to the hides. On the whole, producers were more concerned with loss of production and tick worry than with deaths due to either ticks or tick fevers.

In Argentina [25] a total loss of $ 88 million was calculated for the tick infested zone in 1972, totalling some 12 million heads. In Brasil the loss in meat production in 1974 would be 30 kg per head or a total of 30,000 tons of meat in the abattoir.

The economic feasibility of tick control measures under various conditions and in relation to the damage caused by the ticks can be worked out using the *Boophilus microplus* population model elaborated by Sutherst and Dallwitz [26].

3. Methods for control of babesiosis

Like other arthropod-borne diseases, babesiosis can be controlled by eradication of the vectors, treatment of sick animals and prevention of clinical manifestations by chemoprophylaxis or vaccination. A brief discussion of the present status of the various methods available for control of babesiosis is herewith presented.

4. Chemotherapy

Exhaustive reviews concerning the various aspects of chemotherapy of babesiosis have been published recently [6, 8, 27, 28, 29].

Babesia parasites in the red blood cells of vertebrate hosts are sensitive to several groups of chemical compounds. If the drug is administered early in the infection before heavy damage occurs, recovery usually results.

Currently used drugs for treating clinical babesiosis are derivatives of quinoline (quinuronium sulfate), diamidines (diminazene aceturate, pentamidine) and carbanilides (imidocarb).

Trypan blue, acridine derivatives and other diamidines (stilbamidine, propamidine, and phenamidine) have a relatively limited use in field therapy of babesiosis.

A few cases of resistance of bovine, canine and murine *babesia* strains to quinuronium sulfate and diamidines have been reported [30, 31, 32] but drug resistance does not represent a practical problem in chemotherapy of bovine babesiosis.

The large bovine *Babesia* species (*B. bigemina*) is more sensitive to the commonly used babesicides than the small species (*B. bovis, B. divergens*), but differences in the sensitivity of strains of *Babesia* from various geographical areas also exist. For example multiplication of B. bovis (argentina) is suppressed by quinuronium sulfate [33] while this drug has little effect on B. bovis (berbera) [34].

Chemotherapy can hardly be considered a reliable method for control of babesiosis in cattle. It is rather a means of dealing with emergency situations when long-term routine control methods have failed or have not been applied at all. Unlike routine control methods (chemoprophylaxis, vaccination, vector control) that are planned and applied periodically, chemotherapy requires constant vigilance for detecting and diagnosing sick cattle. In small herds of barn raised cattle there is a good chance of detecting animals during the initial stage of acute babesiosis. In larger groups of cattle kept in paddocks or corrals, outbreaks of babesiosis are usually signalled by morbidity or mortality. This situation is more serious in range-raised cattle spread over vast pasture areas. When outbreaks occur in such large herds the daily identification and treatment of sick cattle is not feasible as a practical measure. In such cases a 'blanket treatment' of infected and non-infected cattle alike is usually administered.

5. Chemoprophylaxis

Babesicidal drugs that are excreted relatively slowly have been used to prevent infection or clinical symptoms in susceptible cattle introduced into enzootic areas. Drugs with a practical protective effect are imidocarb and diminazene. Protection obtained with a given dose appears to last longer against infections with the large Babesia species than with the small ones.

Imidocarb confers the longest protection against infection with both types of Babesia. A dose of 2 mg/kg prevented parasitemia for 40 days following tick-transmitted infection with B. bigemina [35] and 30 to 46 days following needle inoculation of B. bigemina-infected blood. Mild parasitemia without clinical symptoms was observed when cattle were infected 42 to 70 days after treatment [35, 36, 37, 38].

B. bovis types (B. argentina, Francaiella colchica) are less inhibited by imidocarb. In some instances a dose of 5 mg/kg prevented tick infection for 28 days [39] but in others parasitemia occurred in cattle infected 5 and 13 days after receiving 2 or 2.4 mg/kg of drug. However, clinical manifestations were prevented in cattle infected up to 33 days following treatment with the above doses[36, 40]. Similarly a mild B. divergens parasitemia was observed in cattle treated one or two weeks prior to inoculation with 2.4 mg/kg of imidocarb [41, 42].

Diminazene (5 mg/kg) prevented B. bigemina infection 15 days after treatment [43] but did not prevent B. bovis (berbera) infection in splenectomized calves five days after treatment [44].

Since as a practical matter drugs cannot be administered periodically to cattle for their entire lifetime, chemoprophylaxis in enzootic areas makes sense only if a protective asymptomatic infection can be induced during a reasonable period. The epizootiological parameters defined by Mahoney and Ross [45] are valid also when chemoprophylaxis is used i.e. the rate of transmission by ticks should be such as to ensure the infection of all or most of the cattle while they are still protected by a suitable level of babesicides.

6. Effects of drugs on immunity

According to the concept of premunition formulated by Sergent et al. [46] immunity against babesiosis has been regarded as dependent upon the continued presence of parasites in animals recovered from acute infection. A direct implication of this concept is that elimination of the carrier state in a *Babesia*-infected animal will result in loss of immunity. Recent investigations have shown that residual immunity will remain for months and years after cattle have ceased to carry the infection [47, 48, 49, 50]. However, as defined by Löhr [50], a minimal period of contact between the *Babesia* parasites and the host is required for the development of immunity. Trials performed with *B. bigemina* have shown that immunity was dependent upon the length of infection rather than on the level of parasitemia [49].

Since sterile immunity appears to be strain specific [47, 51] it is believed that cattle carrying a latent infection will be better protected against field challenge than cattle cured (sterilized) of the infection.

Most of the presently available drugs may cause *sterilisatio magna* at the recommended therapeutic doses [51]. Destruction of the carrier state of premune cattle can be avoided by using drugs with a relatively large margin between the therapeutic and curative doses. In Israel, highly sensitive dairy cattle which often exhibit a high parasitemia following inoculation with *B. bigemina* vaccine are treated with pentamidine. This drug suppresses parasitemia at a dose of 1 mg/kg, while more than 5 mg/kg are needed to eliminate *B. bigemina* parasites completely [52].

If treatment following vaccination is required the different degrees of sensitivity of the large and small *Babesia* species should be considered. This is important not only when a polyvalent vaccine containing both *B. bigemina* and *B. bovis* [53] is used, but also when single monovalent vaccines are inoculated consecutively. For instance, if cattle are first given *B. bigemina* and then (usually three weeks later) *B. bovis*, the dose of drug needed to suppress excessive multiplication of *B. bovis* may cure (sterilize) the cattle of *B. bigemina* at this relatively early stage of infection. It follows that cattle should be inoculated first with the *Babesia* species that is more resistant to treatment, i.e. *B. bovis*. On the other hand, the residual effect of the drug must be taken into consideration, and a period sufficient for clearance of the drug from the animal's tissues should be allowed to elapse before inoculating the more sensitive *Babesia*. Dairy cattle that were treated with a dose of about 5 mg/kg of diminazene following immunization with *B. bovis* were vaccinated 25 days later with *B. bigemina*. The latter were seen in blood smears in only 43% of the cattle and the remaining animals were susceptible to challenge with blood containing *B. bigemina* [54].

Chemoprophylactic treatment may also lead to asymptomatic infections result-ing in immunity to reinfection. Cattle treated with imidocarb and exposed to *Babesia*-enzootic pastures became infected without showing clinical symptoms [55]. Since there is no evidence that field infection occurs in all animals when a proper prophylactic level of drug is present, it is recommended that cattle be vaccinated while still under the mild influence of the drug. Animals receiving 2 mg/kg of imidocarb and inoculated 1–2 weeks later with *B. divergens* [41] or 21 and 61 days later with *B. bovis* and *B. bigemina* vaccines remain immune to reinfection with homologous species [56]. However, this technique requires further investigation to determine its efficiency in engendering long term protec-tion against field infections.

7. Vaccination

By the end of the 19th century, when epizootics of babesiosis occurred, it became evident that cattle recovered from 'red water' were resistant when reexposed in enzootic areas. Consequently, attempts were made to vaccinate susceptible animals by inoculating them with blood from cattle recovered from babesiosis [57].

This method is effective but has serious drawbacks: (1) An element of danger exists whenever live *Babesia* organisms are injected into cattle; (2) the vaccine has a very short shelf life; (3) the blood may be carrying other pathogens of cattle; and (4) the vaccine contains an overwhelming mass of normal bovine proteins compared to the relatively minute volume of immunizing organisms.

To circumvent some of these drawbacks various experimental vaccines have been tried. Irradiated *B. bigemina* [58, 59], *B. bovis* [60, 61, 62], *B. major* [63, 64, 65] and *B. divergens* [66, 67, 68, 69, 70] caused in most cases a mild parasitemia and various degrees of immunity to challenge with virulent parasites. Killed *B. bigemina* [71, 72, 73] and *B. bovis* [71, 74, 75] and plasma from cattle infected with *B. bigemina*, *B. bovis* and *B. divergens* [71, 76, 77] engendered variable protec-tion against challenge with the homologous species from infected blood or ticks. Since a direct relationship exists between the number of *Babesia* parasites in the vaccine and the intensity of the resulting clinical manifestations [78, 79] minimal infective doses have been tried for vaccinating cattle [80].

The successful propagation of *B. bovis in vitro* [81, 82] opened new possibilities in the search for better immunizing agents against babesiosis. Continuous cultiva-tion has been achieved in microaerophilous stationary phase systems [82] and suspension cultures [83]. Non-viable whole merozoite antigen and a surface coat merozoite antigen from culture supernatant (mixed with adjuvant) induced considerable immunity to challenge with infected blood or ticks [84, 85, 86, 87, 88].

However, the fact remains that the most commonly used method for vaccination against babesiosis in cattle is still inoculation with bovine blood containing living *Babesia* organisms. Despite its drawbacks this product has two advantages over the various experimental vaccines cited above: it can be easily produced in practically unlimited quantities, and it engenders a fair protection against field challenge.

7.1. *Safety of blood-derived vaccines*

The first steps towards developing less virulent parasites were taken by Sergent and his collaborators in the Pasteur Institute in North Africa. They concluded that rapid passages with blood drawn during the acute stage of the infection caused an increase in virulence, while passages with parasites obtained during the chronic stage led to a decrease in virulence. As a result the French investigators recommended vaccination with blood from chronic carriers of *B. bigemina* and *B. bovis* [89]. This method was later modified in that donor calves were splenectomized after recovering from the primary attack and blood was taken for vaccination during the relapse parasitemia [90]. Sergent's conclusions concerning *B. bigemina* have been confirmed in their essentials by Kemron et al. [91] and *B. bigemina* vaccine is presently prepared from splenectomized donor calves inoculated with parasites obtained during relapse parasitemia [92, 93].

On the other hand *B. bovis* parasites that were passaged rapidly in splenectomized calves showed decreased virulence [94] probably due to selection of parasites having a lower affinity for multiplication in the capillaries of internal organs (95, 96). Such parasites cause mild infection in intact (non-splenectomized) calves.

Few data are available in the literature concerning the safety of *B. bigemina* and *B. bovis* vaccine for cattle of different breeds and ages. Laboratories that produce antibabesial vaccines caution farmers about possible illness that may be caused by the vaccine [53, 97]. Generally speaking, healthy young cattle do not suffer post-vaccination disturbances. On the other hand, it appears that cattle with inapparent bacterial or viral infections may experience exacerbations of such infections upon vaccination. Such exacerbation, in turn, may cause decreased resistance to the babesias.

It can be concluded that presently available live babesial vaccines are by no means completely safe for cattle. Type, breed, age and physiological condition should be considered before recommending use of these vaccines. Vaccinated animals should be watched carefully for about 3 weeks post-inoculation.

7.2. Shelf life of vaccines

Babesia parasites survived in defibrinated or citrated blood for 10 to 16 days [89], but the recommended storage time for fresh vaccine was limited to 3–4 days [98].

B. *bovis* vaccine produced in splenectomized calves contains 10^7 parasites per dose. In order to compensate for the die-off of parasites the number is increased by a factor of 1.5 for each additional day of storage up to a maximum of seven days [99]. Erp et al. [83] succeeded in keeping B. *bovis* parasites alive for 30 days in culture medium 199 at a temperature of $4°C$.

The basic parameters for optimal preservation of B. *bigemina* and B. *bovis* in the frozen condition were defined by Dalgliesh [100, 101, 102] and Dalgliesh and Mellors [103]. Dimethyl sulfoxide [DMSO] added to the infected blood to a final concentration of 2M appears to ensure maximal protection against damage during freezing and thawing. However, laboratory and field trials show that relatively high initial numbers of parasites are needed in order for the thawed blood to be infective in all inoculated cattle. Todorovic et al. [104] found that intravenous inoculation of frozen and thawed *Babesia* is more effective than the subcutaneous route. A number of studies have shown that an initial number of 10^7 to 10^8 viable parasites per dose are needed when the vaccine has been stored in the frozen condition [92, 105, 106].

In Israel, only frozen vaccines against B. *bigemina* and B. *bovis* have been supplied since 1978. Splenectomized 10–20 month old bull calves are used as donors. Highly parasitized blood is mixed with DMSO and the blood – DMSO mixture is frozen in 2 ml pellets for B. *bigemina* and 4 ml for B. *bovis*. Pellets are stored in liquid nitrogen. For use they are thawed in isotonic solution (PBS) containing 15% DMSO. Before use in the field, the infectivity of each batch of vaccine is evaluated by inoculating serial dilutions into cattle. Vaccine doses usually contain initially 2×10^8 to 4×10^8 B. *bigemina* and 4×10^8 to 8×10^8 B. *bovis* organisms [92].

7.3. Foreign substances and contaminations

Some bovine cellular elements contained in babesial vaccines may induce an antibody response when inoculated into cattle. For example, lyophilized vaccines prepared from lysed erythrocytes stimulate antibodies against red blood cells when inoculated into cattle together with adjuvants. Presence of these antibodies in the colostrum may provoke hemolytic anemia (neonatal isoerythrolysis) in the suckling calf [107].

In Australia live babesial vaccine provoked hemolytic anemia in newborn calves especially when repeated vaccinations were administered to the dam [108]. Upon diluting the vaccine with balanced salt solution plus glucose and 10% bovine serum instead of with whole blood, no more instances of hemolytic anemia were observed [97].

Similarly, the frozen vaccines used in Israel are diluted in PBS plus 15% DMSO so that a dose contains only about 0.1 to 0.3 ml of packed red blood cells. In South Africa a vaccine dose contains about 0.5 ml of packed red cells. Despite the fact that inoculation of 0.5 ml of packed red cells induced antibodies against red blood cells in cattle [109], manifestations of hemolytic anemia in newborn calves have not been recorded either in South Africa or Israel. One reason for this may be that most cattle in both countries are vaccinated before pregnancy so that only a low level of antierythrocytic antibody is present at calving. However when anti-babesial vaccines are administered to pregnant cows, their offspring should be watched closely for neonetal hemolytic disease.

Early investigators were mainly concerned with the possible contamination of blood-derived vaccines with other hemoparasites (*Anaplasma, Theileria, Eperythrozoon, Trypanosoma* and *Borrelia*). Recently, growing importance has been attributed to latent bacterial and especially viral infections that may be spread by mass inoculation with blood of bovine origin. There are no official international standards for testing and certifying vaccines against babesiosis. In order to reduce the hazard of contaminations, the Kimron Veterinary Institute in Israel has established a testing program for vaccines prepared from bovine blood. After the *Babesia*-infected donor calves are bled for vaccine (1 to 1.5 l of blood per 100 kg body weight) they are treated with babesicides so that they will be available for further testing later on. The vaccines are preserved in liquid nitrogen as described in the previous paragraph. Samples of vaccine are tested for bacterial contaminants according to standard procedures. Thirty to 40 days later the donor calves are tested serologically for antibodies against viral and bacterial infections according to the requirements of the Laboratory for Testing of Vaccines. Blood smears are examined for contaminant parasites 3 times a week during the period the donor is kept in the laboratory. Only vaccines from healthy donors are titrated for infectivity and released for use. Such procedures reduce the risk of contamination in the vaccine but, obviously, the cost of the vaccine is increased considerably.

7.4. *Protection engendered by vaccination*

Vaccination with living erythrocytic merozoites of *Babesia* confers protection against challenge with the infective stages derived from ticks for at least four years [110, 111, 112, 113]. In relatively rare instances a breakdown of immunity may occur under field conditions [54, 99, 114]. Such cases are hard to analyse in a controlled manner. The question of heterologous strain immunity and antigenic variations in *B. bovis* and *B. bigemina* has been discussed by Riek [6], Johnston and Tammemagi [115], Rogers [114], McCosker [116], Thompson et al. [117], Callow [99] and De Vos et al. [118, 119]. Possible immunologic blocking in hyperimmune cattle has been also suggested [99]. However, it must be confessed that the cause of immunologic breakdown in the field remains obscure.

Although revaccination with a heterologous *B. bovis* strain provided slightly improved immunity it is generally accepted that a second vaccination is not necessary in most cases [97, 110, 120].

8. Tick control

Ticks can be controlled by measures directed against them while on or off their bovine hosts. The control of ticks off the host is based on bio-ecological measures and chemical means. Tick control on livestock depends mostly on chemical treatment combined in certain cases with the breeding of tick resistant cattle.

8.1. *Tick control off the host*

In its non-parasitic developmental stages the tick is exposed to environmental conditions, natural enemies, chemical agents and agrotechnical manipulations. These factors should be taken advantage of in the integrated control of ticks in livestock.

8.1.1. *Bio-ecological considerations*
There are four non-parasitic stages in the life cycle of the one-host *Boophilus* tick: engorged female, eggs, freshly moulted larvae and a host-finding stage in which larvae aggregate on the tips of grass in a questing position awaiting a passing host.

Movement of the engorged female is very limited, probably a few meters, and its survival is partly ensured by its circadian rhythm of 'drop-off', detaching mainly at night [121, 122]. Its dispersal is realised through movement of infested animals, mostly bovines and equines, in pasture or among dairy farms and corrals. Larvae survive in pasture from a few weeks to two-three months depending mainly on temperature, relative humidity or saturation deficit and host density. Tick-environment interrelationships have been thoroughly analyzed by the Australian authors [26, 123, 124]. The model elaborated permits assessment of the population dynamics under different natural conditions and forecasts the rate of tick infestation on livestock.

8.1.2. *Ecological control of ticks*
Ecological control of ticks aims at modifying tick habitats and environmental conditions through changes in vegetation and fauna (wild and domestic) in order to decrease tick survival and suppress the tick population below the economic threshold.

Pasture and bush fires. Bush fires are still extensively used over vast areas in

Africa and Latin America. Although this has a certain temporary depressing effect on the tick population pasture burning is not indicated unless advantageous in improving the dry pasture by encouraging grass growth.

Bush clearing. Clearing trees and shrubs, defoliation, removal of grass mat and heavy grazing have a detrimental effect on tick species that are sensitive to solar radiation and desiccation [125].

Crops and plantations. Extensive crops and plantations serve as barriers to the dispersal of ticks, particularly *Boophilus*, through restricting the movement of the host animals and preventing the completion of its non-parasitic life cycle. The dissemination of *Boophilus* ticks by winds and flooding [126], though theoretically possible, could not be demonstrated under field conditions [127].

Control of wild life. The control of rodents and other small mammals might be useful since these animals serve as natural hosts for many species of multi-host ticks [128, 129, 130]. However, no benefit should be expected in the case of *Boophilus*.

Pasture spelling. Pasture spelling might be the most important tool in the control of ticks off the host. This method has been integrated in tick control schemes in beef cattle in Australia [131, 132, 133, 134, 135]. The efficacy of pasture rotation depends on clean musters, conditioned by efficient fencing. The spell period varies according to locality, type of cattle and season, ranging from six to twelve weeks or even more. Pasture spelling has some drawbacks [134, 135]. The grazing area must be sufficiently big, requiring extra fences and water facilities. Pasture spelling reduces stocking rate, affects the pasture quality adversely and increases fire hazards. The technique is not practicable on leased land nor all year round. Furthermore, neighbouring cattle may get into the 'resting' plots. It seems that pasture spelling is often practised for the sake of pasture management while tick control is a secondary though important advantage. However, it is widely accepted that pasture spelling, combined with planned dipping and tick resistant cattle represents an 'integrated approach' to tick control in beef cattle which permits limited use of ixodicides with optimal results [14]. Moreover, the increased cost of acaricides and the occurrence of acaricide resistance will inevitably lead to even more extensive adoption of this method.

8.1.3. *Biological control of ticks*
Various biological methods have been proposed, mostly on academic grounds, for the control of ticks in the ambient.

Parasitoids and predators. *Hunterellus hookeri* was suggested for the control of *Dermacentor andersoni* as long ago as 1933 [136]. However, mass rearing of the insect failed and to this date the use of parasitoids and pathogens for tick control has not crossed the academic barrier. Of more interest might be predators such as wild birds [137], poultry, small mammals and ants [138, 139, 140]. Interestingly enough the cattle egret (*Ardeola ibis*) seems more attracted to insects disturbed by the grazing cattle than to ticks [141].

Sterilizing agents and genetic manipulations. Sterilization of ticks by irradiation or chemical agents has been reported [142, 143, 144, 145] but not put yet into practice as control measures. Little research has been carried out on genetic manipulations of ticks [146]. Crossing *B. microplus* with *B. annulatus* produced genetically sterile males [145, 147]. However, mass rearing of ticks is still not feasible and flooding the environment with sterile males might also pose problems.

Anti-tick grasses. Menendez [148] described the repellent properties of *Melinis minutiflora* for *Margaropus annulatus australis* (Fuller). Similar findings were reported from the Phillipines [149] and Colombia. Recently anti-tick grasses have been suggested as part of a tick control package. Such '. . . anti-tick pastures combined with very limited strategic acaricide application . . . will yield a low cost, efficient tick control and increase beef production for the small livestock producer' [150]. Australian workers [151, 152] described the immobilization and mortality of *B. microplus* larvae on tropical legumes of the genus *Stylosanthes*. These plant species also improve the nutritional value of tropical pastures.

8.1.4. *Chemical control*

Chemical control of ticks in nature or in the corrals should be considered under specific conditions but with due consideration of the possible contamination of the environment and agricultural products. Area control with ixodicides has been little studied in relation to livestock but extensively applied for human protection [153, 154]. The application of stirofos (tetrachlorvinphos) or carbaryl to pasture, 4–6 times a year has been recommended [155]. Such a treatment might reduce pasture spelling time down to 30 days and is applicable in cases where land is limited. The use of an acaricide dust, such as carbaryl or lindane, in *Boophilus* infested corrals has been recommended after removal of litter and manure. New bedding is applied after the dusting, particularly in dairy yards.

8.1.5. *Conclusions*

Pasture spelling seems to be the most important and effective means of tick control off the host in grazing cattle. Pasture spelling can be integrated into a tick control scheme combined particularly with resistant cattle and strategic dipping. Anti-tick grasses, both repelling and killing, should be studied thoroughly under field conditions.

8.2. *Tick control on the host*

The control of *Boophilus* ticks on the host with acaricides is still the most efficient and commonly used technique, accessible to the grazier and dairyman.

8.2.1. *Chemical control of ticks*

For practical purposes control of ticks on livestock depends almost exclusively on ixodicides. The use of tick repellents on animals is still very limited. Chemical warfare against ticks has become complicated due to resistance developed by ticks to the widely used acaricides. It has also become increasingly expensive because of the exceedingly high costs of developing new acaricides. The development of a new agrochemical costs about 12 to 14 million dollars and takes about 7 years from synthesis to marketing. Regulatory agencies maintain a conservative, suspicious attitude towards new compounds. Oversensitivity on the part of the public may shorten considerably the life span of an acaricide as occurred recently when chlordimeform was accused of cancerogenicity. However, 'Adequate food for humanity is a boon that far outweighs the potential health hazards of pesticides' [13]. The activity of the acaricide in the field depends to a large extent on the formulation which is an art on its own merits.

The choice of method and mode of application of ixodicides are as important as the chemical itself, being determined by the economic importance and life cycle of the tick, type and number of cattle, management practices, available equipment and manpower.

Ixodicides. Besides Barnett's manual of tick control [11] the reader is referred to the vast literature dealing with acaricides for single and multi-host ticks [17, 156, 157, 158, 159, 160, 161]. Arsenic trioxide was almost solely used until the late forties when DDT and BHC (Lindane) were introduced. These were followed by other chlorinated hydrocarbons, particularly toxaphene. In most developed countries these compounds were withdrawn from the market due to residue problems and alleged cancerogenicity, to be replaced by the organophosphorous compounds and carbamates. Recently, synthetic pyrethroids, cyclic amidines and other derivatives have been increasingly used. The most widely used acaricides in Australia are (in decreasing order) amitraz, chloromethiuron, trimethicarbon, bromophos ethyl and ethion [24]. In Argentina the list includes amitraz, pyrethroids, and organophosphorous compounds [25], while in East Africa dioxathion (delnav), carbaryl (sevin) and baydip (asuntol & flumetrin) are being mostly used [162]. Dairy cattle present certain difficulties in the choice of ixodicides, mainly due to the problem of residues in milk and milk products. In the USA the only acaricides permitted on milking cows are ciodrin (crotoxyphos) and 0.03% coumaphos (asuntol) [163]. In Australia, South-Africa and some European countries amitraz and synthetic pyrethroids have been released for use on milking cows with no posttreatment withholding periods. Overdosing in such animals should be strictly avoided.

Tick repellents. Studies carried out in the USA established the feasibility of using clothes impregnated with tick repellents for human protection against ticks [164, 165]. Tick repellents have not been tested on livestock but 'The search for an effective and low-cost repellent for use on livestock appears to be a worthwhile objective' [11]. An ideal repellent would keep the animal clean of ticks and prevent 'tick worry' and the transmission of pathogens. Repellents do not expose ticks to a high selective pressure thus the establishment of resistance is delayed. A laboratory model for the study of tick repellents has been developed by Hadani et al. [128] and some preliminary results have been published [166]. Pyrethrum extract showed promising results but proved very short-lived under natural conditions. The new long-lasting pyrethroids and the tickifuge cyclic amidines should be tested. The combined use of a non-residual, highly effective acaricide with a repellent effective for 10–14 days should be also considered.

8.2.2. *Application of ixodicides – techniques, timing and behaviour of ixodicidal washes*

The basic principle underlying the control of ticks by ixodicides is a complete wetting of the animal until run-off. Such an effect can be obtained through dipping, spray dipping or spraying the animals. Under special circumstances systemic acaricides can be used. The frequency and timing of acaricidal treatments play a major role in tick control and are determined by seasonal factors, management schemes, type of animals and tick control strategies.

Plunge dip. This is the most efficient and practical method of controlling ticks on the animal. When constructing dips the site, design, dip management and maintenance and construction materials should be considered. Analysis of ixodicidal fluids, which was simple and quick with arsenical preparations, has become more complicated with the new organic acaricides, but should always dictate the rate of replenishment, preferably a continuous one. At the farmer's level the 'end point' – time to change the dip – is determined arbitrarily, usually according to the physical appearance of the fluids. In government managed installations the dip is changed every 10–15.000 animals [25]. Dipping is the method of choice for grazing beef cattle. It has certain drawbacks [24] such as cost of construction, maintenance and running expenses, injury to the animals, accumulation of contaminants in long standing dips and effect on milk and meat production [24, 134], particularly when cattle are driven long distances to the dipping site. The dipping of dairy cattle and particularly milking cows weighing some 400–500 kg presents difficulties and is not widely applied.

Spray race. The technique consists in the circulation of a high volume of fluid (600–900 litres per minute) at a low pressure (1–1.5 atmospheres) through large orifice nozzles. The method can be applied with dairy as well as with beef cattle and permits proper initial charging, economy of acaricides and accurate replenishment relatively free of contaminants. The animals pass quickly and unstable chemicals such as amitraz can be used with no stabilizers needed. Any number of animals can be treated and the system is adaptable to medium size farms (300–500 animals) as well as small animal holdings. The spray race is transferrable and resists earthquakes better than plunge dips. On the other hand the spray race requires maintenance (the pump, strainer and nozzles) and calls for skill particularly with the filtering system, so as to ensure a thorough treatment. The spray mist can be contaminating for the environment and hazardous to the operators. Stripping might be a problem. However as shown with BHC preparations [167] this can be avoided by starting with 2000 litres, enough for about 500 animals and then preparing fresh fluid. In Australia spray races were found less efficient than either hand spraying or plunge dipping [160]. With the beef cattle in Israel the spray race was superiour to hand spraying [127]. A portable spray dip wagon produced in San Jose, California, USA might also give satisfactory results. This procedure is much slower (60 animals per hour) and requires skill. Non-recirculating spray races are also used. However complete wetting of the animals requires greater volumes of wash fluid.

Hand spray. This technique can give good results if done properly. Spraying should be carried out with a motor driven sprayer, preferrably operated by electricity or by a tractor. The equipment consists of a stirrer, two spraying guns and long hoses, a 100–1000 litres stainless steel or fibreglass tank and a pump providing 10–15 atmospheres. This method is mostly suitable for dairy cattle which should be tied in their stalls. Untied animals and beef cattle should be treated in groups of 5–6 animals in a small corral. Four to six liters of spray wash per head should be used for tied animals and 6–10 litres for untied ones. Hand spraying is the method of choice for the small holders who can get organized, acquire the necessary equipment and hire trained staff to carry out the tick control operations collaboratively. Bucket sprays, hand or motor driven back sprayers should be reserved for special cases i.e. very few animals, horses etc. Hand dressing of ixodicides with swab, cloth, brush, plastic squeeze bottles, aerosoles, foams, dusts, etc. can be used in cases of ticks with predilection sites, such as *Dermacentor nitens*, *Otobius megnini* and *Rhipicephalus evertsi*. Recently eartags impregnated with tickicides have given encouraging results in controlling single and multi-host ticks [168, 169, 170, 171].

Systemic ixodicides. Systemic insecticides have hardly been used for the control of ticks. Treating cattle with ruelene for hypodermosis gave excellent results against ticks. However such treatment is not repeatable and its effect wanes within 5–7 days. Pour-on miscible formulations of amitraz have been effective in controlling *B. microplus*, Biarra strain, on housed calves [172]. Recently avermectin (Merck MK-933) administered in sustained release boluses [173] or injected daily at the rate of 15 Mg/kg per day [174] gave excellent results against various species of ticks. Similar fungal extract insecticides are being studied [175]. Sustained control systems have been reviewed by Miller et al. [176].

Timing of ixodicidal applications. Frequency of ixodicidal applications is determined by the life cycle of the target species, type of chemical used, breed of cattle and its management, and the season. *Boophilus* spp. spend 3–4 weeks on the animal and can be controlled by three week-interval treatments. However, for moulting nymphs that are more resistant to ixodicides, 2-week intervals are preferred. Multi-host ticks can be controlled by a similar schedule. If disease transmission is to be prevented such as in the case of *Rhipicephalus appendiculatus* and *Hyalomma detritum* (theileriosis), or *Ixodes ricinus* (babesiosis), treatments should be carried out more frequently, once in 3–7 days [11]. In grazing beef cattle 10–20 engorged *Boophilus* ticks per animal are well under the economic threshold [177] while immunity is still maintained [21, 45]. This situation can be achieved in *Bos taurus* and low grade *B. indicus* cross cattle by 6–8 treatments per year while two treatments per year will suffice for 50% *B. indicus* infusion cattle [178]. In Australia [24] the number of dippings per year ranges between 3.8–8 or more. Over 33% of the farmers dip more than 10 times per year which is considered excessive. By combining pasture spelling with tick resistant cattle the number of treatments can be reduced further or even totally suspended. The use of residual ixodicides is controversial. Such chemicals are accused of enhancing the establishment of resistance by exposing the ticks to decreasing selective pressure i.e. sparing both the susceptible and heterozygous type [179]. On the other hand residual ixodicides such as DDT, amitraz and perhaps the pyrethroids permit spacing of treatment as well as control of mixed single-and multi-host ticks infestation. Such a situation, while not typical for Australia, prevails in most African, Asian and South American countries.

Deterioration and depletion of ixodicidal washes. Deterioration and depletion of acaricidal formulations, occurring particularly in long standing plunge dip washes, have been reviewed by Barnett [11]. In addition to the physical changes taking place in these unstable systems of emulsions and suspensions one should consider biological and chemical deterioration of the acaricide and its stripping through preferred adsorption on the host's coat. Emulsions are considered more stable and less prone to 'settling out' than suspensions. However cases of intoxication in cattle and particularly in sheep have been attributed to the breakdown of the emulsion fluid in the dip before starting dipping the animals [180]. Dip fluids can be analyzed by chemical methods suggested and often offered as a service by the commercial companies. When such techniques are not practicable bio-assay methods can be used such as the egg laying inhibition of engorged *Boophilus* female ticks, dose response in *Boophilus* larvae [181] or the *Aedes aegypti* larvae method [167]. For further information the reader is referred to a few other publications [182, 183].

8.2.3. *Tick resistant breeds of cattle*

Tick resistance might be defined as the capacity of cattle to limit the number of ticks that survive to maturity. Tick resistant cattle have been reported by many observers [11] and the subject has been reviewed by Francis [184]. Most convincing, perhaps, were Villares experiments in Brazil in which he exposed European, Brazilian (criollo) and Indian breeds to heavy infestations of *B. microplus* [185]. Resistance can result in light tick infestation, failure to complete development, failure to engorge and to lay fertile eggs, delayed life cycle and decrease in mean female weight [186]. Grooming plays an important role but the phenomenon is basically immunological and is expressed by skin reactions and humoral response following an initial exposure to ticks. The mechanism has a high heritability (82%), permitting practical selection in the herd. Some evidence indicates that innate resistance is involved as well [187, 188]. Various aspects of resistance have been studied both in cattle and laboratory animals [186, 189, 190, 191, 192, 193, 194]. Sutherst and Utech [195] layed down the basic principles of the technique of breeding cattle for tick resistance and it's practical applications are discussed by Wharton and Norris [15]. Most studies of host tick resistance involve beef cattle breeds and the tick *B. microplus*. Reduction of tick infestations by the use of resistant cattle has been demonstrated using Brahman × British cattle [193, 196, 197, 198] and Shorthorn dairy cattle [199]. Effect of host resistance on multi-host ticks seems to be much weaker [200]. Sutherst et al. [201] revised the methods used for culling breeders for low tick resistance but such culling in commercial situations still needs further elaboration [135]. Also needed is a simple biological test to determine levels of tick resistance in the animals. Farmers have many constraints against the use of Brahman crosses while certain advantages have been listed as well [15, 134, 135]. On the whole, tick resistant animals appear to offer the most effective tick control method in beef cattle under grazing conditions in Queensland, particularly in combination with pasture rotation [135]. Host resistance is less applicable to dairy cattle and few studies have been conducted in this direction. However the method can be employed with Zebu-Friesian cross heifers in some South American countries.

8.2.4. *Biological control of ticks on the host*

Hormones, sex pheromones and vaccination of cattle with larval extracts have been mentioned as possibilities. The use of hormonal agents has become a subject of intense activity in entomological research. Very little indeed has been done with ticks [197, 198, 202]. On the other hand, sex pheromones, both female and male do present some real, practical interest [203, 204, 205, 206]. Male aggregation hormones have been studies in conjunction with ixodicides for control of 'hard' ticks [207, 208] or used as biological traps [209]. Tick pheromones have been thoroughly reviewed by Sonenshine et al. [210]. The idea of vaccinating cattle against tick larval extract has been suggested by Riek, following his pioneer studies on host:tick relationships [191]. Laboratory animals [211, 212] and cattle

[213, 214] have been vaccinated and followed as to their tick resistance.

In summary, with reference to tick control, one can quote Barnett [215]: 'We hopefully make a list every four years of alternatives or adjuncts to ixodicides: repellents, area control with ixodicides, parasites and predators, genetic and biological control by pasture management and environmental changes' ... of which only the pasture rotation has obvious application and could possibly be combined with tick resistant cattle and anti-tick plants.

8.3. Resistance of ticks to ixodicides

Since tick resistance to chemicals was first reported from South Africa in 1938 [216] the phenomenon has become widespread in most cattle breeding countries and has acquired considerable economic importance, complicating tick control operations.

8.3.1. General considerations
Resistance to ixodicides involves principally the genus *Boophilus*, but multi-host ticks were also shown to develop resistance, though more slowly, to the widely used chemicals [217, 218, 219, 220, 221, 222]. The main factors enhancing the establishment of resistance are misuse of acaricides, excessive application and sub-dosing. As mentioned earlier, any particular ixodicide should be used to the limit of its efficacy, sparing others for future needs. Nevertheless, mixtures of ixodicides were recommended in some cases, particularly those having different physiological mechanisms of resistance in the ticks [161, 223, 224]. The genetic basis of tick resistance to chemicals has been intensively studied in *Boophilus microplus*, being defined as recessive (DDT), dominant (dieldrin and organo-phosphorous compounds) or incompletely dominant [225, 226, 227, 228, 229]. In the last ten years or so tick resistance to chemicals has been accelerating due to more intensive indiscriminate use of ixodicides, often as mixtures casually pre-pared. Furthermore, vigour tolerance, a pre-resistance stage, depending essen-tially on cross-resistance between dissimilar compounds such as DDT and pyre-thrum [230] or pyrethroids, might shorten considerably the life span of a newly introduced acaricide. Occurrence of resistance may be suspected in the field but should be assessed under controlled conditions in the laboratory. Resistance should be diagnosed as early as possible so as not to jeopardise tick control efforts. The reader is referred to the pertinent reviews dealing with tick resistance [231, 232, 233, 234, 235, 236, 237, 238, 239] and its management [179, 240, 241, 242].

8.3.2. Methods for assessment of tick resistance to chemicals
The onset of resistance in the field is generally announced by an unexpected heavy tick infestation on the treated animals. Resistance can reduce tick control

efficiency considerably i.e. from 77% to 14% in arsenicals, 85% to 40% in DDT and 99% to 40% in Coumaphos. Under conditions of sporadic, casual treatments, such as prevail in vast areas in Africa, Asia and South America the recognition of resistance might prove difficult.

Misapplication of the ixodicide should then be discarded and a field test should be carried out for single host [160] and multi-host ticks [220]. Adequate material is sent for assessment in the laboratory. The method used most commonly for *Boophilus* spp. is that of Stone and Haydock [181], adopted as a standard method by FAO 1971 and used by Tatchell [243] on multihost-ticks. Shaw's method [244] uses immersion instead of ixodicide impregnated paper bags. These *'in vitro'* methods call for the availability of a laboratory reference strain of *Boophilus* spp. The method using engorged females [245] was often criticized as being long (four weeks?), not practical due to the large number of engorged females needed and the difficult interpretation of the results. Nevertheless, the method can be used whenever laboratory facilities and skilled manpower are lacking and might supply valuable information as to the existence of resistance and the potency of dip fluids. A similar method using *Hyalomma excavatum* nymphs has been described [246]. The results obtained by these bio-essay methods are compared to those of a susceptible, laboratory maintained strain or to discriminating doses determined previously.

8.3.3. *Monitoring and management of tick resistance*

The establishment of resistance to organophosphorous insecticides took place within 5–7 years of registration. Later, the occurrence of resistance to other compounds proved unpredictable being influenced by 'variable deterministic factors (timing of dippings and concentrations used) and by various chance effects (mutations)'. The build up of resistance in a given tick population can be postponed by moderating the frequency of treatments (strategic applications) and using high concentrations of ixodicides ('saturation strategy') [179]. The same authors disapprove the use of residual ixodicides and favour mixing chemically different acaricides on the grounds of effective synergistic results. Both approaches are debatable. The use of residual ixodicides is indicated in cases such as mixed single – and multi-host tick populations or eradication campaigns of *Boophilus* spp. The application of mixtures – 'cocktails' of acaricides should be considered carefully as a possible approach under specific conditions. When a controlled moderated scheme of applications is not practical one should prefer maximising control means to doubtful prophylactic treatments. The level of susceptibility to acaricides of the economically important ticks should be monitored continuously, preferably by a government laboratory in close collaboration with the agrochemical industry. Such a survey is preceded by the determination of base line data of the susceptibility of the ticks to the main acaricides. Maintenance of laboratory bred reference strains of ticks is also required [210, 244, 247]. Last, but not least, resistance generally appears as a limited, focal event in a herd which if left un-heeded will quickly develop into a regional problem. Quarantine on the movement and transfer of tick-infested animals from such a herd should be installed as soon as possible.

The establishment of the long waited international reference centre for acaricide resistance in ticks [248], sponsored by the FAO, is of crucial importance particularly in the developing countries.

In summary, acaricide resistance in ticks is a global problem rendering tick control campaigns more expensive and complex. However Alexander's pessimism [249] claiming that '. . . the introduction of the new insecticides has coincided with the loss of control of ticks', should by no means be shared by acarologists today. Solid tick control infrastructures, strict control of ixodicides and their mode of application, rigid standards of testing of new acaricides and control of dips will all contribute to the optimal; use of acaricides and delay the onset of resistance.

8.4. Strategies of tick control operations

Anti-tick control measures may be aimed at economic threshold control, eradication, or prevention of disease transmission. Choice of strategy will depend on the target tick (nuisance species), type of cattle and management, climatic factors and socio-economic factors. Models have been elaborated for the analysis of the economic feasibility and efficacy of tick control measures and dynamics of tick infestation under various environmental conditions [26, 179, 201].

8.4.1. Economic threshold control of ticks

This is the method of choice for grazing cattle in *Boophilus* – infested areas, the main purpose being to avoid 'tick worry' and at the same time to maintain a sufficient degree of premunition against tick fevers. The economic threshold control of ticks is achieved either by discretional or strategic tick control operations.

Discretional, opportunistic control of ticks. Control measures are applied when the owner considers necessary, i.e. when tick burden is heavy or when anti-tick treatments conform with other activities of the farm. Such a casual, sporadic scheme, unfortunately widespread, might rapidly lead to the establishment of tick resistance.

Prophylactic, strategic tick control. The schedule of acaricide applications is determined by the life cycle of the target tick species, type of cattle and husbandry, and climatic factors. As mentioned above, strategic dipping or spraying might be combined with resistant cattle, pasture spelling and anti-tick plants. Under these conditions acaricide application can be minimised. Under tropical conditions, with *Boophilus* spp. conducting a continuous life cycle throughout the year, strategic treatments should be planned accordingly. In sub-tropical countries and mountainous areas, winter temperatures are low enough to arrest *Boophilus* development. In such localities treatments are applied in autumn to reduce the number of ticks entering winter inactivity and in spring to reduce tick population build-up in summer and autumn. Multi-host ticks require specific schemes adapted to their life cycles and seasonal distribution.

8.4.2. *Eradication of ticks*

Control of large populations of insects has recently become more feasible, using biological and chemical measures. Nevertheless, programs for tick eradication should be approached rather conservatively. The advantages of eradication are generally obvious enough as to ensure in many cases popular support and funds. Eradication can often be justified with a newly introduced species, e.g. *B. microplus* in Florida, USA. Unfortunately '. . . eradication programs are plagued with a spectacular variety of problems – technical, economic, sociological and political, especially in the ultimate phase from the 99% to the 100% elimination' [22]. The successful eradication of *B. annulatus* from an area of 700.000 square miles in the USA raised expectations in other *Boophilus* stricken areas. Thus in Argentina vast areas south of the 30° parallel south have been cleansed of *B. microplus* by systematic dippings and strict control over movement of bovines and equines. Problems of tick resistance, inaccessible areas and lack of cooperation make this eradication campaign progressively more costly and complicated.

Partial eradication has been achieved in Papua-New Guinea involving some 2500 zebu animals [250]. The successful eradication campaign of *B. annulatus* in the USA stemmed from: (1) The commercial incentive (access to northern markets), ensuring farmers' cooperation, (2) Strict control over movement of animals; (3) Compulsory dipping and (4) The apparent inability of *B. annulatus* to develop resistance to chemicals. In fact acaricide resistance has not yet been described in field strains of this species.

Multi-host ticks have been radically controlled in Southern and Eastern Africa to the point of complete suppression of the transmission of East Coast fever and heartwater by a rigid schedule of compulsory, frequent dipping and inspection of livestock for the presence of ticks [11, 251]. Management of modern zero grazing dairy herds calls for the eradication of *Boophilus* spp. and multi-host tick vectors such as *Hyalomma detritum* and *Rhipicephalus appendiculatus*. This can be achieved rather effectively on the farm level by acaricide treatments and strict control over the newly acquired animals so as to avoid re-infestation. Equines should be treated similarly.

Finally, following McCosker's commentary on control of ticks as opposed to eradication [3] the whole subject should be thoroughly examined possibly in a meeting sponsored by FAO, to be held in a country where tick eradication is being attempted.

284

8.4.3. *Economic analysis and models of tick population dynamics*

As mentioned above, models elaborated by the Australian workers permit cost/benefit analysis of tick control campaigns and prediction of tick burdens under various climatic and husbandry regimes. Recently [123] a model for the survival of *B. microplus* larvae in pasture has been developed. These models permit the planning of an integrated scheme of control analyzed from a cost standpoint against the estimated damage caused by the ticks. The adaptation of these models to the *Boophilus* complex in other countries should be attempted. Similar models can be worked out for multi-host ticks based on a thorough study of their ecological needs and host relationships.

8.5. *Toxicity and safety measures*

This is an integral part of any discussion of pesticides and the reader is referred to the pertinent abundant literature [252, 253, 254].

9. Epizootiological considerations

The planning of control methods and the likelihood of success depend a great deal upon the epizootiological situation in which babesiosis occurs.

Epizootiological factors that are only partially or not at all dependent on man are: (a) passive immunity transferred from dams to their offspring; (b) innate resistance of calves (up to 7–9 months old) resulting in mild babesiosis following infection; (c) relative resistance of some breeds of cattle and high sensitivity of others; and (d) ecological changes that influence the development of vector populations.

Human factors affecting the epizootiological situation are the type of management and husbandry of cattle, specific vector control and prophylactic measures like the use of long-acting babesicides and vaccines.

Systems of cattle management throughout the world can be grouped into three main types.

9.1. *Cattle pastured round the year on the range*

This type of maintenance concerns an important part of the beef cattle population in Australia, Southern and Eastern Africa, South America and Israel. Cattle at risk are grazed on pastures infested with *Boophilus* spp. capable of transmitting *B. bigemina* and *B. bovis*.

The basic studies carried out by Mahoney and coworkers [45, 255, 256, 257] have defined the epizootiological parameters of *Babesia* transmission in this type of cattle. An important factor is the proportion of calves that become infected with *Babesia* before they are nine months of age. A daily probability of infection of 0.01 or higher ensures infection of nearly all calves while they are still protected by passive and innate immunity and results in a stable enzootc situation. Computer models show that enzootic stability is reached when there is an average daily tick infestation of 10 to 20 engorged *B. microplus* ticks per animal [257, 258]. Instability and babesiosis outbreaks were associated with simulated daily infestations of two to eight ticks [258]. Instability also results from the introduction of susceptible cattle into resistant herds.

For practical purposes the enzootic situation can be evaluated by serologic testing of the last generation of cattle in a herd after the waning of the passively transferred antibabesial antibody.

Weather conditions, acaricide treatments affecting the tick population, and chemoprophylaxis that influences the parasitemia in cattle, are all factors that may alter the transmission of babesiosis in range cattle. Management of cattle may also influence the enzootic situation. For example, in Israel most beef calves are born during the autumn and early winter (September to December). On the other hand, the *B. annulatus* population usually decreases during November–May. Consequently, a considerable portion of the new – born calves fail to become infected during their resistant period in the early spring. As a result, the new generations of calves often suffer heavy outbreaks of babesiosis during the following summer when the tick population increases and the natural resistance of the calves has waned.

9.2. *Pastured cattle housed in barns*

This type of management occurs mostly in rural units all over the world. Cattle are sent to pasture daily but spend the night in the barn. Cattle that are not milked may remain on pasture continuously during the whole grazing season.

In Europe the field ticks *Ixodes ricinus* and *Haemaphysalis punctata* transmit *B. divergens* and *B. major* respectively. Donnelly and Pierce [259] demonstrated that *B. divergens* can persist in *I. ricinus* up to the second generation of larvae from an infected female when all the intermediate stages are fed on nonbovine hosts. Since under field conditions *I. ricinus* requires 3 years to complete a generation, *B. divergens* infection may persist in this tick population for 4 years in the absence of cattle. Serologic surveys suggest that *Babesia* infection can be maintained in Red deer independently of cattle [260]. It is obvious that under such conditions it is almost impossible to avoid field infections with *B. divergens*.

According to Joyner and Donnelly [261] bovine redwater in Britain occurs in marginal pastures where the vector has been established for many years, showing a bimodal curve with peaks during the period April–June and August–October. In Austria a peak of positive *B. divergens* blood samples was reported during

May–July while the percentage of positive results from the total number of samples examined remained about the same from March to November [262].

Although high infection rates have been recorded with *B. divergens* [262, 263] it appears that enzootic stability is rarely reached among pasturing cattle in Europe [260, 264].

In temperate areas where *B. annulatus* occurs the tick may become established in barns. In this case a high probability of infection exists and a stable situation is reached with indigenous cattle. However, this situation interferes with livestock development projects, when high grade imported cattle or improved crossbreeds are transferred to family units in order to improve the level of performance of the local herd. Often newly introduced cattle contract hemoparasitic infections after the first few nights in barns in which no clinical cases of tick fevers have been observed for years.

9.3. *Cattle maintained at zero grazing*

This group includes mostly dairy breeds kept in barns, cattle sheds or corrals, and feedlot cattle kept in buildings or open paddocks. Tens to hundreds of cattle may constitute a unit and often adjacent units form agglomerations of thousands of cattle. Such 'closed herds' situated in *Boophilus* infested areas may remain for years free of ticks or babesiosis without special care. However, infected ticks may be introduced into the premises by cattle trading, by stray cattle from pastured herds, or by fresh grass from tick infested fields carrying larval stages of *Boophilus* spp. Relatively few ticks may provoke heavy outbreaks because of the high concentration of cattle in a small area.

Dairy breeds, including young calves, are generally highly sensitive to babesiosis and 'fulminant' infections are often observed. Usually no resistance to babesiosis develops in the majority of these animals since infections are quickly controlled by chemotherapy, often by 'blanket' treatment of all cattle in the unit. This practice leaves little chance for immunity to develop even in those animals that had experienced an infection.

In feedlots *Boophilus* ticks are introduced mainly by animals transferred from pastures. Some feedlots contain mixed populations of relatively resistant calves originating from range herds and highly susceptible calves from dairy breeds. Outbreaks in such feedlots affect mainly the latter type of cattle. The short period during which cattle are kept in feedlots and smaller units and the continuous introduction of new animals into existing groups have an important impact on the control measures that need to be applied.

Although the general considerations mentioned cover most cattle management systems, details in the epizootiology of the same diseases in different regions may vary considerably, and as pointed out by Joyner and Donnelly [261] direct extrapolation from one situation to another is not always valid.

10. Currently applied control techniques in the various systems of cattle management

According to Barnett [215] the situations in which control measures against tick-borne diseases must be considered are: (1) vector and disease agent are present and cause losses; (2) the specific vector is present but the disease is absent; (3) both vector and disease agent are absent but can become established if introduced.

Situation 2 is actually rare so far as the *Boophilus – Babesia* combination is concerned. When situation 3 is state-or nation-wide, the control measures are mainly quarantine regulations and governmental instructions or measures to be taken following known or suspected introduction of babesiosis.

The practical control measures that are applied currently at the farm level in the above 3 epizootiological situations will be discussed here with reference to the various types of cattle management described in section 9.

10.1. *Range cattle*

Vast populations of unselected, poorly producing, indigenous cattle in *Boophilus*-infested areas enjoy enzootic stability. Limited means are invested in veterinary assistance or disease prevention in such herds. Chemotherapy is applied whenever clinical babesiosis is suspected. If prompt vaccination is not practicable, and in areas where vaccines are not available, chemoprophylaxis is used on a relatively small scale with cattle sent to *Boophilus*-infested pastures [97, 265, 266].

In Australia, where *B. bigemina* rarely provokes clinical babesiosis, cattle generally receive *B. bovis* vaccine that has been modified by passages in calves [267]. A single inoculation is recommended since repeated reinoculations did not significantly reinforce the resistance to reinfection [110]. Fresh vaccine is stored up to seven days and a dose of 2 ml is inoculated subcutaneously or intramuscularly. The types of cattle that are candidates for vaccination are: Young animals (4–8 months old) from areas in which tick transmission cannot ensure enzootic stability; cattle from herds in which outbreaks have occured; susceptible cattle being moved through tick-infested areas or cattle introduced into such areas [97].

Tick control is either discretional or strategic in the better managed farms, using mainly plunge dips or spray races. Pasture spelling and tick resistant Zebu crosses significantly reduce frequency of acaricide treatment. Tick resistance to acaricides renders control operations difficult and expensive.

In South Africa a local strain of *B. bovis* and an Australian strain of *B. bigemina*, both modified by passages in calves, are used for preparing vaccines [118, 119]. A 2 ml dose of vaccine contains both species. Vaccine is used mostly for young animals, but susceptible adults are also vaccinated under circumstances similar to those in Australia [120]. Revaccination with *B. bigemina* is advised in cattle receiving babesicidal treatment [53]. Tick resistant beef cattle and crosses of breeds developed from them are also vaccinated though in much lower number [120].

Control of ticks in South Africa follows closely the Australian scheme. Plunge dips are more frequently used than spray races. Heavy infestations with multi-host ticks make frequent treatments necessary.

In Israel modified frozen vaccines against *B. bigemina* and *B. bovis* are used in most range-raised herds [92, 105]. Young cattle are vaccinated at weaning and adult cattle in situations similar to those in Australia and South Africa. Usually *B. bigemina* and *A. centrale* vaccines are inoculated first followed three weeks later by *B. bovis* with *T. annulata* vaccines. Clinical babesiosis caused by the vaccines in beef cattle is rare. The presently available vaccines proved to be safe also for some European breeds of cattle. Thus, about 700, 14–18 month old Charolais and Simenthal bull calves imported from Europe have been vaccinated against tick fevers without losses caused by the vaccines.

Tick control in beef herds is, in general, discretional being dictated by the degree of infestation on the animals. *B. annulatus* constitutes by far the most important species. Spray races, particularly the non-recirculating ones, are mostly used. Resistance to acaricides has not yet been reported.

In Latin America cattle are vaccinated against babesiosis with live vaccines usually on a small scale [10]. Local strains of *Babesia* as well as Australian vaccines strains are used [116]. Since most of the local strains are not adequately modified and may provoke severe parasitemia inoculated cattle are watched and treated when necessary. A few ranches use blood from local cattle infected with *Babesia*. In Uruguay local modified *B. bigemina* and *B. bovis* vaccines are combined with *A. centrale*. An official service for preparing antibabesial vaccines and for vaccinating cattle has been functioning for more than three decades [268].

In Argentina *B. microplus* has been eradicated from vast areas south of the 30° latitude through a severe stubborn tick control campaign, practically in effect since 1906, using compulsory dipping and strict control over livestock transportation. In other parts of South America tick control in beef cattle is in general discretional using plunge-dips, spray races or hand spraying. The use of Brahman crosses reduces the economic impact of tick infestation. However, multi-host ticks, particularly *Amblyomma* spp., are widespread in many parts of the continent and should be controlled as well.

10.2. *Pastured cattle housed in barns*

In *Boophilus*-infested areas this type of management concerns mainly dairy cattle. Large industrial dairy milk herds are usually maintained at zero grazing and only relatively small dairy herds or heifers before first calving are sent to pasture.

Sporadic outbreaks of babesiosis are controlled mainly by chemotherapy. In some cases a few herds may be vaccinated against *B. bovis* and *B. bigemina* before sending them to pasture [54, 120]. In Israel vaccinated cattle are maintained at zero grazing after the first calving, and it is not expected that the immunity induced by the primary vaccination will last for the remainder of the cow's life. In Latin America successful results were reported with controlled vaccination of dairy calves [269]. In Colombia Holstein-Friesian and Brown Swiss calves were vaccinated against *B. bovis* and *B. bigemina* and treated during the patent period with Imidocarb. Further observations showed that the vaccinated animals were protected against infection by ticks in the field [80, 269]. In addition, imidocarb chemoprophylaxis was effective in protecting Friesian-Holstein cattle grazing on *Babesia*-infected pastures [269].

In Europe control of babesiosis is achieved mainly by therapy of clinical cases [270]. It appears that the chemoprophylactic capacity of imidocarb on *B. divergens* [41, 42] has not yet been fully exploited in preventing field babesiosis.

The various types of experimental vaccines against *B. divergens* [66, 67, 68, 69, 70, 77] have not yet been used in field campaigns. On the other hand, live *B. divergens* vaccine has been used in Austria since 1969 to inoculate about 230,000 cattle. However, no significant difference in morbidity caused by babesiosis has been noted in vaccinated (11.38%) vs. non-vaccinated cattle (11.65%) [271].

Information on control of ticks in partially grazing dairy cattle is rather scanty. Unless included in a *Boophilus* eradication campaign, tick control in such herds is directed essentially towards preventing tick worry [270]. To this end strategic or discretional acaricide treatments are applied.

10.3. *Cattle maintained at zero grazing*

Outbreaks or sporadic cases of babesiosis in well-managed dairy herds on zero grazing are relatively rare, and in many areas chemotherapy is the method of choice for controlling the disease. Chemoprophylaxis is not recommended for lactating cows because of drug residues in the milk. However, in some areas long acting drugs like imidocarb are used for chemotherapy of lactating cows.

With few exceptions dairy cattle kept at zero grazing are not vaccinated. Usually the epidemiological situation does not justify such a measure. Moreover, since presently available vaccines are not completely safe for sensitive dairy cattle, the cost of post-vaccination surveillance and possible losses caused by the vaccine makes vaccination impractical.

In feedlots situated in *Babesia*-infected areas, the constant turnover of cattle creates a highly unstable enzootic situation. Although chemotherapy and chemoprophylaxis would seem to be adequate for controlling babesiosis in cattle maintained for few months only, some feedlots prefer to protect their animals by vaccination. Two main reasons guide such a decision: The cost of periodical drug treatments and the desire to avoid problems of drug clearance in treated animals under conditions of unpredictable marketing schedules.

In Israel zero grazing dairy herds and cattle in feedlots are cleansed of *B. annulatus* ticks using acaricides both on the animals and in the corrals. Strict quarantine measures are applied in such areas and newly acquired bovines are maintained in isolated corrals with weekly spraying during 3–4 weeks prior to their integration into the tick-free herd. The corral is heavily dusted to ensure the destruction of the free-living developmental stages of *Boophilus*. Such herds are considered highly susceptible to babesiosis and utmost care is taken to prevent reinfestation.

11. Future prospects

Presently available drugs are effective for treating *Babesia* infections in cattle. Even if new drugs with longer periods of protection are synthesized, the basic problems will still be the cost of the periodic treatments and, more important, public health considerations.

The killed vaccines [73, 74, 75] produced from erythrocytic stages of *Babesia* do not prevent infections, but some of them considerably mitigate clinical manifestations of babesiosis. However, these vaccines have several disadvantages that will need to be overcome before they can be used for vaccination in the field: (a) the need for large quantities of antigen, (b) the need for oil adjuvants, (c) the fact that the final product still contains bovine erythrocytic antigen capable of inducing neonatal isoerythrolysis.

Some irradiated vaccines have given encouraging results in experimental trials [60, 61, 62, 66, 68, 69, 70]. This technique has been tried with various other protozoans but in no case has a commercial vaccine been developed. This suggests that considerable supplementary studies will be required before the practical use of irradiated *Babesia* vaccines can be envisaged.

The infection of cattle with *Theileria* parasites harvested from ticks has stimulated similar investigations with *Babesia*-infected *Boophilus* ticks [273, 274, 275, 276, 277]. A vaccine prepared from *Babesia* parasites derived from ticks would permit immunization with the stages responsible for infection in the field and would provide a vaccine free of bovine erythrocytic antigens. However the presently available methodology cannot supply large quantities of vaccine at a reasonable cost, while attenuation of the highly virulent tick stages of *Babesia* still remains to be done.

Propagation of *Babesia* in tick cell cultures [278, 279] is an attractive approach for possible preparation of vaccine but the feasibility of large scale cultivation of infective *Babesia* stages cannot yet be predicted.

It appears that for the near future at least, immunization with live erythrocytic *Babesia* parasites will still be the procedure of choice in most areas of the world. Cultured *B. bovis* will probably gradually replace parasites derived from infected cattle. Recent investigations show that live *B. bovis* from culture and from infected cattle induced similar degrees of protection against reinfection [54, 88]. The use of cultured *B. bovis* can reduce the hazard of contamination with cryptic infections in vaccine-donnor calves and may allow the selection of more appropriate strains for immunization.

Non-viable vaccines developed from *in vitro* cultures of *B. bovis* possess a higher degree of safety than all presently applied vaccines [280]. When widely available this material will allow extention of vaccination to highly susceptible cattle. An important achievement in this context would be the amelioration of cultivation techniques to facilitate mass production of *B. bovis* antigen at a reasonable cost.

The surface coat merozoite antigen contained in the cultured vaccine engenders a fair protection against arthropod and blood stages of *B. bovis* [84, 85, 86] for a reasonable period of time [87]. At present the degree of protection appears to be inferior to that engendered by live parasites [88]. Nevertheless, a reinforcement of the basic immunity engendered by the non-viable vaccine can be achieved by subsequent inoculation of live parasites before the introduction of the cattle in *Babesia* enzootic areas [54]. Such a double vaccination procedure will confer strong protection while avoiding the hazards related with the direct use of live parasite vaccine for sensitive cattle. The successful cultivation of *B. divergens* [281] suggests that this combined method of immunization might be applicable also to other species of *Babesia* besides *B. bovis*.

At present tick control in livestock depends mainly on the use of acaricides. In zero grazing dairy cattle eradication of ticks at the farm level should be attempted, accompanied by adequate quarantine measures for newly introduced animals. In beef cattle and grazing dairy herds strategic application of acaricides, maintaining enzootic stability, retains its current importance. Pasture spelling and the breeding of tick resistant animals are becoming increasingly popular among graziers. More sophisticated anti-tick measures, like slow release devices, systemic acaricides, pheromones and tick-killing plants may become available in the future. Nation-wide *Boophilus* eradication campaigns need to be evaluated very carefully for their bio-ecological and socio-economic aspects before being undertaken.

References

1. Sergent E, Donatien A, Parrot L, Lestoquard F: Etudes sur les piroplasmoses bovines, Alger. Institut Pasteur d'Algerie. 1945, p 220–236.
2. Stepanova NI: Les piroplasmoses et l'anaplasmose des animaux d'elevage et la lutte contre ces

maladies. Rapport No. 100 XLIV eme session generale du comité de l' O.I.E. Paris, 17–22 Mai, 1976.

3. McCosker PJ: The global importance of babesiosis. In: Babesiosis, Ristic M, Kreier JP (eds). New York. Academic Press. 1981, p 1–24.

4. Hoogstraal H: Biology of ticks. In: Tick-borne diseases and their vectors, Wilde JKH (ed). University of Edinburgh. Center for Tropical Veterinary Medicine. 1978, p 3–14.

5. Riek RF: Immunity to babesiosis. In: Immunity to protozoa, Garnham PCC, Pierce AE, Roitt I (eds). Oxford. Blackwell Scientific Publications. 1963, p 160–179.

6. Riek RF: Babesiosis. In: Infectious blood diseases of man and animals. Diseases caused by Protista, Weinman D, Ristic M (eds). New York. Academic Press. 1968 Vol II, p 219–268.

7. Mahoney DF: Immune response to hemoprotozoa II. Babesia spp. In: Immunity to animal parasites, Soulsby EJL (ed). New York. Academic Press. 1972, p 301–341.

8. Mahoney DF: Babesia of domestic animals. In: Parasitic protozoa, Kreier JP (ed). New York. Academic Press. 1977 Vol IV, p 1–52.

9. Callow LL: Vaccination against bovine babesiosis. In: Immunity to blood parasites of animals and man, Miller LH, Pino JA, Mckelvey JJ, Jr. (eds). New York. Plenum Press. 1977, p 121–149.

10. Lora CA: Methods of immunization against bovine babesiosis used in Latin America. In: Babesiosis, Ristic M, Kreier JP (eds). New York. Academic Press. 1981, p 567–571.

11. Barnett SF: The control of ticks on livestock. Rome. FAO Agricultural studies No. 54. 1961, p 1–115.

12. Beesley WN: The ecological basis of parasite control: ticks and flies. Vet Parasitol 11:99–106, 1982.

13. Rogoff WM: Chemical control of insect pests of domestic animals. In: Advances in pest control research 4, New York. Interscience Publications Inc. 1961, p 153–181.

14. Drummond RO: Current worldwide research on control of ticks involved in animal diseases. Misc Pub Entomol Soc America 6:367–372, 1970.

15. Wharton RH, Norris KR: Control of parasitic arthropods. Vet Parasitol 6:135–164, 1980.

16. Shaw RD: Tick control on domestic animals. II. The effect of modern methods of treatment. Trop Sci 12:29–36, 1970.

17. Wharton RH: Ticks with special emphasis on *Boophilus Microplus*. In: Control of arthropods of medical and veterinary importance, Pal R, Wharton RH (eds). New York. Plenum Press. 1974, p 35–52.

18. Barnett SF: Control of ticks and disease. In: Tick-borne diseases and their vectors, Wilde JKH (ed). University of Edinburgh. Center for Tropical Veterinary Medicine. 1978, p 110–113.

19. Obenchain FD, Galun R (eds): Physiology of ticks, Current Themes in Tropical Science. Vol 1, New York. Pergamon Press. 1983.

20. FAO: Report of the second FAO expert consultation on research on tick-borne diseases and their vectors. Rome, Italy. 12–16 December 1977.

21. Anon: Programming planning and budgeting model for cattle fever tick eradication program. ARS Code 2-45-000-19-004. 1971, p 52–64.

22. Graham OH, Hourrigan JL: Eradication programs for the arthropod parasites of livestock. J Med Entomol 13:629–658, 1977.

23. Beltran LG: Caracteristicas de la campaña nacional mexicana contra la garrapata. Seminario sobre ectoparasitos, Thompson KC (ed). Serie CS-13, 1977. CIAT Cali, Colombia. 25–30 Agosto, 1975, p 77–96.

24. Elder JK, Emmerson FR, Kearnan JF, Waters KS, Dunwell GH, Morris RS, Knott SG: A survey concerning cattle tick control in Queensland. 3. Chemical control. Aust Vet J 56:212–218, 1980.

25. Oria JE: personal communication.

26. Sutherst RW, Dallwitz MJ: Progress in the development of a population model for the cattle tick *Boophilus microplus*. In: Proc 4th Int Cong Acarol. Saalfenden, Austria. 13–18 August, 1974, p 557–563.

27. Dennig HK: Chemotherapy of protozoal tick-borne diseases. Bull Off Int Epiz 81:103–121, 1974.

28. Aragon RS: Bovine babesiosis: A review. Vet Bull 46:903–917, 1976.

29. Kuttler KL: Chemotherapy of babesiosis: A review. In: Babesiosis, Ristic M, Kreier JP (eds). New York. Academic Press. 1981, p 65–85.

30. Beveridge E: Drug resistance in *Babesia rodhaini*. Br J Pharmacol 39:239–240, 1970.

31. Dalgliesh RJ, Stewart NP: Tolerance to imidocarb induced experimentally in tick-transmitted *Babesia argentina*. Aust Vet J 53:176–180, 1977.

32. Fulton JD, Yorke W: Studies in chemotherapy XXVIII – drug resistance in *Babesia* infections. Ann Trop Med Parasitol 35:229–232, 1941.

33. Legg J: The treatment of Babesiellosis (*B. argentina*) with acaprin. Aust Vet J 15:121–123, 1939.

34. Kemron A, Pipano E, Hadani A, Neuman M:Trials with a diamidine compound (M&B 5062A) in the treatment of *Babesiella berbera* infection in cattle. Refuah Vet 17:226–236, 1960.

35. Singh B, Muley AK, Ghafoor MA, Kulkarni MN: Therapeutic and prophylactic activity of imidocarb dipropionate against clinical and experimental *Babesia bigemina* infection in cattle. Haryana Agric Univ J Res 10:130–136, 1980.

36. Callow LL, McGregor W: The effect of imidocarb against *Babesia argentina* and *Babesia bigemina* infections of cattle. Aust Vet J 46:195–200, 1970.

37. Todorovic RA, Vizcaino OG, Gonzalez EF, Adams LG: Chemoprophylaxis (imidocarb) against *Babesia bigemina* and *Babesia argentina* infections. Am J Vet Res 34:1153–1161, 1973.

38. Dwivedi SK, Gautam OP, Banerjee DP: Therapeutic and prophylactic activity of imidocarb dipropionate against *Babesia bigemina* infection in splenectomized bovine calves. Indian Vet J 54:697–702, 1977.

39. Kuttler KL, Graham OH, Trevino JL: The effect of imidocarb treatment on *Babesia* in the bovine and the tick (*Boophilus microplus*). Res Vet Sci 18:198–200, 1975.

40. Li PN, Khamizov KK, Ivanshin YD, Kashezhev ZZ: Chemoprophylaxis of francaiellosis. Veterinariya, Moscow, USSR. (3):41–42, 1982 (russian).

41. Lewis D, Purnell RE, Francis LMA, Young ER: The effect of treatment with imidocarb dipropionate on the course of *Babesia divergens* infections in splenectomized calves, and on their subsequent immunity to homologous challenge. J Comp Path 91:285–292, 1981.

42. Purnell RE, Lewis D, Young ER: Investigations on the prophylactic effect of treatment with imidocarb diproprionate on *Babesia divergens* infections in splenectomized calves. Br Vet J 136:452–456, 1980.

43. Pipano E, Klinger I, Virag R: 'Ganaseg' as a chemoprophylactic in experimental *Babesia bigemina* infection in calves. Refuah Vet 25:116–119, 1968.

44. Pipano E: The treatment of experimental *Babesiella berbera* and *Theileria annulata* infections with 4,4' diazo-amino-dibenzamidine-diaceturate. Refuah Vet 21:247–255, 1964.

45. Mahoney DF, Ross DR: Epizootiological factors in the control of bovine babesiosis. Aust Vet J 48:292–298, 1972.

46. Sergent Ed, Sergent Et: Historique du concept de l'immunite relative ou premunition correlative d'une infection latente. Arch Inst Pasteur d'Algerie 34:52–89, 1956.

47. Callow LL: Strain immunity in babesiosis. Nature 204:1213–1214, 1964.

48. Callow LL, McGregor W, Parker RJ, Dalgliesh RJ: The immunity of cattle to *Babesia argentina* after drug sterilization of infections of varying duration. Aust Vet J 50:6–11, 1974.

49. Pipano E, Weisman Y, Raz A, Klinger I: Immunity to *Babesia bigemina* in calves after successful babesicidal treatment of a previous infection. Refuah Vet 29:1–8, 1972.

50. Löhr KF: Immunity to *Babesia bigemina* in experimentally infected cattle. J Protozool 19:658–660, 1972.

51. Callow LL: Sterile immunity, coinfectious immunity and strain differences in *Babesia bigemina* infections. Parasitology 57:455–465, 1967.

52. Pipano E, Jeruham I, Frank M: Pentamidine in chemoimmunization of cattle against *Babesia bigemina* infection. Trop Anim Hlth Prod 11:13–16, 1979.

53. De Vos AJ: Epidemiology and control of bovine babesiosis in South Africa. J S Afr Vet Assoc 50:357–362, 1979.

54. Pipano E: Unpublished data.

55. Roy-Smith F: The prophylactic effects of imidocarb against *Babesia argentina* and *Babesia bigemina* infections of cattle. Aust Vet J 47:418–420, 1971.

56. Taylor RJ, McHardy N: Preliminary observations on the combined use of imidocarb and *Babesia* blood 'vaccine' in cattle. J S Afr Vet Assoc 50:326–329, 1979.

57. Legg J: The value of the blood of recovered cattle in redwater inoculation. The Aust Vet J 7:70–74, 1931.

58. Castro ER, Canabez F: Propiedades biologicas y caracteristicas de *Babesia bigemina*. Efectos de radiaciones ionicas sorbe la infecciosidad de sangre total infectada. Boletin Chileno de Parasitologia 23:30–33, 1969.

59. Bishop JP, Adams LG: *Babesia bigemina*: immune response of cattle inoculated with irradiated parasites. Exp Parasitol 35:35–43, 1974.

60. Mahoney DF, Wright IG, Ketterer PJ: *Babesia argentina*: The infectivity and immunogenicity of irradiated blood parasites for splenectomized calves. Int J Parasitol 3:209–217, 1973.

61. Wright IG, Goodger BV, Mahoney DF: The irradiation of *Babesia bovis*. I. The difference in pathogenicity between irradiated and non-irradiated population. Z Parasitenk 63:47–57, 1980.

62. Wright IG, Mahoney DF, Mirre GB, Goodger BV, Kerr JD: The irradiation of *Babesia bovis*. II. The immunogenicity of irradiated blood parasites for intact cattle and splenectomized calves. Vet Immunol and Immunopathol 3:591–601, 1982.

63. Brocklesby DW, Purnell RE, Sellwood SA: The effect of irradiation on intra-erythrocytic stages of *Babesia major*. Br Vet J 128:3–5, 1972.

64. Purnell RE, Brocklesby DW, Stark AJ: Protection of cattle against *Babesia major* by the inoculation of irradiated piroplasms. Res Vet Sci 25:388–390, 1978.

65. Purnell RE, Lewis D, Brocklesby DW: *Babesia major*: Protection of intact calves against homologous challenge by the injection of irradiated piroplasms. Int J Parasitol 9:69–71, 1979.

66. Lewis D, Purnell RE, Brocklesby DW: *Babesia divergens*: The immunisation of splenectomized calves using irradiated piroplasms. Res Vet Sci 26:220–222, 1979.

67. Lewis D, Purnell RE, Brocklesby DW: *Babesia divergens*: Protection of intact calves against heterologous challenge by the injection of irradiated piroplasms. Vet Parasitol 6:297–303, 1980.

68. Taylor SM, Kenny J, Purnell RE, Lewis D: Exposure of cattle immunised against redwater to tick challenge in the field: challenge by a homologous strain of *B. divergens*. Vet Rec 106:167–170, 1980.

69. Taylor SM, Kenny J, Purnell RE, Lewis D: Exposure of cattle immunised against redwater to tick-induced challenge in the field: challenge by a heterologous strain of *Babesia divergens*. Vet Rec 106:385–387, 1980.

70. Purnell RE, Lewis D: *Babesia divergens*: Combination of dead and live parasites in an irradiated vaccine. Res Vet Sci 30:18–21, 1981.

71. Todorovic RA, Gonzalez EF, Adams LG: Bovine babesiosis: Sterile immunity to *Babesia bigemina* and *Babesia argentina* infections. Trop Anim Hlth Prod 5:234–245, 1973.

72. Löhr KF: Immunisation of splenectomized calves against *Babesia bigemina* infection by the use of a dead vaccine – a preliminary report. In: Tick-Borne diseases and their vectors, Wilde JKH (ed). University of Edinburgh. Center for Tropical Veterinary Medicine. 1978, p 398–402.

73. Kuttler KL, Johnson LW: Immunization of cattle with a *Babesia bigemina* antigen in Freund's complete adjuvant. Am J Vet Res 41:536–538, 1980.

74. Mahoney DF: Bovine babesiosis: The immunization of cattle with killed *Babesia argentina*. Exp Parasitol 20:125–129, 1967.

75. Mahoney DF, Wright IG: *Babesia argentina*: Immunization of cattle with a killed antigen against infection with a heterologous strain. Vet Parasitol 2:273–282, 1976.

76. Mahoney DF, Goodger BV: *Babesia argentina*: Immunogenicity of plasma from infected animals. Exp Parasitol 32:71–86, 1972.

77. Purnell RE, Brocklesby DW: *Babesia divergens* in splenectomized calves: Immunogenicity of lyophilised plasma from an infected animal. Res Vet Sci 23:255–256, 1977.

78. Kemron A, Hadani A, Egyed M, Pipano E, Neuman M: Studies on bovine piroplasmosis caused by *Babesia bigemina*. III. The relationship between the number of parasites in the inoculum and the severity of the response. Refuah Vet 21:108–112, 1964.

79. Gonzalez EF, Todorovic RA, Thompson KC: Immunization against anaplasmosis and babesiosis. Part I. Evaluation of immunization using minimum infective doses under laboratory conditions. Tropenmed Parasitol 27:427–437, 1976.

80. Todorovic RA, Gonzalez EF, Garcia O: Immunization against anaplasmosis and babesiosis. Part III. Evaluation of immunization under field conditions in the Cauca River Valley. Tropenmed Parasitol 30:43–52, 1979.

81. Erp EE, Gravely SM, Smith RD, Ristic M, Osorno BM, Carson CA: Growth of *Babesia bovis* in bovine erythrocyte cultures. Am J Trop Med Hyg 27:1061–1064, 1978.

82. Levy MG, Ristic M: *Babesia bovis*: Continuous cultivation in a microaerophilous stationary phase culture. Science 207:1218–1220, 1980.

83. Erp EE, Smith RD, Ristic M, Osorno BM: Continuous in vitro cultivation of *Babesia bovis*. Am J Vet Res 41:1141–1142, 1980.

84. Smith RD, Carpenter J, Cobrera A, Gravely SM, Erp EE, Osorno M, Ristic M: Bovine babesiosis: Vaccination against tick-borne challenge exposure with culture-derived *Babesia bovis* immunogens. Am J Vet Res 40:1678–1682, 1979.

85. Smith RD, James MA, Ristic M, Aikawa M, Vega y Murguia CA: Bovine babesiosis: Protection of cattle with culture-derived soluble *Babesia bovis* antigen. Science 212:335–338, 1981.

86. Kuttler KL, Levy MG, James MA, Ristic M: Efficacy of a nonviable culture derived *Babesia bovis* vaccine. Am J Vet Res 43:281–284, 1982.

87. Kuttler KL, Levy MG, Ristic M: Cell culture – derived *Babesia bovis* vaccine: Sequential challenge exposure of protective immunity during a 6-month postvaccination period. Am J Vet Res 44:1456–1459, 1983.

88. Timms P, Dalgliesh RJ, Barry DN, Dimmock CK, Rodwell BJ: *Babesia bovis*: Comparison of culture – derived parasites, non – living antigen and conventional vaccine in the protection of cattle against heterologous challenge. Aust Vet J 60:75–77, 1983.

89. Sergent E, Donatien A, Parrot L, Lestoquard F: Etudes sur les piroplasmoses bovines, Alger. Inst Pasteur d'Algerie. 1945, p 133–140, 178–187, 720–723.

90. Tsur I, Lapinski Z: Immunization trials against bovine babesiosis. II. Vaccination with blood from 'patent' carriers. Refuah Vet 19: 181–183, 1962.

91. Kemron A, Pipano E, Hadani A, Neuman M, Egyed M: Studies on bovine piroplasmosis caused by *Babesia bigemina*. I. The enhancement of the virulence of *Babesia bigemina* by serial passage in non-splenectomized calves using blood collected at the acute stage of the disease. Refuah Vet 19:122–124, 1962.

92. Pipano E: Frozen vaccines against tick fevers of cattle. In: Proc 11th Int Cong on Diseases of Cattle, Mayer E (ed). Haifa P.O.B. 170. Bregman Press. 1980, p 678–681.

93. Dalgliesh RJ, Callow LL, Mellors LT, McGregor W: Development of a highly infective *Babesia bigemina* vaccine of reduced virulence. Aust Vet J 57:8–11, 1981.

94. Callow LL, Mellors LT: A new vaccine for *Babesia argentina* infection prepared in splenectomized calves. Aust Vet J 42:464–465, 1966.

95. Callow LL, Mellors LT, McGregor W: Reduction in virulence of *Babesia bovis* due to rapid passage in splenectomized cattle. Int J Parasitol 9:333–338, 1979.

96. Filipov M, Levy MG, Ristic M: Morphologic and immunologic properties of two *Babesia bovis* populations. In: Proc XIIth World Cong on Diseases of Cattle, The Netherlands. Vol II, Utrecht, Netherlands. 1982, p 1002–1006.

97. Timms P, McGregor W, Dalgliesh RJ: Tick fever vaccines . . . how they are made and how to use them. Queens Agric J 107:311–317, 1981.

98. Sergent E, Donatien A, Parrot L, Lestoquard F: 5e, 6e et 7e campagnes de premunition contre les piroplasmoses bovines dans l'Afrique du Nord (1928–1930). Arch Inst Pasteur d'Algerie 9:193–237, 1931.

99. Callow LL: Vaccination against babesiosis in Australia. In: Workshop on Hemoparasites (Anaplasmosis and Babesiosis), Wells EA (ed). Series CE-12, 1977. CIAT Cali, Colombia. 17–22 March, 1975, p 63–71.

100. Dalgliesh RJ: Dimethyl sulfoxide in the low-temperature preservation of *Babesia bigemina*. Res Vet Sci 12:469–471, 1971.

101. Dalgliesh RJ: Theoretical and practical aspects of freezing parasitic protozoa. Aust Vet J 48:233–239, 1972.

102. Dalgliesh RJ: Effects of low temperature preservation and route of inoculation on infectivity of *Babesia bigemina* in blood diluted with glycerol. Res Vet Sci 13:540–545, 1972.

103. Dalgliesh RJ, Mellors LT: Survival of the parasitic protozoan, *Babesia bigemina*, in blood cooled at widely different rates to $-196°$ C. Int J Parasitol 4:169–172, 1974.

104. Todorovic RA, Gonzalez E, Lopez G: Immunization against anaplasmosis and babesiosis. Part II. Evaluation of cryopreserved vaccines using different doses and routes of inoculation. Tropenmed Parasitol 29:210–214, 1978.

105. Pipano E: Immunization of cattle with *Babesia bigemina* vaccine stored in the frozen state. In: Tick-borne diseases and their vectors, Wilde JKH (ed). University of Edinburgh. Center for Tropical Veterinary Medicine. 1978, p 389–390.

106. Mellors LT, Dalgliesh RJ, Timms P, Rodwell BJ, Callow LL: Preparation and laboratory testing of a frozen vaccine containing *Babesia bovis*, *Babesia bigemina* and *Anaplasma centrale*. Res Vet Sci 32:194–197, 1982.

107. Dennis RA, O'Hara PJ, Young MF, Dorris KD: Neonatal immunohemolytic anemia and icterus of calves. J Am Vet Med Assoc 156:1861–1869, 1970.

108. Dimmock CK, Bell K: Haemolytic disease of the newborn in calves. Aust Vet J 46:44–47, 1970.

109. Osterhoff DR, De Vos AJ: Isoimmune blood group antibodies in cattle after the use of a blood vaccine. J S Afr Vet Assoc 48:137–139, 1977.

110. Emmerson FR, Knott SG, Callow LL: Vaccination with *Babesia argentina* in 5 beef herds in South-Eastern Queensland. Aust Vet J 52:451–454, 1976.

111. Timms P, Steward NP, Dalgliesh RJ: Comparison of tick and blood challenge for assessing immunity to *Babesia bovis*. Aust Vet J 60:257–259, 1983.

112. Mahoney DF, Wright IG, Mirre GB: Bovine babesiosis: The persistence of immunity to *Babesia argentina* and *Babesia bigemina* in calves (*Bos taurus*) after naturally acquired infection. Ann Trop Med Parasitol 67:197–203, 1973.

113. Mahoney DF, Wright IG, Goodger BV: Immunity in cattle to *Babesia bovis* after single infections with parasites of various origins. Aust Vet J 55:10–12, 1979.

114. Rogers RJ: The acquired resistance to *Babesia argentina* of cattle exposed to light infestation with cattle tick (*Boophilus microplus*). Aust Vet J 47:237–241, 1971.

115. Johnston LAY, Tammemagi L: Bovine babesiosis: Duration of latent infection and immunity to *Babesia argentina*. Aust Vet J 45:445–449, 1969.

116. McCosker PJ: Control of piroplasmosis and anaplasmosis in cattle. A practical manual. FAO, Santa Cruz, Bolivia, p 64, 1975.

117. Thompson KC, Todorovic RA, Hidalgo RJ: The immune responses to antigenic variants of *Babesia bigemina* in the bovine. Res Vet Sci 24:234–237, 1978.

118. De Vos AJ, Bessenger R, Fouries CG: Virulence and heterologous strain immunity of South African and Australian *Babesia bovis* strains with reduced pathogenicity. Onderstepoort J Vet Res 49:133–136, 1982.

119. De Vos AJ, Combrink MP, Bessenger R: *Babesia bigemina* vaccine: Comparison of the efficacy and safety of Australian and South African strains under experimental conditions in South Africa. Onderstepoort J Vet Res 49:155–158, 1982.

120. Bigalke RD: Personal communication, 1983.
121. Wharton RH, Utech KBW: The relation between engorgement and dropping of *Boophilus microplus* (Canestrini) (*Ixodidae*) to the assessment of tick numbers on cattle. J Aust Entomol Soc 9:171–182, 1970.
122. Hadani A, Ziv M, Sklar A: In preparation.
123. Utech KBW, Sutherst RW, Dallwitz MJ, Wharton RH, Maywald GF, Sutherland ID: A model of the survival of larvae of the cattle tick *Boophilus microplus,* on pasture. Aust J Agric Res 34:64–72, 1983.
124. Sutherst RW, Utech KBW, Kerr JD, Wharton RH: Density dependent mortality of the tick *B. microplus* on cattle-further observations. J Appl Ecol 16:397–403, 1979.
125. Wilkinson PR: The effect of herbicidal killing of shrubs on abundance of adult *Dermacentor andersoni* (*Acarina, Ixodidae*) in British Columbia. J Med Entomol 13:713–718, 1977.
126. Anon: Cattle tick in Australia. Inquiry by the Cattle Tick Control Commission, 1973. Canberra. The Government Printer of Australia. 1975, p 108.
127. Hadani A, Tsur I: Studies on ticks and attempts at their control in a beef herd. Refuah Vet 17:46–51, 1959.
128. Hadani A, Mer GG, Cwilich R: The rearing of *Rhipicephalus secundus* on the Levant vole (*Microtus guentheri* D&A) and its use as an experimental animal for testing acaricides and repellents. Refuah Vet 18:50–53, 1961.
129. Rubina M, Hadani A, Ziv M: The life cycle of the tick *Hyalomma anatolicum excavatum* Koch, 1844, maintained under field conditions in Israel. Rev Elev Med Vet Pays Trop 35:255–264, 1982.
130. Sonenshine DE, Ziv M: Ecological studies on ticks infesting sheep and small mammals in an un-improved semidesert pasture in Israel. J Med Entomol 8:683–686, 1971.
131. Wilkinson PR: The spelling of pasture in cattle tick control. Aust J Agric Res 8:414–423, 1957.
132. Wharton RH, Harley KLS, Wilkinson PR, Utech KBW, Kelley BM: A comparison of cattle tick control by pasture spelling, planned dipping and tick resistant cattle. Aust J Agric Res 20:783–797, 1969.
133. Powell RT: Project tick control. Queens Agric J 103:443–474, 1977.
134. Elder JK, Waters KS, Dunwell GH, Emmerson FR, Kearnan JF, Morris RS, Knott SG: A survey concerning cattle tick control in Queensland 2. Managerial aspects which indirectly affect tick control. Aust Vet J 56:205–211, 1980.
135. Elder JK, Kearnan JF, Waters KS, Dunwell GH, Emmerson FR, Knott SG, Morris RS: A survey concerning cattle tick control in Queensland 4. Use of resistant cattle and pasture spelling. Aust Vet J 56:219–223, 1980.
136. Cooley RA, Kohls GM: A summary on tick parasites. In: Proc 5th Pacific Cong Canada, (1933) 1934 Vol 5, p 3375–3381.
137. Van Someren VD: The red billed oxpecker and its relation to stock in Kenya. East Afr Agric J 17:1–11, 1951.
138. Wilkinson PR: Factors affecting the distribution and abundance of the cattle tick in Australia: observations and hypothesis. Acarologia 12:492–508, 1970.
139. Wilkinson PR, Garvie MB: Notes on the role of ticks feeding on lagomorphs and ingestion of ticks by vertebrates in the epidemiology of the Rocky Mountain Spotted Fever. J Med Entomol 12:480, 1975.
140. Short NJ, Norval RAI: Tick predation by shrews in Zimbabwe. J Parasitol 68:1052, 1982.
141. Skead CJ: A study of the cattle egret *Ardeola ibis*, Linnaeus. Ostrich Suppl 6:109–139, 1966.
142. Drummond RO, Medley JG, Graham OH: Engorgement and reproduction of Lone Star ticks (*Amblyomma americanum* L.) treated with gamma – radiation. Int J Radiat Biol 10:183–188, 1966.
143. Galun R, Warburg M, Avivi A: Studies on the application of the sterility method in the tick *Ornithodoros tholozani*. Entomol Exp Appl 10:143–152, 1967.

298

144. Oliver JH, Delfin ED: Gynandromorphism in *Dermacentor occidentalis* (*Acari: Ixodidae*). Ann Entomol Soc Amer 60:1119–1121, 1967.

145. Kitaoka S, Mori T: Effects of gamma radiation and chemosterilants on the cattle tick, *Boophilus microplus*. Jap J Sanit Zool 18:126–129, 1967.

146. Pal R, Lachance LE: The operational feasibility of genetic methods for control of insects of medical and veterinary importance. Ann Rev Entomol 19:269–291, 1974.

147. Thompson GD, Osburn RL, Drummond RO, Price MA: Hybrid sterility in cattle ticks (*Acari: Ixodidae*). Experientia 37:127–128, 1981.

148. Menendez R: El Melinitis minutiflora y la garrapata. Rev Agric Puerto Rico 4:219–223, 1924.

149. De-Jesus Z: The repellent and killing effects of Gordura grass on the larvae of the cattle tick, *Boophilus australis*. Phillipines J Anim Indust 1:193–207, 1934.

150. Thompson KC, Roa JE, Romero T: Anti-tick grasses as the basis for developing practical tick control packages. Trop Anim Hlth Prod 10:179–182, 1978.

151. Sutherst RW, Jones RJ, Schnitzerling HJ: Tropical legumes of the genus *Stylosanthes* immobilize and kill cattle ticks. Nature London. 295:320–321, 1982.

152. Gillard P: Beef cattle production from improved pastures. The use of *Stylosanthes* species in the sub-humid tropics of Australia. World Anim Rev 44:2–8, 1982.

153. Drummond RO, Rajagopalan PK, Screenivasan MA, Menor PKB: Tests with ixodicides for the control of the tick vectors of Kyasanur Forest disease. J Med Entomol 6:245–251, 1969.

154. Mount GA, Hirst JM, McWilliams JG, Lofgren CS, White SA: Insecticides for the control of the Lone Star tick tested in the laboratory and as high-and low-volume sprays in wooded areas. J Econ Entomol 61:1005–1007, 1968.

155. Rawlings SC, Mansingh A: Toxicity of acaricidal residues on grass surfaces to larvae of the Southern Cattle tick. J Econ Entomol 72:423–427, 1979.

156. Drummond RO, Davey RB: Acaricide susceptibility of strains of *Boophilus microplus* from Texas, Puerto Rico, and Mexico. The Southwest Entomol 6:335–340, 1981.

157. Enders E, Stendel W, Wollweber H: New compounds active against resistant cattle ticks (*Boophilus* spp.): Relationship between structure and activity within the group of cyclic amidines. Pesticide Science 4:823–838, 1973.

158. Drummond RO, Graham OH, Meleney WP, Diamant G: Field tests in Mexico with new insecticides and arsenic for the control of *Boophilus* ticks on cattle. J Econ Entomol 57:340–346, 1964.

159. Graham OH, Drummond RO: Laboratory screening insecticides for the prevention of reproduction of *Boophilus* ticks. J Econ Entomol 57:335–339, 1964.

160. Wharton RH, Roulston WJ, Utech KBW, Kerr JD: Assessment of the efficiency of acaricides and their mode of application against the cattle tick *Boophilus microplus*. Aust J Agric Res 21:985–1000, 1970.

161. Roulston WJ, Wharton RH, Schnitzerling HJ, Sutherst RW, Sullivan ND: Mixtures of chlorphenamidine with other acaricides for the control of organophosphorus – resistant strains of cattle tick *Boophilus microplus*. Aust Vet J 47:521–528, 1971.

162. Keating MI: Tick control by chemical ixodicides in Kenya: a review 1912 to 1981. Trop Anim Hlth Prod 15:1–6, 1983.

163. Suggested guide for the use of insecticides to control insects affecting crops, livestock, households, stored products, forests, and forest products. Agric Res Serv and Forest Serv USDA, Washington DC. Agriculture Handbook 584. 1982, p 734.

164. Smith CN, Cole MM, Gilbert IH, Gouck HK: Field tests with tick repellents – 1949, 1950, and 1952. J Econ Entomol 47:13–19, 1954.

165. Gouk HK, Gilbert IH: Field tests with new tick repellents in 1954. J Econ Entomol 48:499–500, 1955.

166. Hadani A, Ziv M, Rechav Y: A laboratory study of tick repellents. Entomol Exp Appl 22:53–59, 1977.

167. Cwilich R, Hadani A: The rate of depletion of the gamma isomer of benzene hexa chloride in fluid from a cattle spray race. Refuah Vet 19:241–248, 1962.

168. Davey RB, Ahrens EH Jr, Garza J: Control of the Southern Cattle tick with insecticide – impregnated ear tags. J Econ Entomol 73:651–653, 1980.

169. Ahrens EH, Cocke J: Comparative test with insecticide impregnated ear tags against the Gulf Coast tick. J Econ Entomol 71:764–765, 1978.

170. Ahrens EH, Gladney WJ, McWhorter GM, Deer JA: Prevention of screwworm infection in cattle by controlling Gulf Coast ticks with slow release insecticide devices. J Econ Entomol 70:581–585, 1977.

171. Gladney WJ: Field trials of insecticides in controlled release devices for the control of the Gulf Coast tick and prevention of screwworm in cattle. J Econ Entomol 69:757–760, 1976.

172. Allan K, Palmer BH: The ixodicidal efficacy of a number of 'pour-on' formulations of amitraz against the Biarra strain of the Southern Cattle tick Boophilus microplus (Canestrini) on housed calves. In: Tick-borne diseases and their vectors, Wilde JKH (ed). University of Edinburgh. Center for Tropical Veterinary Medicine. 1978, p 214–218.

173. Drummond RO, Whetstone TM, Miller JA: Control of ticks systemically with Merck MK-933, an avermectin. J Econ Entomol 74:432–436, 1981.

174. Nolan J, Schnitzerling HJ, Bird P: Evaluation of the potential of systemic slow release chemical treatments for control of the cattle tick (Boophilus microplus) using avermectin. Aust Vet J 57:493–497, 1981.

175. Green PF, Connole MD: Screening fungal metabolites for insecticidal activity against the sheep blow fly Lucilia cuprina (Wied.) and the cattle tick Boophilus microplus (Can). Gen Appl Entomol 13:11–14, 1981.

176. Miller JA, Kung SE, Oehler DD: Sustained release systems for livestock pest control. In: Controlled release of pesticides and pharmaceuticals. Lewis DH (ed.) New York, Plenum Pub Corp. 1981, p 311–318.

177. Corlis PL, Sutherland ID: Dipping Brahman crossbred steers in central Queensland. Does it pay? Queens Agric J 102:589–591, 1976.

178. Grant KM: Queensland country life. March 10, 1977.

179. Sutherst RW, Comins HM: The management of acaricide resistance in the cattle tick Boophilus microplus (Canestrini) (Acari: Ixodidae) in Australia. Bull Entomol Res 69:519–537, 1979.

180. Hadani A, Ziv M, Shimshoni A: Intoxication in sheep following dipping in Benzene Hexachloride (BHC) emulsion. Refuah Vet 29:122–126, 1972.

181. Stone BF, Haydock KP: A method for measuring the acaricide susceptibility of the cattle tick Boophilus microplus (Can). Bull Entomol Res 53:563–578, 1962.

182. Schnitzerling HJ, Stone BF: Loss of toxicity to cattle ticks of a wettable powder formulation of coumaphos. Aust Vet J 44:7–10, 1968.

183. O'Neill DK, Alexander AE: The effect of aging on the biological efficiency of some DDT cattle dipping formulations. Aust J Agric Res 12:733–742, 1961.

184. Francis J: Tick resistant cattle in Australia. Br Vet J 122:301–307, 1966.

185. Villares JB: Climatological Zootechny. III. Contribution to the study of genetical resistance and susceptibility of bovines to Boophilus microplus (in Portuguese). Bol Indust Animale 4:60–79, 1941.

186. Campbell RSF: The use of resistant cattle in the control of ticks and vector borne diseases. In: Tick-borne diseases and their vectors, Wilde JKH (ed). University of Edinburgh. Center for Tropical Veterinary Medicine. 1978, p 251–257.

187. Hewetson RW: Selection of cattle for resistance against Boophilus microplus. In: Tick-borne diseases and their vectors, Wilde JKH (ed). University of Edinburgh. Center for Tropical Veterinary Medicine. 1978, p 258–261.

188. Allen JR, Wikel SK: Acquisition of tick-resistance in guinea pigs. In: Tick-borne disease and their vectors, Wilde JKH (ed). University of Edinburgh. Center for Tropical Veterinary Medicine. 1978, p 75–76.

189. Kemp DH: In vitro culture of *Boophilus microplus* in relation to host resistance and tick feeding. In: Tick-borne diseases and their vectors, Wilde JKH (ed). University of Edinburgh. Center for Tropical Veterinary Medicine. 1978, p 95–98.

190. Riek RF: Factors influencing the susceptibility of cattle to tick infection. Aust Vet J 32:204–208, 1956.

191. Riek RF: Studies on the reactions of animals to infestation with ticks. VI. Resistance of cattle to infestation with the tick *Boophilus microplus* (Canestrini). Aust J Agric Res 13:532–550, 1962.

192. Willadsen P: Immunity to ticks. In: Advances in Parasitology, Lumsden WHR, Muller R, Baker JR (eds). London, Academic Press. 1980, Vol 18, p 293–313.

193. Roberts JA: Resistance of cattle to the tick *Boophilus microplus* (Canestrini). II. Stages of the life cycle of the parasite against which resistance is manifested. J Parasitol 54:667–673, 1968.

194. Roberts JA: Acquisition by the host of resistance to the cattle tick *Boophilus microplus* (Canestrini). J Parasitol 54:657–662, 1968.

195. Sutherst MT, Utech KBW: Controlling livestock parasites with host resistance. In: CRC Handbook of Pest Management in Agriculture. II. Pimental D (ed). Boca Raton, Florida. Chemical Rubber Company. 1980.

196. Wharton RH, Utech KBW, Turner HG: Resistance to the cattle tick, *Boophilus microplus* in a herd of Australian Illawarra Shorthorn cattle: its assessment and heritability. Aust J Agric Res 21:163–181, 1970.

197. Francis J, Little DA: Resistance of Droughtmaster cattle to tick infestation and babesiosis. Aust Vet J 40:247–253, 1964.

198. Johnston LAY, Haydock KP: The effect of cattle tick (*Boophilus microplus*) on production of Brahman-cross and British-breed cattle in northern Australia. Aust Vet J 45:175–179, 1969.

199. Wilkinson PR: Selection of cattle for tick resistance, and the effect of herds of different susceptibility on *Boophilus* populations. Aust J Agric Res 13:974–983, 1962.

200. Strother GR, Burns EC, Smart LI: Resistance of pure-bred Brahman, Hereford and Brahman Hereford crossbred cattle to the Lone Star tick, *Amblyomma americanum* (*Acarina: Ixodidae*). J Med Entomol 11:559–563, 1974.

201. Sutherst RW, Norton GA, Barlow ND, Conway GR, Birley M, Comins HN: An analysis of the management strategies for cattle tick (*Boophilus microplus*) control in Australia. J Appl Ecol 16:359–382, 1979.

202. Wright JE: Hormonal termination of larval diapause in *Dermacentor albipictus*. Science 163:390–391, 1969.

203. Berger RS: 2,6-dichlorophenol, sex pheromone of the Lone Star tick. Science 177:704–705, 1972.

204. Wood WF, Leahy MG (Sister), Galun R, Prestwich GD, Meinwald J, Purnell RE, Payne RC: Phenols as pheromones of ixodid ticks. A general phenomenon. J Chem Ecol 1:501–509, 1975.

205. Gladney WJ, Grabbe RR, Ernest SE, Oehler DD: The Gulf Coast tick: Evidence of a pheromone produced by males. J Med Entomol 11:303–306, 1974.

206. Rechav Y, Whitehead GB, Knight MM: Aggregation response of nymphs to pheromones produced by males of the tick *Amblyomma hebraeum* Koch. Nature 259:563–564, 1976.

207. Ziv M, Sonenshine DE, Silverstein RM, West JR, Gingher KH: Use of sex pheromone, 2, 6-dichlorophenol, to disrupt mating by American Dog tick *Dermacentor variabilis* (Say). J Chem Ecol 7:829–840, 1981.

208. Rechav Y, Whitehead GB: Field trials with pheromone acaricide mixtures for control of *Amblyomma hebraeum*. J Econ Entomol 71:149–151, 1978.

209. Rechav Y, Whitehead GB: Assembly pheromones produced by males of *Amblyomma hebraeum* Koch. In: Tick-borne diseases and their vectors. Wilde JKH (ed). University of Edinburgh. Center for Tropical Veterinary Medicine. 1978, p 18–22.

210. Sonenshine DE, Silverstein RM, Rechav Y: Tick pheromone mechanisms. In: Physiology of ticks, Current Themes in Tropical Science. Vol 1. Obenchain FD, Galun R (eds.) New York. Pergamon Press. 1983, p 440–468.

211. Allen JR, Humphreys SJ: Immunization of guinea pigs and cattle against ticks. Nature 280:491–493, 1979.

212. Wikel SK: The induction of host resistance to tick infestation with a gland antigen. Amer J Trop Med Hyg 30:284–288, 1981.

213. Brossard M: Relations immunologiques entre bovins et tiques, plus particulierement entre bovins et *Boophilus microplus*. Acta Trop 33:15–36, 1976.

214. Heller A: Laboratory investigations on the effect of insecticides and host immunization for control of tick infection. Ph.D. Thesis. University of London. 1980, p 318.

215. Barnett SF: Economical aspects of protozoal tick-borne diseases of livestock in parts of the world other than Britain. Bull Off Int Epiz 81:183–196, 1974.

216. Du Toit R, Bekker PM: Resistance to arsenic as displayed by single-host Blue tick *Boophilus decoloratus* (Koch) in a localized area of the Union of South-Africa. J S Afr Vet Med Assoc 12:50–58, 1941.

217. Baker JAF: Resistance to ixodicides by ticks in Africa south of the equator with some thoughts on tick control in this area. In: Tick-borne diseases and their vectors. Wilde JKH (ed). University of Edinburgh. Center for Tropical Veterinary Medicine. 1978, p 101–109.

218. Lourens JHM: Genetic basis for organochlorine resistance in *Amblyomma variegatum* and information on the susceptibility of *Amblyomma lepidum* to organochlorine acaricides. J Econ Entomol 72:790–793, 1979.

219. Lourens JHM: Inheritance of organochlorine resistance in the cattle tick *Rhipicephalus appendiculatus* Neumann (*Acari: Ixodidae*) in East Africa. Bull Entomol Res 70:1–10, 1980.

220. Whitehead GB, Baker JAF: Acaricide resistance in the Red-legged tick *Rhipicephalus evertsi* Neumann. Bull Entomol Res 51:755–764, 1960.

221. Baker JAF, Thompson GE. Miles JO: Resistance to toxaphene by the Bont tick *Amblyomma hebraeum* (Koch). J S Afr Vet Med Assoc 48:59–64, 1977.

222. Wharton RH: Tick-borne livestock diseases and their vectors. 5. Acaricide resistance and alternative methods of tick control. World Anim Rev 20:8–15, 1976.

223. Nolan J, Bird PE: Co-toxicity of synthetic pyrethroids and organophosphorus compounds against the cattle tick (*Boophilus microplus*). J Aust Entomol Soc 16:252, 1977.

224. Blomefield LC: A comparative study of arsenite of soda, benzene hexa chloride, DDT, toxaphene and combinations of these in the control of ticks. J S Afr Vet Med Assoc 23:1–8, 1952.

225. Schunter CA, Roulston WJ, Schnitzerling HJ: A mechanism of resistance to organophosphorous acaricides in a strain of the cattle tick. Aust J Biol Sci 21:97–109, 1968.

226. Stone BF: Brain cholinesterase activity and its inheritance in cattle tick (*Boophilus microplus*) strains resistant and susceptible to organophosphorous acaricides. Aust J Biol Sci 21:321–330, 1968.

227. Stone BF: The inheritance of DDT resistance in the cattle tick *Boophilus microplus*. Aust J Agric Res 13:984–1007, 1962.

228. Stone BF: The inheritance of dieldrin – resistance in the cattle tick, *Boophilus microplus*. Aust J Agric Res 13:1008–1012, 1962.

229. Stone BF: Inheritance of resistance to organophosphorous acaricides in the cattle tick *Boophilus microplus*. Aust J Biol Sci 21:309–319, 1968.

230. Whitehead GB: Pyrethrum resistance conferred by resistance to DDT in the Blue tick. Nature 184:378–379, 1959.

231. Roulston WJ, Wharton RH. Nolan J, Kerr JD, Wilson JT, Thompson PG, Schotz M: A survey for resistance in cattle ticks to acaricides. Aust Vet J 57:362–371, 1981.

232. Spickett AM, Baker JAF: Resistance to organophosphorous ixodicides. J S Afr Vet Med Assoc 52:154, 1981.

233. Baker JAF, Jordaan JO, Robertson WD: Ixodicidal resistance in *Boophilus microplus* (Canestrini) in the Republic of South-Africa and Transkei. J S Afr Vet Med Assoc 50:296–301, 1979.

234. Crampton PL, Gichanga MM: A survey of resistance to acaricides in economically important

Ixodidae (Acari) of the major cattle raising areas of Kenya. Bull Entomol Res 69:427–439, 1979.

235. Polyakov DK, Smirnova OI: Development of resistance to chlorofos (trichlorphon) in the ticks *Hyalomma anatolicum* and *Rhipicephalus bursa* (in Russian). Prob Vet Sanit 61:54–57, 1978.

236. Polyakov DK, Smirnova OI: Cross resistance to acaricides in *Hyalomma anatolicum* and *Hyalomma detritum* (in Russian). Prob Vet Sanit 61:58–60, 1978.

237. Brown AWA, Pal R: Insecticide resistance in arthropods. Monog Ser WHO No 38, 1971.

238. Whitehead GB: Resistance in the *Acarina:* Ticks. In: Advances in Acarology, Naegele JA (ed). Ithaca, NY. Cornell Univ Press. 1965, Vol 2, p 53–70.

239. Drummond RO: Resistance in ticks and insects of veterinary importance 1977. In: Pesticide management and insecticide resistance. Watson DL, Brown AWA (eds). New York. Academic Press. 1977, p 303–319.

240. Solomon KR, Baker MK, Heyne H, Van Kleef J: The use of frequency diagrams in the survey of resistance to pesticides in ticks in Southern Africa. Onderstepoort J Vet Res 46:171–177, 1979.

241. Comins HN: The management of pesticide resistance. J Theor Biol 65:339–420, 1977.

242. Georghiou GP, Taylor CE: Operational influences in the evolution of insecticide resistance. J Econ Entomol 70:653–658, 1977.

243. Tatchell RJ: The use of the packet test for detecting acaricide resistance in African ticks. In: Proc 3rd Int Cong Parasitol 1974, Munchen 25–31 August, 1974, p 993–994.

244. Shaw RD: Culture of an organophosphorous – resistant strain of *Boophilus microplus* (Can.) and an assessment of its resistance spectrum. Bull Entomol Res 56:389–405, 1966.

245. Whitnall ABM, Bradford B: An arsenic resistant tick and its control with gammexane dips. Bull Entomol Res 38:353–372, 1947.

246. Hadani A, Cwilich R, Rechav Y: Laboratory study of ixodicides using nymphs of *Hyalomma excavatum*. Refuah Vet 25:119–125, 1968.

247. Matthewson MD, Hughes G: The establishment of cultures of two and three host ticks in the laboratory and their use in the screening of candidate ixodicides. In: Tick-borne diseases and their vectors. Wilde JKH (ed). University of Edinburgh. Center for Tropical Veterinary Medicine. 1978, p 231–240.

248. Bram RA: Tick borne livestock diseases and their vectors. 1. The global problem. World Anim Rev 16:1–5, 1975.

249. Alexander RD: The role of the veterinarian in public and animal health. 1. Research. J S Afr Vet Med Assoc 21:147–153, 1955.

250. Anderson JL: Cattle tick (*Boophilus microplus*) – its occurrence and attempted eradication in the territory of Papua and New Guinea. The Papua and New Guinea Agric J 15:91–104, 1962/3.

251. Matson BA: Epizootiology and control of tick-borne diseases of cattle in Rhodesia. Rhod Agric J 63:118–122, 1966.

252. Barns JM: Control of health hazards associated with the use of pesticides. Adv Pest Control Res 1:1–38, 1957.

253. Hayes WJ: Pesticides in relation to public health. Ann Rev Entomol 5:379–404, 1960.

254. Clarke ML, Harvey DG, Humphreys DJ: Veterinary toxicology. London. 2nd edition. Bailliere Tindall. 1981.

255. Mahoney DF: Bovine babesiosis: A study of factors concerned in transmission. Ann Trop Med Parasitol 63:1–14, 1969.

256. Mahoney DF, Mirre GB: Bovine babesiosis: estimation of infection rates in the tick vector *Boophilus microplus* (Canestrini). Ann Trop Med Parasitol 65:309–317, 1971.

257. Mahoney DF: The diagnosis of babesiosis in Australia. In: Workshop on Hemoparasites (Anaplasmosis and Babesiosis). Wells EA (ed). Series CE-12, 1977. CIAT Cali, Colombia. 17–22 March, 1975. p 49–62.

258. Smith RD: *Babesia bovis*: Computer simulation of the relationship between the tick vector, parasite, and bovine host. Exp parasitol 56:27–40, 1983.

259. Donnelly J, Peirce MA: Experimental transmission of *Babesia divergens* to cattle by the tick *Ixodes ricinus*. Int J Parasitol 5:363–367, 1975.

260. Adam KMG, Beasley SJ, Blewett DA: The occurrence of antibody to *Babesia* and to the virus of louping-ill in deer in Scotland. Res Vet Sci 23:133–138, 1977.
261. Joyner LP, Donnelly J: The epidemiology of babesial infections. Adv Parasitol 17:115–140, 1979.
262. Hinaidy HK: Die Babesiose des Rindes in Österreich. II. Untersuchung von Blutproben natürlich erkrankter Rinder. Wien tierärztl Mschr 68:188–191, 1981.
263. Donelly J, Joyner LP, Crossman PJ: The incidence of *Babesia divergens* infection in a herd of cattle as measured by the indirect immunofluorescent antibody test. Res Vet Sci 13:511–514, 1972.
264. Taylor SM: Assessment of prevalence of clinical babesiosis in cattle in Northern Ireland. The Vet Rec 12:247–250, 1983.
265. Todorovic RA: Bovine babesiosis: Its diagnosis and control. Am J Vet Res 35:1045–1052, 1974.
266. Benitez MT, Boyer RL. Leon RCE: Estudio serologico de un rebaño de bovinos importados tratado con imidocarb (droga profilactica contra la babesiosis). Veterinaria Tropical 2:91–101, 1977.
267. Callow LL: Some aspects of the epidemiology and control of bovine babesiosis in Australia. J S Afr Vet Assoc 50:353–356, 1979.
268. Nari A, Solari MA, Cardozo H: Hemovacuna para el control de *Babesia* spp y *Anaplasma marginale* en el Uruguay. Veterinaria, Montevideo, (Uruguay) 15:137–148, 1979.
269. Todorovic RA, Lopez LA. Lopez AG, Gonzalez EF: Bovine babesiosis and anaplasmosis: Control by premunition and chemoprophylaxis. Exp parasitol 37:92–104, 1975.
270. Barnett SF: Economical aspects of tick-borne diseases control in Britain. Bull Off Int Epiz 81:167–182, 1974.
271. Hinaidy HK: Die Babesiose des Rindes in Österreich. I. Verbreitung und Vorkommen. Wien tierärztl Mschr 68:52–57, 1981.
272. Cunningham MP, Joyner LP, Brown CGD, Purnell RE, Bailey KP: Infection of cattle with East Coast fever by inoculation of the infective stage of *Theileria parva* harvested from the tick vector *Rhipicephalus appendiculatus*. Bull Epiz Dis Afr 21:235–238, 1973.
273. Mahoney DF, Mirre GB: *Babesia argentina*: The infection of splenectomized calves with extracts of larval ticks (*Boophilus microplus*). Res Vet Sci 16:112–114, 1974.
274. Dalgliesh RJ, Stewart NP: Stimulation of the development of infective *Babesia bovis* (*B. argentina*) in unfed *Boophilus microplus* larvae. Aust Vet J 52:543, 1976.
275. Morzaria SP, Young AS, Hudson EB: *Babesia bigemina* in Kenya: Experimental transmission by *Boophilus decoloratus* and the production of tick-derived stabilates. Parasitology 74:291–298, 1977.
276. Dalgliesh RJ, Stewart NP: The extraction of infective *Babesia bovis* and *Babesia bigemina* from tick eggs and *B. bigemina* from unfed larval ticks. Aust Vet J 54:453–454, 1978.
277. Ronald NC, Cruz D: Transmission of *Babesia bovis*, using undifferentiated embryonic cells from *Boophilus microplus* tick-eggs. Am J Vet Res 42:544–545, 1981.
278. Bhat UKM, Mahoney DF, Wright IG: The invasion and growth of *Babesia bovis* in tick tissue culture. Experientia 35:752–753, 1979.
279. Droleskey RE, Holman PJ, Craig TM, Wagner GG, Mollenhauer HH: Ultrastructure of *Babesia bovis* sexual stages as observed in *Boophilus microplus* cell cultures. Res Vet Sci 34:249–251, 1983.
280. Smith RD, Ristic M: Immunization against bovine babesiosis with culture-derived antigens. In: *Babesiosis*, Ristic M, Kreier JP (eds). New York. Academic Press. 1981, p 485–507.
281. Vayrynen R, Tuomi J: Continuous *in vitro* cultivation of *Babesia divergens*. Acta Vet Scand 23:471–472, 1982.

Subject index

Announcement

The Laveran International Foundation was established on September 7th, 1984, according to the recommendation approved by the Second International Conference on Malaria and Babesiosis which took place in Annecy, France, in September 1983.

The aim of the Foundation is to contribute to research, training and distribution of information relative to the control of malaria and babesiosis. The council is composed of 16 members. Its president is Professor L.J. Bruce-Chwatt (UK), the vice-presidents are Professor M. Ristic (USA) in charge of the American branch of the Foundation, and Professor P. Ambroise-Thomas (France). The treasurer is Dr L. Valette (Fondation Marcel Mérieux, Lyon).

The address of the main office is Les Pensières, 55 Route d'Annecy, 74290 Veyrier du Lac, France.